QUALITY OF LIFE TECHNOLOGY HANDBOOK

REHABILITATION SCIENCE IN PRACTICE SERIES

Series Editors

Marcia J. Scherer, Ph.D.

President
Institute for Matching Person and Technology

Professor
Orthopaedics and Rehabilitation
University of Rochester Medical Center

Dave Muller, Ph.D.

Executive
Suffolk New College

Editor-in-Chief
Disability and Rehabilitation

Founding Editor
Aphasiology

Published Titles

Assistive Technology Assessment Handbook, *edited by Stefano Federici and Marcia J. Scherer*

Assistive Technology for Blindness and Low Vision, *Roberto Manduchi and Sri Kurniawan*

Multiple Sclerosis Rehabilitation: From Impairment to Participation, *edited by Marcia Finlayson*

Paediatric Rehabilitation Engineering: From Disability to Possibility, *edited by Tom Chau and Jillian Fairley*

Quality of Life Technology Handbook, *Richard Schultz*

Forthcoming Titles

Ambient Assisted Living, *edited by Nuno M. Garcia, Joel Jose P. C. Rodrigues, Dirk Christian Elias, Miguel Sales Dias*

Computer Systems Experiences of Users with and without Disabilities: An Evaluation Guide for Professionals, *Simone Borsci, Masaaki Kurosu, Stefano Federici, Maria Laura Mele*

Neuroprosthetics: Principles and Applications, *Justin C. Sanchez*

Rehabilitation Goal Setting: Theory, Practice and Evidence, *edited by Richard Siegert and William Levack*

QUALITY OF LIFE TECHNOLOGY HANDBOOK

EDITED BY
RICHARD SCHULZ

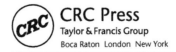

CRC Press
Taylor & Francis Group
Boca Raton London New York

CRC Press is an imprint of the
Taylor & Francis Group, an **informa** business

CRC Press
Taylor & Francis Group
6000 Broken Sound Parkway NW, Suite 300
Boca Raton, FL 33487-2742

First issued in paperback 2017

© 2013 by Taylor & Francis Group, LLC
CRC Press is an imprint of Taylor & Francis Group, an Informa business

No claim to original U.S. Government works

ISBN-13: 978-1-4665-0534-6 (hbk)
ISBN-13: 978-1-138-07513-9 (pbk)

Library of Congress Cataloging-in-Publication Data

Quality of life technology handbook / editor, Richard Schulz.
    p. ; cm. -- (Rehabilitation science in practice)
  Includes bibliographical references and index.
  ISBN 978-1-4665-0534-6 (alk. paper)
  I. Schulz, Richard, 1947- II. Series: Rehabilitation science in practice series.
  [DNLM: 1. Self-Help Devices. 2. Aged. 3. Biomedical Enhancement. 4. Disabled Persons--rehabilitation.
  5. Quality of Life. 6. Rehabilitation--instrumentation. WB 320]

617'.033--dc23
                                    2012015409

Visit the Taylor & Francis Web site at
http://www.taylorandfrancis.com

and the CRC Press Web site at
http://www.crcpress.com

Contents

Part I   Introduction and Conceptual Foundations

Part II   Design, Development, and Evaluation

Part III   Core Technologies and Their Application

Part IV   Transforming Education and the Market Place

Preface: Introduction and Overview—What Do We Mean by Quality of Life Technologies?

Richard Schulz, Scott R. Beach, Annette DeVito Dabbs, Judith T. Matthews, Karen L. Courtney, Katherine D. Seelman, and Laurel Person Mecca

P.1 Introduction*

We are in the midst of a technological revolution that is changing lives in fundamental ways. Virtually everything we do from how we learn, work, and communicate to how we spend our leisure time has been touched by the digital revolution. Although much has been achieved, we are still in the early stages of this revolution. There exists a vast untapped potential for technology to improve the quality of life (QoL) of human beings of all ages worldwide. This book is about harnessing this potential for the health and well-being of older and disabled adults.

Imagine technologies that can monitor individuals' behavior; understand their needs, preferences, and intentions; identify and manipulate objects in natural environments; navigate enclosed as well as external environments; and instantly transmit information about a person's health and functioning to professionals or family members. Such a system could know how well you slept last night, identify potential health problems before they become serious or catastrophic, know whether you are able to carry out daily routines, assist with tasks you have trouble completing such as meal preparation or taking medications, motivate you to do your exercises, get you to an appointment at the right place and time, and assure your daughter who lives in a distant city that you are doing well today. Parts of this scenario are already a reality, and the rest is achievable in the not-too-distant future.

One of the great success stories of the last century is the increased survival and longevity of children and adults with disability as well as the growth of the elderly population worldwide. This has fueled the demand for and sophistication of assistive technologies. It is our strong belief that we are now at the brink of a revolution in QoL technologies that will bring about intelligent, person-aware systems that provide the right kind of assistance at the right time to maximize the functioning and autonomy of individuals with disability. Drawing on cutting-edge expertise from multiple disciplines, the goal of this book is to describe our approach to realizing this goal.

Interest in QoL technologies is driven by multiple converging trends: the rapid pace of technological development, particularly in consumer electronics and communication; the unprecedented growth of the aging populations in the United States and worldwide; the increase in the number and survival of persons with disability; the growing interest on the part of business, industry, and government agencies in addressing health-care needs with technology; and the growing and unsustainable costs of caring for the elderly. Taken together, these trends have contributed to the strong conviction that technology can play an

---

* Portions of this preface appear in *Proceedings of the IEEE* (Schulz et al., in press).

important role in enhancing QoL and independence of individuals with impaired functioning due to trauma, chronic disorders, illness, or aging. Moreover, this can be achieved with high levels of efficiency, potentially reducing individual and societal costs of health care.

As we shall see in Chapter 1, the rapid growth of the elderly population worldwide in the next four decades poses immense challenges to formal health care and social service systems as well as informal caregivers. Maintaining the health, functioning, and QoL of this growing segment of the population will require fundamental changes in our approach to addressing their needs. New technologies will be key ingredients in finding a solution to these challenges.

P.2 Defining Quality of Life

QoL is an elusive construct connoting a multidimensional appraisal of a variety of important aspects of life. Its assessment typically includes both objective and subjective measures of multiple domains such as physical health and functioning, emotional health, cognitive functioning, role performance, work productivity, and life satisfaction. It differs from related constructs such as subjective well-being or life satisfaction, which emphasize people's evaluations of what is happening in their lives, including emotions such as happiness (Diener et al. 2003).

There is no single, universally accepted instrument for measuring QoL. Instruments are available for assessing global QoL and health-related QoL (HRQoL), with the latter categorized as either generic or condition specific. The World Health Organization QoL instrument (The WHOQoL Group 1994) is a 28-item global measure that is widely used to assess physical, functional, and psychological well-being as well as satisfaction and social relationships. Among the most widely used generic tools for measuring HRQoL in the United States and worldwide is the SF-36, a 36-item scale measuring all of the domains listed earlier (Ware et al. 1993). The EQ-5D (Brooks 1996), another generic HRQoL instrument developed by the EuroQoL Group, is a five-item, utility-based scale that taps the domains of mobility, self-care, usual activities, pain/discomfort, and anxiety/depression.

Disease-specific QoL instruments are designed to provide a more nuanced assessment of individuals with a specific disease or functional disability. For example, an instrument for assessing QoL in cancer patients might include items that assess common symptoms of the disease or its treatment such as dyspnea, loss of appetite, fatigue, nausea and vomiting, insomnia, constipation, and diarrhea in addition to items measuring broader constructs like physical, cognitive, emotional, and social functioning. Both types of scales are valuable and have been widely used to assess the effects of treatment, facilitate communication between patients and health-care providers, assess patient preferences, and inform medical decision making (Fayers and Machin 2000).

All of these instruments have several features in common. They are completed by the respondent as opposed to having an external observer rate the status of the individual; they are all multidimensional in that they assess multiple life domains; and there is considerable overlap in the domains assessed. For example, the SF-36 assesses physical, social, and emotional functioning while the EuroQol captures physical, mental, and social functioning with items assessing mobility, self-care, usual activities, pain/discomfort, and anxiety/depression.

As the name implies, QoL technologies are designed to impact the QoL of individuals who use them. Thus, at a general level we would expect these technologies to maintain or enhance the physical, social, or emotional functioning of humans, and like medical interventions, their impact could be evaluated using QoL instruments to assess both generic effects as well as the specific domains targeted by a particular technology. For example, the effects of a technology such as a reminder or coaching system aimed at enhancing cognitive functioning of older individuals with cognitive impairment would be assessed with a generic instrument such as the EuroQol as well as targeted instruments designed to provide a detailed account of the user's cognitive functioning abilities. Table P.1 shows how different QoL technologies are related to QoL domains and their associated measurement strategies. As shown in Table P.1, a wheelchair has its primary impact on the mobility of the user, which is part of physical functioning domain of QoL. At the same time, we would expect improved mobility to have secondary impacts on the emotional well-being and social functioning of the user inasmuch as increased mobility would also enable increased social activities, which may improve the psychological well-being of the user. In this book, we discuss in greater detail evaluation strategies for assessing the impact of QoL technologies.

Although the focus of our discussion has been on specific measures designed to assess QoL, typically based on individual self-report, this is not the only method for assessing the impact of a technology. Self-report measures are often supplemented with more objective assessments such as functional abilities, performance tests, or the utilization of health-care services. These types of outcomes might be particularly important to insurance companies that need to be convinced that a technology improves functioning based on objective assessments and/or saves money because of reduced health-care utilization.

TABLE P.1

Examples of QoL Technologies and Their Impact on QoL Domains

Major QoL Domains	Indicators of Impact	Existing QoLTs
Physical function	Mobility, self-care, pain, discomfort	Wheelchair/scooter: Primary impact is to enhance mobility; secondary impacts include enhanced emotional well-being and social functioning
Emotional function	Depression, anxiety	Telehealth cognitive-behavioral therapy: Primary impact is on treatment of mental disorder such as depression; secondary impacts are on social functioning and physical functioning
Social function	Social integration, social role functioning	Social networking tools: Primary impact is on integrating the individual into a community of like-minded persons and supportive social networks; secondary impacts include enhanced emotional functioning
Cognitive function	Intelligence, neurological performance tests, decision-making ability	Medication management devices: Primary impact is on monitoring medication-taking behavior and providing reminders to carry out scheduled regimens; secondary impacts are on physical and/or emotional functioning and symptom control

P.3 Classifying QoL Technologies

There are hundreds of technologies that could be classified as QoL systems. Making sense of, or organizing, families of technologies into coherent categories is an important but as yet unmet goal in this area. An agreed-upon classification system for QoL technologies would facilitate communication among researchers, clinicians, and other stakeholders or end users, enable appropriate comparisons between competing technologies, identify gaps in existing technologies, and help guide policy decisions about eligibility for the use of and reimbursement for technologies.

Traditionally, the term "assistive technologies" has been used to describe products, devices, or equipment that are used to maintain, increase, or improve the functional capabilities of people with disabilities. The Assistive Technology Act of 1998 extended this definition to include "any item, piece of equipment, or product system, whether acquired commercially, modified, or customized, that is used to increase, maintain, or improve the functional capabilities of individuals with disabilities." This is an extremely broad definition and would include products such as Velcro and microwave ovens that are useful to people with disabilities but were not specifically designed for them. For the purposes of our discussion, a defining characteristic of QoL technologies is their ability to enhance the functioning of an individual.

The most widely used standard for classifying assistive technologies is the International Standard ISO 9999, developed by the International Organization for Standardization (Bougie 2008). In this system, assistive products are classified according to their function using a three-level hierarchical strategy. The major classes of aides described include products for personal medical treatment, skills training, personal care and protection, personal mobility, housekeeping, communication, information and signaling, handling objects and devices, environmental improvements, tools and industrial machinery, furnishing and adaptations to homes, recreation, and orthoses and prostheses.

The U.S. Food and Drug Administration (FDA) has also weighed in on technologies for enhancing health, safety, and QoL in the home environment, although their focus is limited to medical devices, broadly defined to include devices used to prevent, mitigate, and treat disease in home settings. These devices are viewed as improving QoL because they allow patients to remain ambulatory and independent by receiving care in the comfort and convenience of their own homes (Center for Devices and Radiological Health 2010).

The ISO approach to classifying assistive technologies by their intended function is reflected in numerous other more recent classification systems. For example, in a recent survey of older individuals and family caregivers, the American Association of Retired Persons (AARP) identified categories such as "home safety devices," "personal health and wellness devices," "telepharmacy and telemedicine," and "personal computers" (Barrett 2008). This classification system emphasizes specific functional goals of the technology (e.g., safety, health, wellness, and taking medications).

The Center for Aging Services Technologies (CAST), a subsidiary of the American Association of Homes and Services for the Aging (AAHSA), identifies four broad categories addressed by technologies: safety, health and wellness, social connectedness, and electronic documentation. In their Briefing Paper on Technologies to Help Older Adults Maintain Independence (2009), the Center for Technology and Aging takes a similar approach and identifies seven categories of technologies, including systems designed to help manage medication information, dispensing, adherence, and tracking (medication optimization); technologies designed to monitor and manage health conditions such as glucometers and blood pressure monitors (remote patient monitoring); assistive technologies, which compensate for sensory, physical, and cognitive impairments; technologies that assess and improve cognitive fitness such as thinking games and challenging puzzles; and social networking technologies that enable individuals to communicate, organize, and share information and resources with each other.

Taken together, these classification systems appropriately emphasize the functional domain addressed by the technology as the primary organizing heuristic. However, this strategy leaves out several other attributes that are also important, including (a) whether the technology serves to compensate for declining functional abilities, prevent adverse outcomes, or maintain or improve functioning in nonimpaired persons; (b) how passive or interactive it is; and (c) how intelligent or adaptive the system is to the user's needs and preferences and the user's natural environment. Each of these attributes is discussed in some detail below.

A highly specialized technology such as a glucose monitor may have very narrow goals (i.e., monitor blood glucose levels) whereas a kitchen robot might carry out multiple tasks from preparing a meal to loading a dishwasher. An important starting point for the development of any QoL technology is a clear specification of the domains the technology will address.

Technologies may compensate, maintain, or improve functioning depending on who is using it. For example, an individual with mild cognitive impairment may use a medication reminder system to compensate for lost cognitive abilities, while a normal functioning individual might benefit from such a device because of the cognitive complexity of his or her medication regimen. One of the underlying themes to our approach to technology development is that it be adaptable to the needs, preferences, and abilities of individuals, thereby enhancing its functionality as well as the size of the end user pool and the potential market for the technology.

A third distinction the earlier examples illustrate is that technology can be either passive or highly interactive with the individual. Monitoring systems that unobtrusively gauge the behavior or functional ability of an individual in order to identify persons who are at risk for adverse health outcomes such as falling are examples of passive systems. They monitor the environment and/or the behavior of the individual, generate user status information and alerts, and may even provide instructions or advice to the user based on the data collected. Technologies that require conscious user input such as using a glucose monitoring device, operating a power wheelchair, or a robotic arm are examples of interactive systems. The user plays an active role in directing the technology.

The amount of user input required by a technology may vary as a function of its intelligence or adaptability, the fourth general attribute of QoL technologies. System intelligence can serve as a substitute for human input. For example, a power wheelchair that automatically detects and adapts to differences in terrain would require less user input than one that does not have this capability. Intelligent systems have the capacity to make fine-grained assessments of individuals in their environment, learn and reason based on these observations, and provide the correct type of assistance, at appropriate levels, at the right time.

To summarize, we have identified four relatively orthogonal QoL attributes that can be used to characterize QoL systems:

1. *Functional domain targeted*: Technologies typically address a specified need, which may be narrow (e.g., monitoring glucose levels) or broad (e.g., enhancing mobility). Identifying the need being addressed is critical for at least two reasons: (1) it helps define the significance or potential value of the technology and (2) it helps identify appropriate outcome measures for assessing its effectiveness.

2. *Compensatory, preventive and maintaining, or enhancing*: Technologies can be viewed as existing along a continuum where they compensate for diminished functioning

at one end and enhance normative functioning at the other. In between, they may prevent decline or maintain functioning, or serve to alert the individual or an observer to an impending threat to functional ability. Highly adaptive or intelligent technologies will have the ability to address the needs of individuals throughout this continuum.

3. *Passive or interactive*: This dimension characterizes the extent of user involvement in operating the technology. One of the trade-offs between passive and interactive systems is that passive systems generally require more intelligence to achieve the same goal.

4. *System intelligence*: Technologies vary in the extent to which they perceive, reason, learn, and act in the service of addressing individual needs and desires regarding their QoL. Most existing technologies have limited capacity to adapt to user abilities, needs, preferences, and environments. The development of intelligent systems is a fundamental goal of the next generation of QoL technologies and a guiding theme for this book.

Although we tend to think of most QoL technologies as being compensatory or assistive, it is worth noting that even technologies that have little direct functional impact, such as those that entertain or stimulate, could be viewed as QoL technologies because they meet the criterion of improving some aspect of an individual's QoL. By this definition, technologies that elevate mood or improve psychological well-being through auditory or visual stimulation, for example, could be considered QoL technologies. However, for the purposes of this book, we concentrate on those technologies that provide direct functional benefit to the user and that are of particular value to individuals with existing or emerging functional disability due to trauma, congenital defect, chronic disorder, or aging. It is our belief that the next generation of QoL technologies will need to have the ability to monitor individuals in their natural environments, intelligently adapt to the capacity and needs of the individual, and provide appropriate levels of assistance that significantly improve functioning while maintaining high levels of individual autonomy.

P.4 Overview of This Book

This book represents a collaborative effort of a diverse interdisciplinary team, including engineers, computer scientists, clinicians, social scientists, and policy experts. Our intent is to describe not only emerging new QoL technologies but also the process of developing them. The book is divided into four parts. Part I, comprised of Chapters 1 through 3, provides an introduction and conceptual foundation for quality of life technologies (QoLTs). In Chapter 1, we focus on the intended end users of QoLTs to address the question, who might benefit from QoLTs? A broad range of data sources are described that characterize potential markets for QoLTs, including older individuals, persons with disability, informal caregivers, and professional health-care providers. Chapters 2 and 3 focus on facilitators and barriers of technology uptake at both the individual end-user level (Chapter 2) and organizational societal level (Chapter 3).

These chapters describe the interplay of three key factors determining technology uptake: (a) characteristics, needs, and preferences of end users; (b) features of the technology; and (c) societal factors, including social and health policy and the regulatory environment.

Part II, comprised of Chapters 4 through 8, describes the design and development process for QoLTs. Methods for assessing needs and preferences of end users are described in Chapter 4. The process of turning an idea into a testable and useful product is described in Chapter 5, while Chapter 6 focuses on the importance of universal design in the design and development process. Developing successful QoLT products invariably requires interdisciplinary teamwork and community partners. Thus, Chapter 7 describes how to organize and manage interdisciplinary teams and foster relationships with community partners who can provide evaluative input and testbeds for new technologies. Chapter 8 focuses on evaluation strategies for assessing QoLTs, describing both formative and summative approaches, including randomized clinical trials as a means for gauging the cost–benefits of QoLTs.

Core technologies and their applications are discussed in Part III, comprised of Chapters 9 through 13. Chapter 9 explores key technologies in the general area of visual sensing, that is, systems that can automatically extract information from images and videos from cameras. Understanding the user's environment is a key feature of intelligent systems designed to augment the user's capability, for example, to help older adults and people with disabilities in their daily activities. Chapter 10 focuses on robots designed to perform useful everyday tasks in the home with and around people. It addresses the important question, what is different about designing robots for factories versus robots in the home? Chapter 11 deals with virtual coaches, technology systems that continuously monitor users and their environment, detect situations where intervention would be desirable, and offer prompt assistance. Environmentally embedded sensing systems are described in Chapter 12. These systems have the capacity to monitor human behavior 24/7 and thereby provide valuable diagnostic information about the health and functioning of frail older individuals who are at risk for adverse health events. Chapter 13 demonstrates how existing communication technologies can be used to improve the quality of lives of both older disabled individuals and family members who are involved in their care.

Part IV, comprised of Chapters 14 and 15, makes an argument for transformations needed in education and the marketplace if QoLTs are to flourish. Students will need to develop new competencies, and developers will need to acquire new perspectives on the innovation and commercialization process if this enterprise is to succeed and grow.

References

Barrett, L. L. 2008. *Healthy@home Research Report*. Washington, DC: American Association of Retired Persons Foundation.

Bougie, I. T. 2008. ISO 9999 assistive products for persons with disability—Classification and terminology. In *The Engineering Handbook of Smart Technology for Aging, Disability and Independence*, eds. A. Helal, M. Mokhtari, and B. Abdulrazak, Chapter 6. Hoboken, NJ: John Wiley & Sons, Inc.

Brooks, R. 1996. EuroQol: The current state of play. *Health Policy* 37(1): 53–72.

Center for Devices and Radiological Health: U.S. Food and Drug Administration (FDA). 2010. *Medical Device Home Use Initiative*. Washington, DC: FDA, April.

Center for Technology and Aging. 2009. Briefing paper: Technologies to help older adults maintain independence: advancing technology adoption. Oakland, CA: SCAN Foundation and Public Health Institute, July.

Diener, E., S. Oishi, and R. E. Lucas. 2003. Personality, culture, and subjective well-being: Emotional and cognitive evaluations of life. *Annual Review of Psychology* 54: 403–425.

Fayers, P. M. and D. Machin. 2000. *Quality of Life: Assessment, Analysis, and Interpretation*. Chichester, U.K.: John Wiley & Sons, Inc.

Schulz, R., S. R. Beach, J. T. Matthews et al. 2012. Designing and evaluating quality of life technologies: An interdisciplinary approach. In *Proceedings of the IEEE* 100: 2397–2409.

The WHOQoL Group. 1994. The development of the World Health Organization quality of life assessment instrument (the WHOQoL). In *Quality of Life Assessment: International Perspectives*, eds. J. Orley and W. Kuyken. Heidelberg, Germany: Springer-Verlag.

Ware, J., K. Snow, M. Kosinski, and B. Gandek. 1993. *SF-36 Health Survey Manual and Interpretation Guide*. Boston, MA: The Health Institute, New England Medical Center.

Editor

Richard Schulz is professor of psychiatry and director of the University Center for Social and Urban Research at the University of Pittsburgh, Pittsburgh, Pennsylvania. He also serves as associate director of the Aging Institute of UPMC Senior Services and the University of Pittsburgh and as director of the Person and Society Core of the Quality of Life Technology (QoLT) Engineering Research Center, which is responsible for infusing individual end-user and societal perspectives in the development and evaluation of technologies for older persons and persons with disability.

Dr. Schulz received his AB in psychology from Dartmouth College and his PhD in social psychology from Duke University. He has spent most of his career doing research and writing on adult development and aging. His work has focused on social–psychological aspects of aging, including the impact of disabling late life disease on patients and their families, and he has been funded by the National Institutes of Health for more than three decades to conduct descriptive, longitudinal, and intervention research on diverse older populations representing illnesses such as cancer, spinal cord injury, stroke, Alzheimer's disease, heart disease, and arthritis.

He has been a leading contributor to the literature on the health effects of family caregiving, Alzheimer's disease caregiving, and intervention studies for caregivers of persons with Alzheimer's disease. This body of work is reflected in more than 280 publications, which have appeared in major medical, psychology, aging, and engineering journals, including the *New England Journal of Medicine*, the *Journal of the American Medical Association*, *Archives of Internal Medicine*, and *IEEE*. He is also the author of numerous books, including the fourth edition of the *Encyclopedia of Aging* and the *Handbook of Alzheimer's Caregiver Intervention Research*. In the last decade, Dr. Schulz has become interested in supportive interventions, including technology-based approaches to enhance patient functioning and quality of life of both patients and their family caregivers.

Dr. Schulz is the recipient of numerous honors, including the Kleemeier Award for Research on Aging from the Gerontological Society of America and the Developmental Health Award for Research on Health in Later Life from the American Psychological Association.

Contributors

Gregory L. Alexander
Sinclair School of Nursing
University of Missouri
Columbia, Missouri

Scott R. Beach
Survey Research Program
and
University Center for Social and Urban
    Research
University of Pittsburgh
Pittsburgh, Pennsylvania

Shelly Brown
Human Engineering Research
    Laboratories
VA Pittsburgh Health System
Pittsburgh, Pennsylvania

Diane Collins
School of Health and Rehabilitation
    Sciences
University of Pittsburgh
Pittsburgh, Pennsylvania

Karen L. Courtney
School of Health Information Science
University of Victoria
Victoria, British Columbia, Canada

Sara J. Czaja
Miller School of Medicine
University of Miami
Miami, Florida

Annette DeVito Dabbs
School of Nursing
University of Pittsburgh
Pittsburgh, Pennsylvania

Anind Dey
Human-Computer Interaction
    Institute
Carnegie Mellon University
Pittsburgh, Pennsylvania

Dan Ding
School of Health and Rehabilitation
    Sciences
VA Pittsburgh Health System
Pittsburgh, Pennsylvania

Mary Goldberg
Human Engineering Research
    Laboratories
VA Pittsburgh Health System
Pittsburgh, Pennsylvania

Rainer Dane Guevara
Department of Electrical and
    Computer Engineering
University of Missouri
Columbia, Missouri

Martial Hebert
School of Computer Science
Carnegie Mellon University
Pittsburgh, Pennsylvania

James F. Jordan
H. John Heinz III College
Carnegie Mellon University
Pittsburgh, Pennsylvania

Takeo Kanade
The Robotics Institute
Carnegie Mellon University
Pittsburgh, Pennsylvania

Richelle J. Koopman
Curtis W. & Ann H. Long Department
    of Family and Community Medicine
University of Missouri
Columbia, Missouri

Chin Chin Lee
Miller School of Medicine
University of Miami
Miami, Florida

Judith T. Matthews
University Center for Social and Urban
    Research
University of Pittsburgh
Pittsburgh, Pennsylvania

Laurel Person Mecca
University Center for Social and Urban
    Research
University of Pittsburgh
Pittsburgh, Pennsylvania

Steve J. Miller
Sinclair School of Nursing
University of Missouri
Columbia, Missouri

Maria Milleville
Human Engineering Research
    Laboratories
VA Pittsburgh Health System
Pittsburgh, Pennsylvania

Lorraine J. Phillips
Sinclair School of Nursing
University of Missouri
Columbia, Missouri

Marilyn J. Rantz
Sinclair School of Nursing
University of Missouri
Columbia, Missouri

Richard Schulz
School of Medicine
and
University Center for Social and Urban
    Research
University of Pittsburgh
Pittsburgh, Pennsylvania

Katherine D. Seelman
Department of Rehabilitation Science
    and Technology
University of Pittsburgh
Pittsburgh, Pennsylvania

Daniel P. Siewiorek
Department of Electrical and
    Computer Engineering and
    Computer Science
Carnegie Mellon University
Pittsburgh, Pennsylvania

Reid Simmons
The Robotics Institute
Carnegie Mellon University
Pittsburgh, Pennsylvania

Marjorie Skubic
Center for Eldercare and Rehabilitation
    Technology
and
Department of Electrical and Computer
    Engineering
University of Missouri
Columbia, Missouri

Asim Smailagic
Institute for Complex Engineered Systems
Carnegie Mellon University
Pittsburgh, Pennsylvania

Roger O. Smith
Department of Occupational Science
    and Technology
University of Wisconsin–Milwaukee
Milwaukee, Wisconsin

Siddhartha S. Srinivasa
The Robotics Institute
Carnegie Mellon University
Pittsburgh, Pennsylvania

Edward Steinfeld
School of Architecture and
    Planning
University at Buffalo
Buffalo, New York

Part I

Introduction and Conceptual Foundations

1

Who Can Benefit from Quality of Life Technology?

Richard Schulz and Scott R. Beach

CONTENTS

1.1 Introduction

Understanding who the intended end users are and their needs and preferences is a first step in the technology development process (Stanton et al. 2005). Both quantitative and qualitative methods can be used to identify needs and preferences for quality of life technology (QoLT) including (a) population-based epidemiologic studies, (b) surveys assessing preferences for QoLT, (c) field observations, and (d) focus groups.

Identifying prevalence rates from population-based or epidemiological surveys is one of the most fundamental ways to understand the potential market for QoLT. These surveys not only provide estimates of how many adults are living with disabilities of various types (e.g., physical, sensory, cognitive, self-care, and mobility), they also constitute a rich source of data on the sociodemographic and health-related correlates of such disability. In this chapter, we identify and characterize the major target populations for QoLTs.

1.2 Older Persons and Adults with Disability

The majority of the world's increasingly older adult population requires some degree of formal and/or informal care due to loss of function as a result of congenital defect, injury, or failing health. Persons with disability are the primary candidates for QoL technologies, although defining what is meant by disability remains a matter for debate: As a result, prevalence rates of disability vary widely depending on which of the more than 20 definitions of disability are used for purposes of entitlement to public or private income support programs, government services, or statistical analysis (Mashaw and Reno 1996). The World Health Organization (WHO) has adopted the International Classification of Functioning, Disability and Health (ICF) definition of disability which emphasizes the interactional nature of disability: "disability is a complex phenomena that arises from an interaction between attributes of the person and the overall physical, human-built, attitudinal, and social environment in which the person lives and acts" (Bickenbach 2008). At the heart of this definition is the idea that disability is not exclusively the result of impairments in body function or structure but may also be the result of activity restrictions or participation restrictions. This nuanced perspective on disability is consistent with other conceptualizations of disability that explicitly recognize the interaction of environment and pathologies or impairments to cause disability (Nagi 1969; Jette and Badley 2001; Institute of Medicine 2007).

In practice, most surveys on disability simply ask questions about having difficulty in doing activities such as dressing, bathing, or getting around the home, learning, remembering, or concentrating "because of physical, mental, or emotional conditions lasting 6 months or more" (U.S. Census 2000). The primary sources of disability data in the United States are the U.S. Census 2000, American Community Survey (ACS), Current Population Survey (CPS), National Health Interview Survey (NHIS), Medical Expenditure Panel Survey (MEPS), Panel Study of Income Dynamics (PSID), Survey of Income and Program Participation (SIPP), and the Health and Retirement Study (HRS).

Three of the most widely used sources for disability statistics—U.S. Census 2000, CPS, ACS—report disability rates ranging from 8.4% to 10.4% of adults aged 21–64. Among persons aged 65 and higher, the ACS reports disability rates of 38% or 14.2 million persons, with slightly higher rates reported by the U.S. Census 2000. In 20 years, the United States will have 72 million people over the age of 65, a significant proportion of whom will have physical and cognitive disabilities. Table 1.1 provides an example of prevalence estimates from several surveys for various types of disability (Gould and Lewis 1985; Goodhue 1995; Crandall et al. 2006).

It should be noted that there is some variability in disability rates depending on the specific question asked and whether institutionalized, noncivilian populations are included; nevertheless, across all surveys, there is strong consensus that disability rates increase dramatically with age.

There are many other sources of disability statistics (see review in Institute of Medicine 2007), including the Behavioral Risk Factor Surveillance System (BRFSS) and the National Health and Nutrition Examination Survey (N-HANES), which are both repeated cross-sectional surveys as well as the following panel surveys:

- The Medicare Current Beneficiary Survey (MCBS)
- The National Long-Term Care Survey (NLTCS)
- Medical Expenditure Panel Survey (MEPS)
- Panel Study of Income Dynamics (PSID)
- Survey of Income and Program Participation (SIPP)
- Health and Retirement Study (HRS)

These surveys provide not only prevalence estimates, but the ability to track trends over time. In addition, the sociodemographic (e.g., age, gender, race, education, income) and

TABLE 1.1

Examples of Population-Based Disability Prevalence Surveys

Survey/Source	Disability Questions	Prevalence Estimate(s) and Number (Million)
American Community Survey (ACS) 2008	*Hearing*: Is this person deaf or does he/she have serious difficulty hearing?	3.5% (10.4 million) 2.2% (age 21–64; 4.1)
Noninstitutionalized U.S. population (cross-sectional)	*Visual*: Is this person blind or does he/she have serious difficulty seeing even when wearing glasses?	15.7% (age 65+; 5.8) 2.3% (6.8 million) 1.8% (age 21–64; 3.4)
Replaced the Census "Long Form"	*Cognitive*: Because of a physical, mental, or emotional condition, does this person have serious difficulty concentrating, remembering, or making decisions?	7.7% (age 65+; 2.9) 4.8% (13.4 million) 4.1% (age 21–64; 7.7)
	Ambulatory: Does this person have serious difficulty walking or climbing stairs?	9.9% (age 65+; 3.7) 6.9% (19.2 million) 5.1% (age 21–64; 9.6)
	Self-Care: Does this person have difficulty dressing or bathing?	24.8% (age 65+; 9.2) 2.6% (7.2 million) 1.8% (age 21–64; 3.3)
	Independent living: Because of a physical, mental, or emotional condition, does this person have difficulty doing errands alone such as visiting a doctor's office or shopping?	9.2% (age 65+; 3.4) 5.5% (13.2 million) 3.5% (age 21–64; 6.5)
	Any disability	17.2% (age 65+; 6.4) 12.1% (36.1 million) 10.1% (age 21–64; 19.1) 38.2% (age 65+; 14.2)
U.S. Census 2000 (Long form)	Does this person have any of the following long-lasting conditions: *Sensory*:	
Noninstitutionalized U.S. (population age 21–64 reported here)	Blindness, deafness, or a severe vision or hearing impairment? *Physical activity*:	2.4% (3.9 million)
	A condition that substantially limits one or more basic physical activities such as walking, climbing stairs, reaching, lifting, or carrying? Because of a physical, mental, or emotional condition lasting 6 months or more, does this person have any difficulty in doing any of the following activities: *Mental*:	6.8% (10.9 million)
	Learning, remembering, or concentrating? *Self-care*:	3.8% (6.0 million)
	Dressing, bathing, or getting around inside the home?	
	Any disability	1.9% (3.0 million) 10.2% (16.2 million)
Current Population Survey (CPS) 2009 Noninstitutionalized U.S. (population age 21–64 reported here) (panel survey)	*Disability-related work limitations*: Does anyone in this household have a health problem or disability which prevents them from working or which limits the kind or amount of work they can do?	8.4% (14.8 million)

(continued)

TABLE 1.1 (continued)

Examples of Population-Based Disability Prevalence Surveys

Survey/Source	Disability Questions	Prevalence Estimate(s) and Number (Million)
National Health Interview Survey (NHIS) 2009	By yourself, and without using any special equipment, how difficult is it for you to	7.0% (15.9 million)
Noninstitutionalized U.S. population age 18 and older (cross-sectional)	*Walk ¼ mile*	2.0% (age18–44; 2.2) 7.8% (age 45–64; 6.2) 13.1% (age 65–74; 2.7) 28.0% (age 75+; 4.8) 15.7% (35.6 million)
	Any of the following:	
	• Walk ¼ mile	6.0% (age18–44; 6.6)
	• Climb up 10 steps without resting	18.8% (age 45–64; 14.9) 27.9% (age 65–74; 5.8)
	• Stand for 2 h	48.3% (age 75+; 8.3)
	• Sit for 2 h	
	• Stoop, bend, or kneel	
	• Reach over head	
	• Grasp or handle small objects	
	• Lift or carry 10 pounds	
	• Push or pull large objects	
	Because of a physical, mental, or emotional problem, do you need the help of other persons with *Personal care needs* such as eating, bathing, dressing, or getting around inside the home? *(ADL)*	1.9% (4.4 million) 0.5% (age18–44; 0.6) 1.8% (age 45–64; 1.4) 3.1% (age 65–74; 0.6) 10.3% (age 75+; 1.8)
	Because of a physical, mental, or emotional problem, do you need the help of other persons in handling *routine needs* such as everyday household chores, doing necessary business, shopping, or getting around for other purposes? *(IADL)*	4.0% (9.2 million) 1.3% (age18–44; 1.5) 3.7% (age 45–64; 2.9) 6.4% (age 65–74; 1.3) 20.3% (age 75+; 3.5)

Source:　Gould, J.D. and Lewis, C., *Commun. ACM*, 28(3), 300, 1985; Goodhue, D.L., *Manag. Sci.*, 41(12), 1827, 1995; Crandall, B. et al., *Working Minds: A Practitioner's Guide to Cognitive Task Analysis*, MIT Press, Cambridge, MA, 2006.

other health-related correlates or contributing conditions to disability can be derived from these sources. For example, data from the 2002 and 2003 NHIS show that arthritis or other musculoskeletal conditions were the most frequent cause of disability among those aged 65–84, followed by heart/other circulatory conditions and diabetes. Among those aged 85 and older, vision and hearing difficulties and dementia/senility were additional major contributors to disability (Institute of Medicine 2007; Altman and Bernstein 2008).

Data from many of these national surveys is publicly accessible for download, enabling the user to carry out customized secondary data analysis. It should be noted that secondary analysis requires some level of statistical sophistication to deal with issues surrounding the analysis of complex survey data (e.g., statistical weighting and variance estimation). Fortunately, there are web-based resources available to the public that simplify the generation of disability statistics. One of the best is the Cornell Center on Disability Demographics and Statistics (http://www.ilr.cornell.edu/edi/disabilitystatistics). The site allows users to access disability-related data from the ACS, U.S. Census 2000, and the CPS via interactive menus allowing specification of type of disability (e.g., hearing, cognitive, self-care, physical activity; for ACS, U.S. Census 2000), along with demographic subgroup(s) of interest, including gender and age (all three surveys) and race and education level for the ACS. The demographic variables can be looked at either individually (e.g., males, females of all ages, race, and education levels) or in specific combinations with other variables (e.g., males, age 65+, African-American with a high-school education or less). This tool allows precise targeting of disability data on potential subpopulations who may be candidates for QoLT.

In sum, there is a wide variety of population-based/epidemiological disability-related data available in the United States to help identify the potential market for QoLT, which is fairly large and likely to continue increasing. The data are publicly available and there are tools available to help researchers access it in an efficient and targeted manner. Gathering this data is essential in the early stages of defining the target populations and ultimately the need for QoLT applications.

An example of using epidemiologic data to define potential target populations for various technologies is presented in Table 1.2. The CMU/Pitt QoLT ERC has defined four broad system areas within which specific technologies are being developed—virtual coaches, QoLT bots, home and community health and wellness, and safe driving. These systems, including envisioned specific applications, key capabilities, and targeted populations, are summarized in Table 1.2.

The development of these systems is an ongoing process that involves input from various stakeholders—end users, caregivers, clinical practitioners, industry—working with engineers and computer scientists to arrive at common understandings of requisite system capabilities that will ultimately have a positive impact on quality of life. Various aspects of this iterative QoLT system development process will be described in detail in this and other chapters of this book. The main point here is the final column showing potential target populations, which were derived from various data sources like those described in this section. Note that the proposed systems include both broadly applicable (fitness coach; activity monitoring) and more narrowly targeted (HERB; PerMMA) markets. Extraction of these statistics served to both define the potential size of the target population market and to suggest required functionalities of the QoLT systems.

1.3 Persons with Traumatic Brain Injury

Traumatic brain injury (TBI) is damage to the brain which occurs as a result of violent blows to the head or when an object pierces the skull. The symptoms of TBI can be mild, moderate, or severe and may include loss of consciousness, headache, confusion, dizziness, convulsions or seizures, behavioral and mood changes, and trouble with memory, concentration, attention, or thinking. Depending on the extent and location of the brain damage, persons with TBI may suffer lifelong physical, cognitive, behavioral, and emotional consequences such as decreased problem-solving and decision-making ability, increased impulsivity, and memory and language impairments. The leading causes of TBI are falls, motor vehicle crashes, being struck by or against objects, and assaults. Blasts are a leading cause of TBI among active duty military personnel in war zones. The relatively high prevalence of TBIs among veterans of the wars in Iraq and Afghanistan has stimulated the development of supportive technologies for persons with TBI.

TABLE 1.2

Sample QoLT ERC Systems, Capabilities, Technologies, and Target Populations

	Envisioned Systems	Key Capabilities	Targeted Populations (Size)
Virtual Coach	Households Affairs Coach	• Manage home inventory	• Older adults living alone (4 M)
Cognitive and reasoning assistance wherever a person goes and whatever he or she does			• People with Alzheimer's (5.3 M) • People with mild cognitive impairment (>6 M older adults)
	Personal Safety Coach	• Assess risk of falling • Assess IADL performance	• Survivors of stroke (2.5 M) • People with TBI (5.3 M)
	Fitness Coach	• Assess fitness • Assess diet	• All adults
QoL Tbots	TransferBot	• Assist caregiver with transfers between chairs, beds, etc.	• People with mobility impairments (10 M) • Frail elderly (4 M)
Physical assistance combined with a perceptive environment that provides for diminished manipulation and mobility in and out of the home	HERB-Kitchen Robot	• Prepare meals • Find and fetch personal items	• Wheelchair users (2.7 M) • Wheelchair users with dexterity impairment (0.2 M) • Wheelchair user with cognitive impairment (0.2 M) • Arthritis sufferers (19 M+)
	PerMMA	• Feed, groom person, recognize discomfort • Learn personal preferences	• Wheelchair users with dexterity impairment (0.2 M) • Wheelchair users with cognitive impairment (0.2 M)
Home and Community Health and Wellness	Activity and Behavior Monitoring	• Continuous assessment of physical function and emotional state	• Aging adults (39 M) • Sufferers of chronic illness (>133 M) • People with cognitive decline (12 M)
Smart home and community technologies and infrastructure for independence and health maintenance	Health Kiosk Home Medical Device Monitor	• Identify changes in physiology/activity/ behavior that portend impairment • Cognitive orthotics	
	Self-tuning Environment	• Smart/safe home medical instruments • Remote caregiving • Self-adapting environmental conditions	
Safe Driving	DriveCap Advisor	• Assess a person's capability • Provide advice	• Drivers with vision (>3 M) or hearing impairments (24 M) • People with mild cognitive impairment (>6 M)
Ways to make driving safer for older adults and people with disabilities	Virtual Valet	• Auto park • Semi-autonomous control	• Wheelchair users (2.7 M) • Walker/cane users (9 M)

In the United States, about 1.4 million TBIs occur each year with 1.1 million emergency department visits, 235,000 hospitalizations, and 50,000 deaths (Langlois et al. 2006). It is estimated that about 5.3 million Americans are living with long-term or lifelong disability resulting from TBI involving hospitalization. The total prevalence of long-term disability from TBI is likely to be considerably higher since not all TBIs result in hospitalization.

1.4 Informal Caregivers

Older adults and persons with disability are not the only potential beneficiaries of QoL technologies. They can also benefit caregivers (both professional and informal), health care providers, and aging/disability services providers by improving the quality of care and enhancing the caregivers' experiences, efficiencies, and cost-effectiveness. Of these, the largest group, by far, is comprised of informal caregivers. These are typically family members who provide care to a child with disability or an older individual who needs assistance or supervision because of declining functional ability.

1.4.1 Informal Caregivers of Adults with Disability

There are no exact estimates of the number of informal caregivers in the United States. Prevalence estimates vary widely depending on definitions used and populations sampled. At one extreme are estimates that 28.5% of the U.S. adult population, or 65.7 million Americans, provided unpaid care to an adult relative in 2009, with the majority (83%) of this care being delivered to people age 50 years or older (National Alliance for Caregiving and American Association for Retired Persons 2009). This number approximates the estimated 59 million adults with a disability in the United States, based on the BRFSS survey (Centers for Disease Control and Prevention 2006). At the other extreme, data from the National Long-Term Care survey suggest that as few as 3.5 million informal caregivers provided instrumental activities of daily living (IADL) or activities of daily living (ADL) assistance to people age 65 and over. Intermediate estimates of 28.8 million caregivers ("persons aged 15 or over providing personal assistance for everyday needs of someone age 15 and older") are reported by the Survey on Income and Program Participation (National Family Caregivers Association and Family Caregiver Alliance 2006). A recent national survey of individuals age 45 and older yielded a caregiving rate of 12% or 14.9 million adults (Roth et al. 2009).

These differences are in part attributable to when the data were collected, the age range of the population sampled, and care recipient populations targeted, but most importantly to the definition of caregiving. Thus, the high-end estimates are generated when broad and inclusive definitions of caregiving are used (e.g., "Unpaid care may include help with personal needs or household chores. It might be managing a person's finances, arranging for outside services, or visiting regularly to see how they are doing.") (National Alliance for Caregiving and American Association for Retired Persons 2009), and low-end estimates are generated when definitions require the provision of specific ADL or IADL assistance (e.g., Wolff and Kasper 2006). A related issue is that definitions of caregiving do not clearly distinguish caregiving for chronic disability from caregiving for acute care episodes that might follow a hospitalization event. However, most definitions used emphasize chronic disability; intermittent episodes of caregiving are not well represented in the existing data.

Although there are some encouraging signs that age-related disability is declining in the United States, this will be offset by the rapid growth of the senior population to an estimated 70 million in 2035. It is projected that the number of older adults with functional deficits will grow from 22 million in 2005 to 38 million by 2030, assuming no changes in disability rates from current levels (Institute of Medicine 2007). The challenges posed by this demographic shift will be exacerbated by the decreasing ability of existing formal care systems to care for older adults because of a shortage of nurses and other health care workers, and increasing costs of hospitalization and long-term care (Talley and Crews 2007).

Recent historical events have added one additional unanticipated caregiving challenge. Young adults are returning from our ongoing wars with multiple, interacting injuries, or polytrauma, that they may be coping with for the rest of their lives. Posttraumatic stress is a common sequel of service in wartime, as well. The need for sustained informal caregiving for these young veterans is potentially immense, and the nature of the challenges for their informal caregivers warrants thorough investigation.

1.4.2 Long-Distance Caregivers

Approximately 15% of caregivers to older adults live at least an hour away from their relatives, and as such provide care at a distance. Long-distance caregivers tend to be more educated and affluent, and are more likely to play a secondary helper role when compared to in-home caregivers. Distant caregivers spend on average 3.4 h/week arranging services and another 4 h/week checking on the care recipient or monitoring care. One-third of long-distance caregivers visit at least once a week and provide on average 34 h of I/ADL assistance per month (National Alliance for Caregiving 2004).

Because distance and time are limiting factors to providing direct support to the care recipient, long-distance caregivers have the added challenges of identifying relevant resources in the recipient's local environment at a distance, hiring individuals to provide needed care, and monitoring the care providers' performance as well as the status of the care recipient. From a human factors perspective, performing these tasks requires sophisticated search skills, the ability to screen and evaluate professional care providers, and systems for monitoring care recipient status which may range from contact via telephone to sophisticated electronic monitoring and communication devices. These caregivers also may have to be able to cope with psychological distress associated with being unable to do more for their distant loved ones who need care.

1.4.3 Caregivers for Children

All children are care recipients under a broad definition of caregiving. Human beings require nearly two decades to acquire the necessary knowledge and skills to function independently. Throughout this developmental period, virtually all children also experience multiple acute illnesses which require support and care from their parents. More extraordinary levels of care occur when a child suffers from a chronic disability that requires intensive and long-term support from their parents. The 2005–2006 National Survey of Children with Special Health Care Needs estimates that 13.9% of children under age 18 have special health care needs, defined in terms of use of services, therapies, counseling, or medications, or functional limitations at least a year in duration (U.S. Department of Health and Human Services-Health Resources and Services Administration-Maternal and Child Health Bureau 2008). According to this survey, 21.8% of households with children in this country have a child with special needs.

The leading chronic health conditions reported as causing activity limitations among children up to the age of 18 include learning disabilities; attention deficit or hyperactivity disorder; other mental, emotional, or behavioral problems; mental retardation or other developmental problems; asthma or breathing problems; and speech or language problems (Institute of Medicine 2007). These conditions have developmental trajectories such that speech problems are more prevalent at young ages and learning disabilities at later ages. Not included in this list are illnesses or conditions such as childhood cancers, diabetes, heart disease, and cerebral palsy, which are less common among children than adults but create high caregiving demands when present. Other examples of low prevalence conditions with outsized demands for care and particularly high levels of family stress are autism spectrum disorder and cystic fibrosis.

Many children with a disability will carry the burden of chronic illness and disability into middle and old age and require support from informal care providers throughout their lives. This means that some individuals will spend their entire adult lives as caregivers. The ability to survive with disability into late life will add to the already growing number of people who acquire disability as adults, increasing demands for support and care. The growing prevalence of obesity and related disorders among both children and adults in the United States is expected to further raise disability rates and increase the demand for care.

1.4.4 Episodic Caregiving

Because most caregiving data are based on care for chronic illness and disability, we know little about the prevalence of episodic care. Episodic caregiving is typically provided after discharge from an acute care hospital for events such as hip fracture, stroke, cancer, or trauma. In 2007, the United States had nearly 40 million hospital discharges (Agency for Healthcare Research and Quality 2007), and many of these individuals likely required care from a family member postdischarge. We know little about the intensity, duration, or type of care provided or about the characteristics of informal caregivers in this instance. Because episodic events are often characterized by acute onset without warning, they entail different challenges than chronic caregiving. Episodic caregivers have to quickly acquire skills related to performing in-home medical procedures, operating medical equipment, monitoring patient status, and coordinating care. Technologies that help monitor patients, provide coaching to carry out complex medical procedures, and guide how and when to access needed services would be very beneficial to this group.

Although we tend to view technologies as being most beneficial to individuals with long-term or permanent disability, Table 1.3 shows that they may be beneficial as well to individuals with short-term needs, such as the 40 million persons discharged from hospitals in the United States each year who may not be able to function independently and/or require assistance to carry out complex medical regimens, or the 7.6 million individuals in the United States who receive formal home healthcare services annually (National Association for Home Care & Hospice 2008). In addition, persons with chronic disease but no disability might benefit from technologies that assist them with managing conditions such as diabetes or heart disease.

These data provide only crude guidance about broad categories of individuals that might be targeted for technology development. As we shall see in later chapters of

TABLE 1.3

Recipients and Providers of Informal Care

Recipients of Care	Providers of Care	Prevalence of Informal Caregiving
Adults with chronic health/disability problems	Middle-aged and older parents and spouses	12%–22% adult population
Children with chronic health/disability problems	Young to middle-aged parents, grandparents	22% of households with children
Hospital discharge patients—children and adults	Adults of all ages	40 million discharges per year

this book, determining who might benefit from a specific QoL technology requires a much finer grained understanding of potential end users and their needs. Methods for obtaining more in-depth user preferences and needs are described in subsequent chapters.

1.5 Health Care Providers (Professional Caregivers)

The third potential beneficiaries of QoL technology are health care providers of all types who benefit indirectly through technologies that affect patient behaviors and outcomes and directly through technologies that facilitate or enhance diagnosis, prescribing, care management, and treatment delivery. Many types of technology are currently available including home and office/hospital telemedicine systems that substitute face-to-face medical diagnosis and treatment and assistive devices such as medication reminders and dispensers. While ultimately benefiting the patient, these technologies often serve as extenders for human health care providers. A growing literature reporting interventions utilizing assistive technology applications demonstrates successful adoption of various low- and high-tech strategies by older adults with stroke (Mann et al. 1996; Gosman-Hedström et al. 2002; Chiu and Man 2004; Hitchcock 2006); arthritis (Mann et al. 1995); multiple sclerosis (Finlayson et al. 2001; Verza et al. 2006); Parkinson disease (Stewart et al. 2004); cognitive impairment (Mann et al. 1996; Yang et al. 1997); chronic back pain (Polly 2005); intellectual disabilities (Hammel et al. 2002); generalized frailty (Chen et al. 2000; Doughty and Williams 2001; Mann et al. 2004); and a range of mobility, physical, and sensory impairments (Mann et al. 1993; Watzke 1997; Dahlin-Ivanoff and Sonn 2004), including individuals at specific risk of falls (Aminzadeh and Edwards 1998). Health care providers are often in position to prescribe these technologies and typically play an active role in overseeing their functioning, reviewing data generated by these systems, and adapting their diagnosis or care plans based on results obtained. Health care providers also play an active role in the system-wide application of emerging technologies. For example, the Veterans Administration has adopted numerous telemedicine programs based on patient outcomes and provider input.

The number and types of professionals who might use these technologies is vast, ranging from primary care physicians and medical specialists to nurses, physical, occupational, rehabilitation, and speech therapists.

1.6 Integrated Systems for Multiple Different End Users

Most older persons and their caregivers enter the health care system through their primary care provider and remain with that provider throughout the long-term course of an illness or disability. Thus, primary health care is the major entry point into the greater health and social service system and has the potential of being the central coordinating system for the provision of ongoing support for both older patients and informal caregivers. In a more perfect world, technology would facilitate support and communication among all three potential beneficiaries of new QoL technologies. For example, technology that directly benefits the person with disability by enhancing personal care functioning might at the same time communicate patient status and functioning to family members and health care providers who could adapt their interactions with the patient based on feedback they receive. The health care provider could additionally coordinate with and support the role of the informal caregiver to maximize their ability to support the patient and maintain their own well-being.

Figure 1.1 illustrates how an optimal system that involves the three key member of the triad involved in supporting the health and well-being of a person with disability or older person. One can imagine technology that supports the functioning of each member of the triad while at the same time facilitating communication among them. Such a system would likely be more efficient than systems that target only one individual in the triad and, importantly, has the potential of enhancing the quality of life of all three members of the triad.

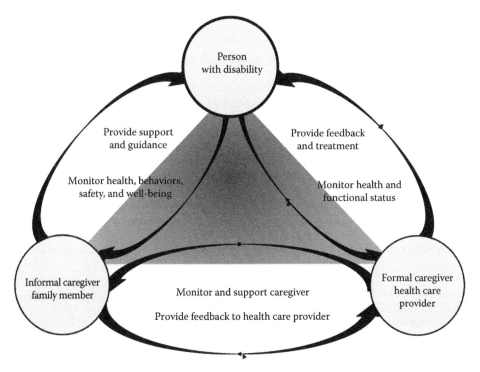

FIGURE 1.1
Integrated system of multiple different end users.

References

Agency for Healthcare Research and Quality (AHRQ). 2007. *Acute Care/Hospitalization* Rockville, MD: AHRQ. http://www.ahrq.gov/research/dec07/1207RA12.htm

Altman, B. and Bernstein, A. 2008. *Disability and Health in the United States, 2001–2005*. Hyatsville, MD: National Center for Health Statistics.

Aminzadeh, F. and Edwards, N. 1998. Exploring seniors' views on the use of assistive devices in fall prevention. *Public Health Nursing* 15 (4): 297–304.

Bickenbach, J.E. 2008. Assistive technology and the international classification of functioning, disability and health. In *The Engineering Handbook of Smart Technology for Aging, Disability and Independence*, eds. A. Helal, M. Mokhtari, and B. Abdulrazak, pp. 81–100. Hoboken, NJ: John Wiley & Sons, Inc.

Centers for Disease Control and Prevention (CDC). 2006. *Disability and Health State Chartbook, 2006: Profiles of Health for Adults with Disabilities*. Atlanta, GA: Centers for Disease Control and Prevention.

Chen, T.Y., Mann, W.C., Tomita, M.R., and Nochajski, S.M. 2000. Caregiver involvement in the use of assistive devices by frail older persons. *Occupational Therapy Journal of Research* 20 (3): 179–199.

Chiu, C.W.Y. and Man, D.W.K. 2004. The effect of training older adults with stroke to use home-based assistive devices. *OTJR: Occupational, Participation and Health* 24 (3): 113–120.

Crandall, B., Klein, G., and Hoffman, R.R. 2006. *Working Minds: A Practitioner's Guide to Cognitive Task Analysis*. Cambridge, MA: MIT Press.

Dahlin-Ivanoff, S. and Sonn, U. 2004. Use of assistive devices in daily activities among 85-year-olds living at home focusing especially on the visually impaired. *Disability and Rehabilitation* 26 (24): 1423–1430.

Doughty, K. and Williams, G. 2001. Towards a complete home monitoring system. Paper presented at the *RoSPA Conference on Safety in the Home Stratford-Upon-Avon*, November 12–13, Warwickshire, U.K.

Finlayson, M., Guglielmello, L., and Liefer, K. 2001. Describing and predicting the possession of assistive devices among persons with multiple sclerosis. *American Journal of Occupational Therapy* 55 (5): 545–551.

Goodhue, D.L. 1995. Understanding user evaluations of information systems. *Management Science* 41 (12): 1827–1844.

Gosman-Hedström, G., Claesson, L., Blomstrand, C., Fagerberg, B., and Lundgren-Lindquist, B. 2002. Use and cost of assistive technology the first year after stroke. A randomized controlled trial. *International Journal of Technology Assessment in Health Care* 18 (3): 520–527.

Gould, J.D. and Lewis, C. 1985. Designing for usability: Key principles and what designers think. *Communications of the ACM* 28 (3): 300–311.

Hammel, J., Lai, J.S., and Heller, T. 2002. The impact of assistive technology and environmental interventions on function and living situation status with people who are ageing with developmental disabilities. *Disability and Rehabilitation* 24 (1): 93–105.

Hitchcock, E. 2006. Computer access for people after stroke. *Topics in Stroke Rehabilitation* 13 (3): 22–30.

Institute of Medicine (IOM). 2007. *The Future of Disability in America*. Washington, DC: The National Academies Press.

Jette, A. and Badley, E. 2001. Conceptual issues in the measurement of work disability. In *Survey Measurement of Work Disability*, eds. N. Mathiowetz and G. Wonderlich, pp. 4–27. Washington, DC: National Academy Press.

Langlois, J.A., Rutland-Brown, W., and Wald, M. 2006. The epidemiology and impact of traumatic brain injury: A brief overview. *Journal of Head Trauma Rehabilitation* 21 (5): 375–378.

Mann, W.C., Hurren, D.M., Charvat, B.A., and Tomita, M.R. 1996. Changes over one year in assistive device use and home modifications by home-based older persons with Alzheimer's disease. *Topics in Geriatric Rehabilitation* 12 (2): 9–16.

Mann, W.C., Hurren, D., and Tomita, M.R. 1993. Comparison of assistive device use and needs of home-based older persons with different impairments. *American Journal of Occupational Therapy* 47 (11): 980–987.

Mann, W.C., Hurren, D., and Tomita, M.R. 1995. Assistive devices used by home-based elderly persons with arthritis. *American Journal of Occupational Therapy* 49 (8): 810–820.

Mann, W.C., Llanes, C., Justiss, M.D., and Tomita, M. 2004. Frail elder adults' self-report of their most important assistive device. *OTJR: Occupation, Participation and Health* 24 (1): 4–12.

Mashaw, J.L. and Reno, V. 1996. Balancing security and opportunity: The challenge of disability income policy. Report of the Disability Policy Panel, National Academy of Social Insurance, Washington, DC.

Nagi, S. 1969. *Disability and Rehabilitation: Legal, Clinical and Self-Concepts of Measurement.* Columbus, OH: Ohio State University Press.

National Alliance for Caregiving (NAC). 2004. *Miles Away: The MetLife Study of Long-Distance Caregiving.* Bethesda, MD: NAC. http://www.caregiving.org/data/milesaway.pdf

National Alliance for Caregiving (NAC) and American Association of Retired Persons (AARP). 2009. *Caregiving in the U.S.* Bethesda, MD: NAC.

National Association for Home Care & Hospice. 2008. *Basic Statistics About Home Care.* Washington, DC: National Association for Home Care & Hospice. http://www.nahc.org/facts/08HC_stats.pdf

National Family Caregivers Association (NFCA) and Family Caregiver Alliance (FCA). 2006. *Prevalence, Hours and Economic Value of Family Caregiving, Updated State-by-State Analysis of 2004 National Estimates,* ed. P.S. Arno. Kensington, MD: NFCA.

Polly, D.W. 2005. An internet-delivered cognitive-behavioral intervention with telephone support improved some coping skills in patients with chronic low back pain. *The Journal of Bone and Joint Surgery (American)* 87: 1169.

Roth, D.L., Perkins, M., Wadley, V.G., Temple, E.M., and Haley, W.E. 2009. Family caregiving and emotional strain: Associations with quality of life in a large national sample of middle-aged and older adults. *Quality of Life Research* 18 (6): 679–688.

Stanton, N.A., Salmon, P.M., Walker, G.H., Baber, C., and Jenkins, D.P. 2005. *Human Factors Methods: A Practical Guide for Engineering and Design.* Aldershot, U.K.: Ashgate Publishing.

Stewart, F., Worrall, L.E., Egan, J.N., and Oxenham, D. 2004. Addressing internet training issues for people with Parkinson's disease. *International Journal of Advanced Speech-Language Pathology* 6 (4): 209–220.

Talley, R.C. and Crews, J.E. 2007. Framing the public health of caregiving. *American Journal of Public Health* 97 (2): 224–228.

U.S. Department of Health and Human Services (U.S. DHHS), Health Resources and Services Administration (HRSA), Maternal and Child Health Bureau (MCHB). 2008. *The National Survey of Children with Special Health Care Needs: Chartbook 2005–2006.* Washington, DC: U.S. DHHS-HRSA-MCHB. http://mchb.hrsa.gov/cshcn05/

Verza, R., Lopes de Carvalho, M.L., Battaglia, M.A., and Uccelli, M.M. 2006. An interdisciplinary approach to evaluating the need for assistive technology reduces equipment abandonment. *Multiple Sclerosis* 12 (1): 88–93.

Watzke, J. 1997. Older adults' responses to an automated integrated environmental control device: The case of the remote gateway. *Technology and Disability* 7 (1): 103–114.

Wolff, J.L. and Kasper, D.J. 2006. Caregivers of frail elders: Updating a national profile. *The Gerontologist* 46 (3): 344–356.

Yang, J.J., Mann, W.C., Nochajski, S., and Machiko, T.R. 1997. Use of assistive devices among elders with cognitive impairment: A follow-up study. *Topics in Geriatric Rehabilitation* 13 (2): 13–31.

Survey Resources on the Web

U.S. Census 2000

U.S. Census 2000. http://www.census.gov/main/www/cen2000.html

American Community Survey (ACS) 2008

American Community Survey (ACS). 2008. http://www.ilr.cornell.edu/edi/disabilitystatistics/reports/

Current Population Survey (CPS) 2009

U.S. Census Bureau. 2009. *Current Population Survey (CPS)*. http://www.census.gov/cps/

National Health Interview Survey (NHIS), 2009

Centers for Disease Control and Prevention. 2009. *National Health Interview Survey (NHIS)*. http://www.cdc.gov/nchs/nhis/nhis_2009_data_release.htm

Medical Expenditure Panel Survey (MEPS)

Agency for Healthcare Research and Quality (USDHHS). *Medical Expenditure Panel Survey (MEPS)*. Available at: http://www.meps.ahrq.gov/mepsweb/

Panel Study of Income Dynamics (PSID)

Institute for Social Research, University of Michigan. *Panel Study of Income Dynamics (PSID)*. http://psidonline.isr.umich.edu/

Survey of Income and Program Participation (SIPP)

U.S. Census Bureau. *Survey of Income and Program Participation (SIPP)*. Washington, DC: U.S. Census Bureau, Demographics Survey Division, Survey of Income and Program Participation Branch. http://www.census.gov/sipp/

Health and Retirement Study (NIA/USDHHS, March 2007)

National Institute on Aging and U.S. Department of Health and Human Services. 2007. *Growing Older in America: The Health and Retirement Study*. Bethesda, MD: National Institutes of Health (Publication No. 07-5757), March. http://www.nia.nih.gov/ResearchInformation/ExtramuralPrograms/BehavioralAndSocialResearch/HRS.htm

2

Facilitators and Barriers to Technology Uptake: Individual End-User Perspectives

Richard Schulz

CONTENTS

2.1 Introduction

Technology needs to be adopted and used if it is to have an impact on quality of life. This may seem obvious, but there are numerous examples of assistive and other health-related technologies that, while based on sound engineering, have limited uptake in the community at large. Despite the proliferation of technologies and the large number of published studies on technology-based health care (*cf. Journal of Telemedicine and Ecare, Journal of Telemedicine and Telecare*), they have limited uptake in the community at large. For example, it is estimated that 50,000 households were using telecare services in 2006, but this represents a small fraction of the eligible population that might benefit from such services (Hersch et al. 2006; Smith 2008). Fewer than 200 of the 7000 Medicare-certified home health agencies regularly use telecare (Whitten 2006).

The success of a technology depends on the interplay of three important factors: characteristics, needs, and preferences of the end user; features of the technology; and societal factors including social and health policy and the regulatory environment. The interplay of these three factors is illustrated in Figure 2.1.

Our model of user uptake shows that the combination of system characteristics and user capabilities define system–user fit. When system features are closely matched to the sensory, cognitive, and motor capabilities of the potential user, system–user fit is high and

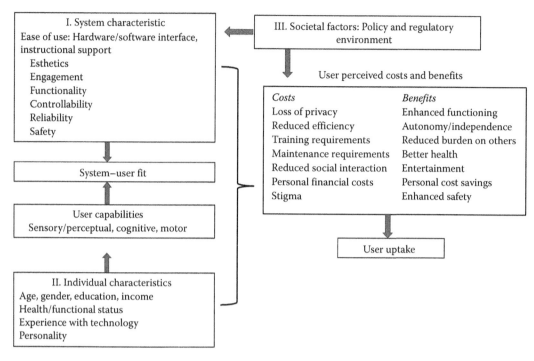

FIGURE 2.1
Model of technology uptake: system, individual, and societal factors.

the probability of uptake is enhanced. User capabilities are in part determined by individual characteristics including demographic characteristics, health and functional status, experience with technology, and personality. From the individual user's perspective, uptake ultimately depends on the perceived costs and benefits of a particular system. Costs might include factors such as loss of privacy; reduced efficiency relative to alternative solutions such as human assistance, training, and maintenance requirements; personal financial costs; and stigma, while benefits include enhanced functioning and independence, reduced burden on others such as a family caregiver, improved health, entertainment value of the technology, personal cost savings, and enhanced safety. The third factor illustrated in Figure 2.1 identifies the policy and regulatory environment that affect uptake. Some technologies may require the approval of Federal regulatory agencies such as the Food and Drug Administration (FDA) before they can be made publicly available. Similarly, technologies may be too costly for individuals to afford and, therefore, require approval of insurance companies or Medicare/Medicaid if they are to be widely disseminated.

Each of the three factors contributing to technology uptake is discussed as follows.

2.2 System Characteristics

Any technology system will vary on a number of dimensions that ultimately will play a role in its adoption. For example, interface design determines how the individual will interact with the technology. A computer-based system might require users to interact via touchscreen, keyboard, mouse, voice command, or some combination of these. Decisions about which input device to use should be guided by the capabilities of the targeted end user. Another key system factor concerns ease of learning to use the system. What type of instructional support is provided to learn how to operate the system? How quickly can the user become proficient in its use? Usability out of the box is increasingly becoming the standard for system uptake. Technologies that rely on complex instruction manuals are likely to generate little interest among potential users. A related factor is how engaging the technology is for the end user; put another way, what is the fun factor for technology use? A system may be cognitively stimulating or provide entertainment while it is doing its job; it may provide feedback to the user that makes them feel good about themselves, empowered, or raise their self-esteem. The aesthetic qualities of a technology may also impede uptake. Historically, technologies such as hearing aids have had limited uptake because they are perceived to be obtrusive, unattractive, and stigmatizing. Researchers interested in developing assistive robots may have to decide how anthropomorphic or "humanlike" the technology should be. Human beings are inherently motivated to control their environment, and this would apply to technology devices as well. Even with intelligent systems with sophisticated capabilities, humans still like to be in charge. Thus, controllability is another key feature of technology. Minimally, humans need to have the ability to turn a technology on or off, and ideally the technology should enable a level of participation and control that is matched to the abilities and preferences of the user. Finally, technologies have to be reliable and safe. For some technologies, a single failure may forever doom uptake by users. For example, an emergency call system that fails, even a small percent of the time, would be deemed unacceptable by most individuals. For those technologies that have catastrophic consequences for the individual should they fail, the bar for reliability and safety needs to be extremely high to garner the acceptance of users.

2.3 Individual Characteristics and User Capabilities

A broad range of background characteristics shape the individuals capabilities and motivation to adopt new technology. As we shall see in Chapter 3, the age, gender, and education level of an individual help shape attitude toward new technologies and their level of motivation to adopt them. These same factors may also profoundly affect the capabilities of an individual to learn and use certain technologies. The most obvious example is the role of age and education, which, along with the health status of an individual, can affect sensory, perceptual, cognitive, and motor abilities required to operate a particular system. Since older individuals are a primary target for quality of life technologies (QoLTs), we review in the following some of the key age-related changes that need to be considered when designing technology for this population.

2.3.1 Memory and Cognition

Although there is a great deal of variability in memory at all ages, increased age is often associated with lower levels of performance in tests of memory. Furthermore, the age differences are not limited to a particular type of material because older adults have been found to remember fewer items than young adults with unrelated words, meaningful paragraphs and new stories, faces, displays of spatial information, and activities performed in the past. Occasional memory lapses are normal, and merely because someone is concerned about his or her memory, it does not necessarily mean that a pathological condition exists. Memory and other cognitive problems are usually considered serious when the scores on several different types of tests are low for one's age (typically defined as the 5th percentile or lower), when the change from a previous higher-functioning state has been fairly rapid, and when the problems begin to interfere with independent living. However, even under these circumstances, the diagnosis will not necessarily be irreversible dementia because depression and metabolic disorders caused by malnutrition and drug interactions can also affect memory.

Adult age differences in cognitive and intellectual abilities have been well documented in large standardized mental ability tests since World War I. However, not all types of intelligence decline with increasing age because measures of acquired information and knowledge, sometimes known as crystallized intelligence, tend to remain stable across most of the adult years, while measures of the efficiency of solving novel problems, sometimes known as fluid intelligence, gradually declines beginning as early as the late 20s. Even with the fluid intelligence measures, however, there is a great deal of variability at every age, and consequently it is difficult to make accurate predictions on the basis of one's age. The reasons for age-related decline in measures of fluid intelligence are still not understood, and the existing evidence is not completely consistent with expectations based on health, education, general environmental change, or disuse. For example, although impressive increases in scores on standardized intelligence tests have been reported over historical time by people of the same age, the reasons for these increases are not yet known, nor are their implications for understanding relations between age and cognition. Also, the "use it or lose it" view in which declines are attributed to disuse remains popular despite a surprisingly small amount of positive evidence.

The term dementia (or dementing illness) refers to a disease that leads initially to the loss of cognitive functioning and, in later stages, to the loss of motor and physical functioning. In particular, the symptoms of dementia can include the following:

- A decline in intellectual ability severe enough to interfere with the sufferer's work and social life
- Impairments in memory, judgment, and abstract thinking
- Language problems due to brain damage (aphasia)
- An inability to carry out a requested action, even though the sufferer understands the request and is physically able to perform it (apraxia)
- A failure to recognize or identify familiar objects despite good vision and sense of touch (agnosia)

Several different types of dementia have been identified depending on the etiology or cause of the symptoms. Dementia of the Alzheimer's type is the most prevalent of the dementias, followed by dementias due to vascular disease or stroke, dementia due to HIV disease, dementia due to head trauma, and so on. More than 70 different conditions can cause dementia. Of these, the two most common among elderly persons are Alzheimer's disease and vascular dementia.

Mild cognitive impairment (MCI) is a condition characterized by cognitive decline greater than expected for an individual's age and education level but does not interfere significantly with activities of daily life. Thus, it is an intermediate condition between normal aging and dementia, and in about half of the cases it converts to dementia within

5 years after initial diagnosis. It is estimated that from 3% to 19% of the adults older than 65 years suffer from this condition. There is currently a great deal of interest in this condition because its identification could lead to treatment strategies that prevent the emergence of full-blown dementia. Individuals with MCI might also be excellent targets for QoLTs because they still have the capabilities to use technology systems and could potentially benefit from systems that provide cognitive support.

2.3.2 Vision

Long before old age, the eyes begin to undergo significant change. For example, the pupillary reflex responds more slowly after age 50, and the pupils do not dilate as completely. The lens becomes larger, more yellow, and less flexible after age 40. And the cornea, the transparent covering of the iris, decreases in luster by age 40 and increases in curvature and thickness past age 50. Some of these anatomical changes have important functional consequences.

As we grow older, the eyes adapt to the dark less rapidly and less effectively (dark adaptation). Middle-aged and elderly adults have considerably more difficulty dealing with sudden and pronounced decreases in illumination, as when going from bright sunlight into a darkened movie theater. Sudden increases in illumination are also troublesome, such as encountering the headlights of an oncoming car while driving at night. When designing environments for older adults, therefore, it is important to avoid abrupt transitions in light intensity, shadows, and glare (as might result from shiny floors or the chrome on wheelchairs).

The process of accommodation also deteriorates with increasing age, particularly between ages 40 and 55. This reduced ability to focus on nearby objects (presbyopia) may well necessitate corrective measures, such as reading glasses or bifocals. Tasks like driving an automobile will also be more difficult, since we must often shift our focus back and forth from points far down the road to the gauges directly in front of us.

The ability to identify stationary objects (static visual acuity) shows a decided drop with age; the percentage of adults with 20/20 vision declines markedly after age 45, and the ability to identify moving objects (dynamic visual acuity), such as credits on TV or road signs while driving, also decreases appreciably as we grow older, though not necessarily at the same rate as static visual acuity.

Color sensitivity also changes with age. The yellowing of the lens after age 40 affects our ability to see certain colors, notably those at the blue green end of the spectrum. The effect is somewhat like viewing the world through yellow sunglasses: Older adults can discern yellows, oranges, and reds more easily than violets, blues, and greens. This is not a serious defect, but it can cause problems under some conditions (e.g., a tennis court illuminated at night with bluish light, or a white soup bowl on a white place mat). For this reason, the color controls on television sets in homes for the elderly may be set at atypical values in order to make the hues appear more realistic.

The elderly have somewhat more difficulty recognizing shapes, numbers, letters, and words (Kline and Scialfa 1996). As a result, reading a sign or locating someone in a crowd may be more troublesome. The differences between younger and older adults are rather small, however, indicating that age is a relatively minor factor insofar as the quality of visual information processing is concerned.

Numerous studies show that the speed of visual information processing declines as people age. In studies of critical flicker frequency, for example, subjects are typically shown a rapidly flashing light. Older adults require a significantly longer interval between the flashes in order to perceive that the light is not on continuously, indicating that the sensitivity of the visual system declines with age. Some studies require the subject to locate a target object in a field of distracting stimuli as quickly as possible, a task that depends on both sensory processes and decision making ability. Adults age 60 and older perform such visual scanning tasks significantly more slowly than do young adults. This is especially true if the subject must concentrate on other tasks simultaneously, as when the driver of an automobile must pick out the relevant information from a lengthy road sign while continuing to guide the car.

Aging is also associated with several pathological conditions that affect vision. Cloudy or opaque areas may develop in part or all of the lens, inhibiting the passage of light and causing a significant decline in vision. These cataracts usually form gradually, without pain, redness of the eye, or excessive tears; they are most common after age 60. Some recent research evidence suggests that cataract formation may be linked to enzyme modifications, or to changes in the characteristics of lens protein. Some cataracts remain small enough to be safely ignored. Those large enough to cause significant problems can be surgically removed, a safe procedure that is almost always successful.

Glaucoma occurs when the fluid pressure in the eye becomes excessive, causing internal damage and gradually destroying one's vision. If glaucoma is detected in its early stages, however, it can usually be controlled well enough to prevent blindness. Common methods for this purpose include prescription eye drops, oral medication, laser treatments, or perhaps surgery. As with cataracts, the initial stages of glaucoma seldom involve any pain or discomfort, so routine eye examinations of adults over 35 typically include a test for eye pressure.

Most serious of all are the retinal disorders, which are the leading causes of blindness in the United States. In senile macular degeneration, a specialized part of the retina that is responsible for sharp central and reading vision (the macula) loses its ability to function effectively. Warning signs include blurred vision when reading, a dark spot in the center of one's field of vision, and distortion when viewing vertical lines. If detected early enough, senile macular degeneration may be amenable to laser treatments. Diabetic retinopathy occurs when small blood vessels that normally nourish the retina fail to function properly. As the name implies, this disease is one of the possible complications resulting from diabetes. The early stages of diabetic retinopathy are denoted by distorted vision, the later stages by serious visual losses. Retinal detachment, a separation between the inner and outer layers of the retina, has a more favorable prognosis: Detached retinas can usually be surgically reattached well enough to restore good, or at least partial, vision. This is probably the best known of the retinal disorders, due to media coverage of cases involving famous athletes (e.g., champion boxer Sugar Ray Leonard).

2.3.3 Audition

Most often, methods for measuring hearing use pure tones as the test stimuli. Losses in our ability to detect these tones begin to occur by about age 40, although pronounced changes are not evident until sometime later. For example, the typical 30 year old male can detect a 6 kHz tone (6000 Hz) at a volume of about 4 dB, which is softer than the rustling of leaves. Yet the same tone must be presented to the average 65 year old man at approximately 40 dB, the level of normal conversation, in order to be heard. The greatest declines occur at frequencies above 2.5 kHz, due primarily to atrophy and degeneration of the hair cells and supporting mechanisms in the cochlea. To the extent that a task requires the detection and/or discrimination of middle to high-frequency tones, many middle-aged and elderly adults may well be at a significant disadvantage.

Our ability to perceive and understand speech also declines with increasing age, although the magnitude of this loss depends to a considerable extent on prevailing listening conditions as well as other cognitive demands placed on the individual.

If we were to consider only our own culture, we might erroneously conclude that substantial declines in hearing with increasing age are an inescapable part of the human condition. In actuality, however, both aging and our environment contribute to the hearing losses commonly found among middle-aged and elderly Americans. The atrophy of our auditory system is one price that we pay for living in a noise-ridden, industrialized society.

A substantial number of older Americans report that they suffer from hearing impairments, men more so than women. Some 13% of Americans over the age of 65 show advanced signs of presbycusis. This disorder involves a progressive loss of hearing in both ears for high-frequency tones, which is often accompanied by severe difficulty in understanding speech. Presbycusis results from the deterioration of mechanisms in the inner ear; this may be caused by aging, long-term exposure to loud noises, certain drugs, an improper diet, or genetic factors. The onset of this disorder is gradual, and it typically becomes pronounced after age 50.

Hearing aids alone are unlikely to resolve this problem. They serve to amplify sounds in the external world, yet speech will remain distorted because of the inner ear degeneration. Speech reading, informational counseling, and hearing aid orientation are important aspects of comprehensive aural rehabilitation with patients suffering from presbycusis. Conductive hearing loss occurs when sound waves are unable to travel properly through the outer and middle ear. This disorder is caused by impediments in the ear, such as dense wax, excessive fluid, an abnormal bone growth, or an infection. Sufferers experience external sounds and other people's voices as muffled, but their own voices appear louder than normal. This disorder is less common than presbycusis and can usually be resolved through flushing of the ear, medication, or surgery. Those who suffer from central auditory impairment have great difficulty understanding language. However, the ability to detect external sounds is not affected. This rare disorder is caused by damage to the nerve centers within the brain, which typically results from an extended illness with a high fever, lengthy exposure to loud noises, the use of certain drugs, head injuries, vascular problems, or tumors. Unlike presbycusis, central auditory impairment may occur at any age; it may also interact with presbycusis in older adults. There is no cure for central auditory impairment, although rehabilitation by an audiologist or speech language pathologist may be helpful in some instances.

It has been estimated that 30% of all adults between the ages of 65 and 74, and 50% of those between 75 and 79, suffer some degree of hearing loss. In fact, hearing impairments rank second only to arthritis among the leading health problems of those over the age of 75. Hearing disorders have significant practical consequences: failing to understand what other people are saying, which may significantly affect relationships with family and friends; letting a ringing telephone or doorbell go unanswered, and missing an important call; being unable to enjoy movies, plays, concerts, and television programs without closed captions; and having to give up driving an automobile because the warning signal of an ambulance or fire engine cannot be heard. In addition, stimuli such as the plumbing sounds from another room provide an important auditory background that helps us to keep in touch with our surroundings. When hearing impaired persons cannot detect these background stimuli, they may well become afraid to venture out into all but the most familiar environments. As a result, hearing losses have caused elderly people to be incorrectly diagnosed as confused, unresponsive, uncooperative, or even pathologically depressed, thereby denying them help that would have been readily available.

Hearing impairments may even lead to true depression, with sufferers becoming so frustrated at their inability to communicate with other people (or so suspicious because others always seem to mumble incoherently) that they withdraw from social interactions.

2.3.4 Tactile Abilities

The importance of our sense of touch is easily taken for granted. Nevertheless, this sense is involved in many important behaviors: judging the smoothness of a piece of wood or the closeness of a shave or identifying a switch on the automobile console without taking one's eyes off the road. Although studies examining age-related changes in touch and vibratory sensitivity are still relatively rare, existing evidence suggests that our sensitivity to touch and pressure decrease with age, our ability to discriminate small distances between two points exerting pressure on the skin declines, as does our ability to identify objects through touch alone. Changes in vibratory sensitivity are helpful in diagnosing and assessing disorders of the nervous system. Older adults are significantly less sensitive than young adults to vibratory stimuli, particularly in the lower extremities. Age-related declines are most apparent after the age of 65 and are typically greater among men than women.

The temperature sensitivities and preferences of older adults do not appear to differ in any significant way from those of younger subjects. But the ability to cope with cold temperatures and maintain bodily warmth, and the ability to cope with hot environments, declines with increasing age. This may explain in part why mortality rates increase among the elderly when there are sudden and extreme changes in ambient temperature.

Pain is defined as an unpleasant sensory and emotional experience associated with actual or potential tissue damage. Given the increased likelihood of pathology among the elderly, any age-related changes in pain sensitivity would have important practical consequences. Perhaps for this reason, pain is the skin sense most often subjected to age-related studies. Unfortunately, these data are highly contradictory: Many studies report a marked decline in pain sensitivity with increasing age, numerous others find no such decrements and a few even report increased pain sensitivity among older adults. The best conclusion we can draw at this point in time is that there is no strong evidence that age itself reduces pain sensitivity or that age affects the qualitative properties of pain. We can, however, be confident in concluding that the frequency and intensity of chronic pain is higher among older persons when compared to younger persons. Moreover, chronic pain is likely to be an important source of depression in the elderly.

2.3.5 Proprioception and Kinesthesia

An important problem faced by the elderly is their susceptibility to falls, and the sometimes fatal complications that result. Such falls may be caused by dizziness, by muscular weakness, or by decreased input from the proprioceptive and kinesthetic receptors that detect movements or strain in the muscles, tendons, and joints. Proprioception refers to the sensations generated by the body that let you know the location of your limbs in space, and kinesthesia refers to one's sense of location while moving through space. It is well known that older persons exhibit increased postural sway, and have an increased tendency to lose their balance. But it is not clear to what extent these problems are due to aging of the proprioceptive system as opposed to factors such as deconditioning of muscles or illness. Nevertheless, current thinking holds that there are some declines in proprioception and kinesthetic function. An important functional consequence of these declines is that it affects the ability to maintain posture.

2.3.6 Taste and Smell

The senses of smell and taste are essential to survival and our ability to enjoy life. They help us select food, get the right nutrients, and they help protect us from toxins that might be fatal. Our senses of taste and smell are closely interrelated. For example, both of these senses play an essential role in determining the desirability of various foods. It is therefore difficult to study these senses separately, although some researchers have sought to do so.

Sensory researchers have identified four primary qualities of taste: sweet, bitter, sour, and salty. Taste sensitivity experiments typically present the subject with a solution based on one primary quality (e.g., a sucrose solution in the case of sweetness), and a separate quantity of water. The keener the subject's sensitivity to, say, sweetness, the smaller the concentration of sucrose that can be differentiated from plain water.

Several studies suggest that adults past age 50 have more difficulty detecting all four primary taste sensations, although the declines in sensitivity are relatively small. In one recent study, researchers found that even centenarians could reliably discriminate the four primary tastes, although they were not quite as good at doing this as younger persons. Like our sense of hearing, the ability to taste is affected by both normal aging processes as well as other factors such as medications, medical conditions, and possibly environmental pollutants. Thus, it is difficult to know the extent to which observed changes within any one person are due to normal aging or health-related conditions.

Several studies have found that our ability to detect various odors declines with age. In one large study, 1955 volunteers ranging in age from 5 to 99 were tested with 40 chemically simulated scents that included cinnamon, cherry, pizza, gasoline, tobacco, mint, soap, grass, lemon, motor oil, and root beer. The results suggested that olfactory ability is usually at its best between the ages of 20 and 40, begins to diminish slightly by age 50, and declines rapidly after age 70. Among subjects aged 65–80, some 60% suffered severe losses in olfactory sensitivity, and about 25% lost all ability to smell. For those over 80, the proportion with severe olfactory losses was 80%, and nearly one half could not smell anything.

2.3.7 Motor Skills

Motor skills refer to the ability to control muscles in order to produce movement. Fine motor skills involve small movements such as writing and tying shoes, while gross motor skills are large movements like walking and kicking. During early development, infants learn to control their heads to stabilize their gaze and track moving objects and learn how to sit without support and ultimately walk, run, and jump. Both gross and fine motor skills continue to develop throughout childhood, adolescence, and early adulthood. In as much as motor performance is dependent on multiple factors including cognition, sensory, perceptual, and proprioceptive abilities as well as physical attributes such as muscle mass and strength, it is not surprising that motor abilities tend to decline in late life. However, the rate of decline in motor skills in old age depends to some extent on the amount and type of activity people engage in, and researchers have shown that older persons can acquire skills such as improving their gait in order to minimize falls.

Motor disability is a common characteristic of old age, as noted in the previous chapter. Many older individuals have difficulty walking, climbing stairs, reaching, lifting, or carrying objects. As a result, they must rely on the assistance of others or use technology that facilitates these activities. To a lesser extent, older individuals may also suffer from a number of pathological conditions which affect movement. Persons suffering from Parkinson's disease may have tremors in the hands, fingers, forearms, or feet, and have poor balance and a distinctive unsteady gait. Essential tremor is a more common movement disorder of late life that is characterized by rhythmic shaking which occurs during voluntary movement such as lifting a spoon to one's mouth. Developing technologies for such individuals poses unique challenges as it requires careful attention to the interface design.

2.4 Perceived Costs and Benefits

Having a good fit between a technology and a user is a necessary but not sufficient condition for user uptake. A technology system has to be operable before it will be used; however, users also consider a host of other of factors before deciding to adopt a particular technology. On the cost side of the ledger, users may consider issues such as loss of privacy, the amount of time and effort involved in learning to use and to maintain a technology, whether or not it reduces social interaction with other humans, how expensive it is, and whether or not it is stigmatizing to the individual. On the benefit side of the ledger we have enhanced functioning and independence of the user, which are likely to carry a great deal of weight in the adoption decision. Users may also favor a technology because it reduces the burden on family members who would otherwise need to assist the user or it makes them feel safer, healthier, and/or saves money. Finally, technology may have entertainment value, that is, it might simultaneously enhance functioning and provide enjoyment and stimulation to the user. As we shall see in the next chapter where we present data on many of these factors, user uptake is a complex multifactorial process.

2.5 Social and Health Policy and the Regulatory Environment

Technologies that address important needs such as the health and functioning of older individuals and persons with disability are rarely implemented in isolation. They are subject to organizational, regional, and national policy constraints. At the local level, clinicians working with elderly clients or persons with disability are in a position to promote the use of technology, but they face significant challenges to doing so; they have limited time per client and often little training in the evaluation and selection of appropriate technologies. Acquiring technologies for clients often takes multiple appeals, and there is a paucity of evidence justifying the implementation of particular technologies. At broader policy levels, organizations such as private insurers, which often follow the lead of Medicare, are reluctant to pay for technology without compelling cost-benefit and cost-effectiveness data; yet they are not willing to make the investments in research and demonstration projects that might generate such data. Small companies and universities involved in technology development rarely have the resources to carry out major translational research programs without external support. The role that organizational and policy environments play in the development and marketing of technology are discussed in detail in later chapters.

Fortunately, there is growing interest in the potential of technology to address the challenges posed by an aging society, and both private and public investment in technology development and testing is on the rise. Organizations such the National Institutes of Health and the National Science Foundation are increasingly supporting innovative programs to develop and test new technologies that will enhance or maintain the quality of life of individuals with disability.

References

Hersch, W.R., Hickam, D.H., Severance, S.M. et al. 2006. Diagnosis, access and outcomes: Update of a systematic review of telemedicine services. *Journal of Telemedicine and Telecare* 12 (2 Supplement): 3–31.

Kline, D.W. and Scialfa, C.T. 1996. Visual and auditory aging. In *Handbook of the Psychology of Aging* (4th edn.), eds. J.E. Birren and K.W. Schaie, pp. 181–203. New York: Academic Press.

Smith, C. 2008. Technology and web-based support. *American Journal of Nursing* 108 (9 Supplement): 64–68.

Whitten, P. 2006. Telemedicine: Communication technologies that revolutionize healthcare services. Simple applications now, virtual reality and simulation soon. *Generations* 30 (2): 20–24.

3

Facilitators and Barriers to Technology Uptake: Organizational and Societal Perspectives

Katherine D. Seelman

CONTENTS

3.1 Introduction

In the previous chapter, we examined issues related to technology uptake from the perspective of the individual end user. In this chapter, we focus on the public policy framework for advanced technology to improve the quality of life of older adults and people with disabilities, which plays an equally important role in determining whether or not a technology is adopted. In the course of this examination, facilitators and barriers to innovation, commercialization, and availability to end users are identified.

Public policy for these advanced technologies is in a state of flux. New and advanced technology to improve quality of life of people with disabilities across the age span does not fit easily into existing policies that guide research and development (R&D), commercialization, regulation, and reimbursement. The policy framework is buffeted by external conditions such as new U.S. health care legislation, skyrocketing cost of health care, and the aging demographic.

In general, public policy is based on formal authority such as laws and regulations which engender a far more opaque set of informal forces that are brought to bear on complex technology. Informal forces involve stakeholders such as industry, the scientific community, clinicians, and patients who educate and lobby Congress, regulatory agencies, and each other. Policies are routinely implemented by government entities, often regulatory agencies that have the expertise to implement highly complex supervisory and oversight tasks. Some regulations and measurement tools for safety and efficacy, such as those used by the U.S. Food and Drug Administration (FDA), were established prior to the development of advanced medical device technologies which are characterized by sophisticated electronics and software, communications capability, robotics, and artificial intelligence. As a result, respected scientific agencies, such as the Institute of Medicine (IOM) of the National Academy of Sciences, have questioned whether or not the FDA clearance process to evaluate the safety and effectiveness of earlier and less complex medical devices is appropriate to evaluate the safety and effectiveness of newer advanced medical devices (Institute of Medicine (U.S.) Committee on the Public Health Effectiveness of the FDA 510(k) Clearance Process 2011; Silverstein 2011).

The term "advanced technology" is used throughout this chapter to refer to quality of life technology (QoLT) for older adults and persons with disabilities. These technologies are characterized by features such as advanced computation and communications capability and robotics. They include a wide range of products such as wheelchairs, coaches, and monitoring devices, the purpose for which is to advance wellness, prevention, rehabilitation, individual function, and participation in society.

This chapter begins with an overview of the markets for advanced technologies such as those developed by the Center for Aging Services Technology (CAST), Center for Research and Education on Aging and Technology Enhancement (CREATE), Johnson and Johnson's Independence Technology, and Quality of Life Technology Engineering Research Center (QoLT ERC) (CREATE 2011; Independence Technology, L.L.C. 2011; Independence Technology—A Johnson & Johnson Co. Ibot (Power Wheelchairs)—USA Techguide 2011; LeadingAge: Center for Aging Services Technologies 2011; Quality of Life Technology Center 2011). It then provides government agency definitions for a particular group of advanced technologies often referred to as medical devices. Medical devices occupy a large market share of advanced technology for older adults and people with disabilities. Following the definitions section, stages in technology development are introduced. In contrast to Chapter 15, which focuses more on the private sector, this chapter provides researchers, developers, and other interested readers with guidance about when and how to be more proactive in complying with key public sector laws and regulation. Subsequent sections of the chapter elaborate on regulation and the technical standards organizations relevant to advanced technologies. Next, the complexities of reimbursement policy for medical devices are examined with respect to payment models, stakeholders, and the Centers for Medicare and Medicaid Services (CMS). Medicare coverage, coding, and payment policies are closely scrutinized in order to identify enablers such as policies that cover medical devices and barriers such as medical necessity and in-the-home use criteria which restrict coverage. The final sections address assistive technology (AT) and conclusions. The conclusion section describes some technology and policy trends and identifies needs in health policy research which would advance the study of the process of innovation and adoption of advanced technology for quality of life.

3.2 Advanced Technology Markets

A single market for advanced QoLT has not yet emerged. Multiple industries and regulatory agencies are associated with these advanced technology products. For example, pharmacies and drug stores may sell orthopedic shoes with sensors to accurately measure force, pressure, acceleration, and other physical parameters. The main regulating body for pharmacies and drug stores is the FDA (U.S. Food and Drug Administration 2011), an independent regulatory agency. Companies that use large numbers of vehicles may be a market for products such as Drive Cap, a system developed by the QoLT ERC. Drive Cap analyzes and learns distinct driver behaviors in order to improve driver safety (Quality of Life Technology Center 2011). The main regulating body for Drive Cap is the National Highway Traffic Safety Administration in the U.S. Department of Transportation.

Many products for older adults and people with disabilities will be marketed by the medical device industry, which includes medical device manufacturing, medical instrument and supply manufacturing, home care providers, and AT (Market Research Reports & Analysis | IBISWorld US 2010). These global industries generate billions of dollars in revenue. The medical device industry has identified FDA regulation and CMS reimbursement as very important to their companies. CMS is located in the U.S. Department of Health and Human Services. Industry trade associations such as the Medical Device Manufacturing Association represent industry interests and are among the most important informal forces in the medical device policy and regulatory arena. Many products, such as the iBot (iBOT—Wikipedia, the Free Encyclopedia 2011) and Personal Mobility and Manipulation Appliance (PerMMA) wheelchairs, virtual coaches, and health kiosks (LeadingAge: Aging Services Technologies 2011; Quality of Life Technology Center 2011), will be designated either as medical devices or fall in a gray area of FDA regulation. Gray areas are generated when the FDA does not clearly state through regulation whether a technology is a medical device or a device used in areas that are not necessarily subject to FDA clearance, such as health and wellness. Gray areas cause confusion for developers who are unsure whether or not they must have FDA clearance before marketing their products.

3.3 Definition of Terms Used to Characterize QoL Technologies

Government agencies use a variety of terms to refer to advanced technology products for quality of life of older adults and people with disabilities. It is useful to recognize terms used by various agencies because these terms correspond to agency law and policy. Table 3.1

TABLE 3.1

Definitions of Selected Terms in U.S. Law and Regulation and the WHO

Term	Agency	Definition	Law
Medical device	U.S. Food and Drug Administration	An instrument, apparatus, implement, machine, contrivance, implant, in vitro reagent, or other similar or related article, including a component part, or accessory which is (a) recognized in the official National Formulary, or the U.S. Pharmacopoeia, or any supplement to them; (b) intended for use in the diagnosis of disease or other conditions, or in the cure, mitigation, treatment, or prevention of disease, in man or other animals; or (c) intended to affect the structure or any function of the body of man or other animals, and which does not achieve any of its primary intended purposes through chemical action within or on the body of man or other animals and which is not dependent upon being metabolized for the achievement of any of its primary intended purposes	Section 201(h) of the Federal Food Drug and Cosmetic Act
Durable medical equipment	Centers for Medicare and Medicaid Services, U.S. Department of Health and Human Services	Equipment that (a) can withstand repeated use; (b) is primarily and customarily used to serve a medical purpose; (c) generally is not useful to a person in the absence of an illness or injury; and (d) is appropriate for use in the home	Section 18 of the Social Security Act of 1965
Assistive technology	Office of Special Education and Rehabilitation Services, U.S. Department of Education; U.S. Access Board	Any item, piece of equipment, or system, whether acquired commercially, modified, or customized, that is commonly used to increase, maintain, or improve functional capabilities of individuals with disabilities	Technology-Related Assistance to Individuals with Disabilities Act (1988) and Assistive Technology Act (1994)
Medical device	World Health Organization (WHO) as proposed by the Global Harmonization Task Force (Cheng 2003)	"Medical device" means any instrument, apparatus, implement, machine, appliance, implant, in vitro reagent or calibrator, software, material, or any other similar or related article intended by the manufacturer to be used, along or in combination, for human beings for one or more of the specific purposes of • Diagnosis, monitoring, treatment, or alleviation of disease • Diagnosis, monitoring, treatment alleviation of or compensation of an injury • Investigation, replacement, modification, or support of the anatomy or of a physiological process • Supporting or sustaining life • Control of conception • Disinfection of medical devices	

TABLE 3.1 (continued)

Definitions of Selected Terms in U.S. Law and Regulation and the WHO

Term	Agency	Definition	Law
		• Providing information for medical purposes of in vitro examination of specimens derived from the human body and which does not achieve its primary intended action in or on the human body by pharmacological, immunological, or metabolic means but which may be assisted in its function by such means	
		Note: An accessory is not considered to be a medical device. However, where an accessory is intended specifically by its manufacturer to be used together with the "parent" medical device to achieve its intended purpose, it should be subject to be same procedures and GHTF guidance documents as apply to the medical device itself.	
		Note: The definition of a device for in vitro examination includes, for example, reagents, calibrators, sample collections, and related equipment	
Assistive Device	World Health Organization (Björn 2009)	Assistive device: Equipment that enables an individual who requires assistance to perform daily activities essential to maintain health and autonomy and life as full a life as possible. Such equipment may include, for example, motorized scooters, walkers, walking sticks, grab rails, and tilt-and-lift chairs	
Assistive Technology	World Health Organization (Björn 2009)	Assistive technology: An umbrella term for any device or system that allows individuals to perform tasks they would otherwise be unable to do or increases the ease and safety with which tasks can be performed	

Source: Björn, F., *Programme for Health Technologies: Call for Innovative Technologies Background and Process*, World Health Organization, Geneva, Switzerland, 2009; Cheng, M., *Medical Device Regulations: Global Overview and Guiding Principles*. World Health Organization, Geneva, Switzerland, 2003.

presents definitions of medical devices, durable medical equipment (DME) and AT, and their locations in U.S. law. It also provides definitions of terms used by the World Health Organization (WHO).

The FDA uses the term "medical device" for advanced technology subject to its regulation. The FDA definition places heavy emphasis on intended use, diagnosis of disease or other condition, and cure, mitigation, treatment, or prevention of disease and to a lesser extent on bodily function. The CMS uses DME (Centers for Medicare & Medicaid Services, 2008). The CMS definition is restricted to medical purpose and use in-the-home. These medically oriented definitions are in contrast to the definition of AT included in the Assistive Technology Act of 1998, which emphasizes the capacity of a device or system to increase, maintain, or improve functional capabilities. This definition of AT is more easily associated with activities of daily living, participation in society, prevention, and wellness. It has been adopted and integrated into a number of other laws such as the Older Americans Act (OAA) (Unofficial Compilation of the Older American Act of 1965 as amended in 2006 [Public Law 109–365]). The international community has its own terminology. WHO, in particular, has embarked on activities to "globalize" regulation of medical devices, focusing its efforts in under-resourced countries which lack both devices and the regulatory framework to assure their safety and effectiveness (Cheng 2003). WHO uses terms such as medical device to emphasize more medical use and assistive device to emphasize individual function. The International Organization for Standardization (ISO), which is harmonizing its classification with that of WHO, uses the term "assistive products" (Heerkens et al. 2000; National Institute for Public Health and the Environment 2010).

Advanced technologies may also be distinguished by the market, payment, and reimbursement pathways they travel. Drive Cap, described earlier, is a nonmedical device which may be introduced into the auto supply market and will be paid for out-of-pocket. "Leaning" edge software from Lean & Zoom is another example of a product that may be sold in the electronics marketplace and paid for out-of-pocket. Lean & Zoom is an aid not only for people with visual disabilities but also for mainstream computer users. It uses a computer's camera to magnify the screen as users move forward (Schwartzel 2011). Medical devices, such as advanced wheelchair technology, if cleared by FDA and CMS, will enter the medical device market and be reimbursed by public insurance programs, such as Medicare, Medicaid, and private insurance. Medicare rates of payment are determined prospectively, often a year or more in advance (Foster 1982). Medical devices that are not determined reimbursable by CMS can also be introduced into the competitive marketplace, but they often do not survive. The AT industry may also turn to state-level Offices of Vocational Rehabilitation (OVR) for reimbursement for work-related AT.

3.4 Enablers and Barriers to Innovation Including Research and Development, Commercialization, and End-User Availability

The overview, definitions, and markets sections provide hints of tensions in the health policy and regulatory arenas. Tensions can develop with the introduction of new health care legislation that alters coverage or reimbursement guidelines for medical and nonmedical devices. Tensions have surfaced with the emergence of advanced technologies that are radically different in technical and use characteristics from those existing at the time regulations were established. These emerging technologies may include robotics, bio-nano-genetics, materials, information and communication technology (ICT), human–computer interface, human augmentation, smart/anticipatory living spaces, networked intelligence, and personalization/user involvement (Timmers 2011).

It is too early to evaluate the impact of new health legislation and regulatory reform on innovation, commercialization, and end-user availability. This is not the case for medical devices where the existing legal, regulatory, and reimbursement framework is highly enabling of devices that serve medical purposes such as diagnosis. However, barriers exist for advanced technology intended to support people with disabilities across the age span to maintain their health, prevent onset of conditions and injuries, and perform daily-living activities independently. Barriers to availability and accessibility also exist for caregivers who help patients and consumers to delay or prevent the manifestation of functional impairment. As will be shown in subsequent sections on regulation and reimbursement, these policy barriers generate huge problems for innovators, marketers, and end users of advanced technologies.

3.4.1 Stages in the Development of Advanced Technology

Both medical and nonmedical devices advance through multiple stages of development. For nonmedical devices, these stages include innovation and R&D and commercialization. Medical devices have two additional stages: service delivery and reimbursement, both of which are examined in a later section.

Figure 3.1 illustrates stages in the development of advanced technology for older adults and individuals with disabilities. At the research stage, activities involve idea formulation. Development is the stage in which research is converted from a theoretical construct into a practical application and transitioned to technology development (Lane 1997, 2003). A proof of concept prototype marks the transition from R&D to commercialization. Commercialization is the process of bringing products to market, a stage in which the private sector is very much involved with activities such as finance and marketing. Each stage of development is structured by a number of public laws and regulations but also expertise, stakeholders, location, and financing. Arrows in Figure 3.1 suggest dynamic, interdependent relationships between and among stages of development. For example, the arrow to and from R&D and finance suggests that the level of finance affects the amount of resources invested in R&D. Public policy aspects of the various stages of development are examined and enablers and barriers in technology development are discussed. Guidance is provided about when and how to navigate the policy framework so that researchers and developers may move their products to the marketplace.

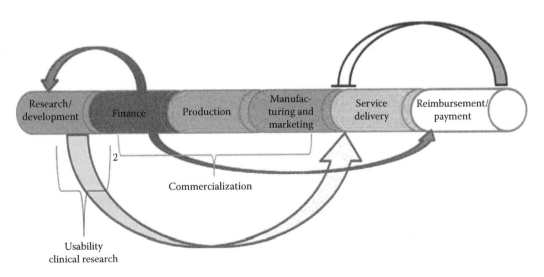

FIGURE 3.1
Technology development pipeline.

3.4.2 Innovation and Research

Research is supported mainly by public research agencies, corporations and corporation consortia, and foundations. The CREATE is sponsored by the National Institute on Aging and the Quality of Life Technology Engineering Research Center (QoLT ERC) is supported by the National Science Foundation (NSF). The iBOT, an advanced mobile powered wheelchair, was developed by inventor Dean Kamen in a partnership between his company, DEKA, and Johnson and Johnson's Independent Technology Division. The Center for Aging Services Technologies (CAST) is a consortium—an international coalition of more than 400 technology companies, aging-services organizations, businesses, research universities, and government representatives (Sirat 2011). CAST is focused on development, evaluation, and adoption of emerging technologies that will transform the aging experience.

Publicly funded research exists within a framework of laws that legitimize agency policy and programs, facilitate innovation, and provide protections for the rights of human subjects. Based on their missions, agencies such as the National Institutes of Health (NIH) generate priorities and funding opportunities and upon receipt of proposals make funding decisions using criteria such as intellectual merit and technical approach.

The NSF supports approximately 15 ERCs (Engineering Research Centers Association 2010). These centers are multi-university collaborations, funded to do transformative R&D, spawn new industry segments, and train the people who will grow them. One NSF ERC, QoLT, focuses on advanced technology for the disability and aging population. R&D, especially basic research, is routinely conducted by research personnel who are located in research facilities.

Major federal sponsors of disability-focused research are the National Institute on Disability and Rehabilitation Research in the U.S. Department of Education (USDE), the National Center for Medical and Rehabilitation Research in the National Institute of Child Health and Human Development, the U.S. Department of Health and Human Services, and the Rehabilitation Research and Development Services in the U.S. Department of Veteran Affairs (Field et al. 2007). While many federal departments and agencies provide services to older Americans, four agencies are particularly significant sponsors of aging-related research. They are the National Institute on Aging, the Administration on Aging, and the Centers for Medicare and Medicaid Services (all within the U.S. Department of Health and Human Services) and the Social Security Administration (an independent agency) (U.S. Congress Senate Special Committee on Aging 2008). The size, budget, and mission of each of these agencies differ substantially. The Defense Advanced Research Projects Agency (DARPA) bioengineering program provides an example of the Department of Defense (DOD) in involvement in rehabilitation research (Beard 2008).

3.4.3 Development

The development stage begins when research is converted into a practical idea or an application. Development may occur in various domains including academia, government institutions, existing companies or by a new group of individuals (Jordan 2010). Researchers and developers will concern themselves with product safety and efficacy in the early development stage at which time usability and clinical research are initiated and prototypes developed. Research results may be used as part of an investigation of whether or not the device must undergo FDA clearance or for eventual submission to FDA if the product must undergo FDA clearance. Researchers may also begin investigating the potential for reimbursement by Medicare and private insurers by looking at the experience of products similar to the ones being developed. Research grant administrators initiate processes, such as agreements with site managers, to have products deployed from research locations to sites such as senior housing and independent living centers for people with disabilities, homes and workplaces which are the natural environments of older adults and people with disabilities.

Later in the development stage, researchers begin the process of protecting their intellectual property. Before transferring to or collaborating with the private sector at the late development and early commercialization stages, they use strategies such as patents, trademarks, and copyrights to protect their property. In the case of university-based R&D, university-based intellectual property offices serve as resource specialists for identifying, protecting, marketing, licensing, transferring, and commercializing the university's intellectual property. During this stage, researchers may begin in earnest to investigate the possibilities for public reimbursement, if applicable to their products. The transfer process from R&D to market may involve incorporating private sector experts who are familiar with the FDA and CMS processes and personnel because medical device companies interact regularly with government agencies. If seeking to transfer a product directly into the market, researchers may seek out entrepreneurs because researchers often lack expertise in finance and the development of viable business models. Commercialization is largely a private sector process, and thus, its examination belongs to another chapter. However, as Table 3.2 shows, the product transfer process proceeds within a framework of law and policy.

TABLE 3.2

Federal Laws on Privacy and Promotion of Technology Transfer from Research to Market

Law	Description
The Health Insurance Portability and Accountability Act of 1996	Establishes a nationwide federal standard concerning the privacy of health information and how it can be used and disclosed. Researchers must comply; universities must establish a process through an IRB (or privacy board) for a HIPAA review of research protocols
Technology Innovation Act (1980) also known as Stevenson-Wydler Act	Establishes technology transfer as a mission of the federal government
Patent and Trademark Amendment Act (1980; also known as Bayh-Dole Act)	Gives nonprofit organizations including universities exclusive rights to patent their inventions and makes it possible for these entities to receive royalties and other compensation in return
Small Business Innovation Research Act (1982)	Requires federal government departments to set aside funds to stimulate technological innovation in the private sector, increase the role of small businesses in meeting federal R&D needs, and increase private sector commercialization of innovations derived from federally supported R&D effort
Federal Technology Transfer Act (1986) and National Competitiveness Technology Transfer Act (1989)	Allows federal labs to implement cooperative agreements, usually with manufacturers
Small Business Technology Transfer Act (1992)	Mandates that five federal departments and agencies provide R&D funding to support R&D partnerships
Patient Protection and Affordable Care Act (2010)	Establishes Cures Acceleration Network (CAN) at NIH to bridge the early commercialization period for biotech products when finance and sales are limited; authorizes the Access Board to issue accessibility standards for medical diagnostic equipment

Table 3.2 introduces a law pertaining to privacy and many laws related to technology transfer. The Health Insurance Portability and Accountability Act (HIPAA) addresses issues such as protection of privacy for human subjects involved in research, especially privacy in electronic communications and health records. Increasingly, medical devices may be equipped with wireless transmission and cameras that can receive and transmit sensitive user information, such as personal health records. Patient data may then become vulnerable to use for unscrupulous practices such as identity theft and insurance denial.

Table 3.2 shows laws which provide incentives for transferring technology to the market-place. Realizing that products spun-off from the federal laboratories would not be sufficient to maintain U.S. industrial preeminence, beginning in 1980, Congress passed legislation aimed at improving supply-side transfer and later to improve demand-side technology transfer (Bauer 2003). Supply-side is based on the assumption that economic growth can be most effectively created by lowering barriers for people to produce (supply) goods and services, such as lowering income tax and capital gains tax (http://en.wikipedia.org/wiki/Capital_gains_tax rates), and by allowing greater flexibility by reducing regulation.

The Small Business Administration (SBA) manages a supply-side grant program authorized under the Small Business Innovation Research (SBIR) Act and the Small Business Technology Transfer (STTR) Act which provides financial support to companies for transfer and commercialization of products. The purpose of the program includes increasing the role of small businesses in innovation and the economy. As Table 3.3 shows, the SBIR program typically is composed of three phases. Phase 1 is meant to establish product feasibility and commercialization potential; Phase 2, development to prototype, is meant to establish scientific and technical merit and commercial potential; and Phase 3, commercialization, is non-SBIR-funded follow-up support for R&D and manufacturing from the private sector. Each year, federal agencies with extra-mural R&D budgets that exceed $100 million are required to allocate 2.5% of their R&D budget to these programs. Eleven federal agencies participate in the program (SBIR). Each agency administers its own individual program within guidelines established by Congress. These agencies designate R&D topics in their solicitations and accept proposals from small businesses.

TABLE 3.3

Small Business Administration Innovation Research Program

Phase 1	The objective of Phase I is to establish the technical merit, feasibility, and commercial potential of the proposed R/R&D efforts and to determine the quality of performance of the small business awardee organization prior to providing further federal support in Phase II. SBIR Phase I awards normally do not exceed $150,000 total costs for 6 months
Phase 2	The objective of Phase II is to continue the R/R&D efforts initiated in Phase I. Funding is based on the results achieved in Phase I and the scientific and technical merit and commercial potential of the project proposed in Phase II. Only Phase I awardees are eligible for a Phase II award. SBIR Phase II awards normally do not exceed $1,000,000 total costs for 2 years
Phase 3	The objective of Phase III, where appropriate, is for the small business to pursue commercialization objectives resulting from the Phase I/II R/R&D activities. The SBIR program does not fund Phase III. Phase III may involve follow-on non-SBIR-funded R&D or production contracts for products, processes, or services intended for use by the U.S. Government

Source: SBIR, Small Business Innovation Research, U.S. Government [cited August 2011], retrieved August 2011, from www.sbir.gov/about/about-sbir

Awards are made on a competitive basis after proposal evaluation. SBIR and STTR funding may make a product more attractive to private sector funders because it has been reviewed by scientists and a panel of experts which has evaluated its commercial value (Jordan 2010).

In 2010, *Assistive Technology Outcomes and Benefits* published an evaluation of the impact of the SBIR and STTR grant programs of five agencies, NIH, NSF, and U.S. Departments of Education, Agriculture, and Transportation, on AT development (Bauer and Arthanat 2010). The study used the International Classification of Functioning, Disability and Health (ICF) (The WHO Family of International Classifications 2011) framework as a basis for its inclusion/exclusion criteria and assignment for AT. Study conclusions indicated that policy lacked critical data, such as data about commercial success and constructs such as the ICF to evaluate SBIR and STTR programs and to provide oversight and guidance to agencies managing these programs. The authors concluded that the NIH and the USDE are the key SBIR funders for AT development. However, the study also indicated that NIH, which has a mission in biological research and is cure oriented, is unlikely to commit more than a low percentage of its total NIH SBIR funding to advanced technologies for quality of life. The NIH is the key STTR funder for AT but the program is underutilized by AT manufacturers. The USDE had the smallest SBIR program, yet was second in importance as an SBIR funder only to the NIH.

An IOM study shows that publicly supported research for rehabilitation enjoys minimal funding (Field et al. 2007). At the research stage, there is some evidence that the large federal research agencies, such as NIH and NSF, do not commit a significant proportion of their budgets to advanced technology for quality of life (Brandt et al. 1997). At the development stage, this situation seems to continue. The SBIR and STTR programs are enablers of small business innovation and findings from SBIR- and STTR-sponsored research can provide evidence useful to potential financiers about the quality of the science and commercialization potential of a product. However, while the U.S. government has the authority to set national research priorities and enable advanced AT development for older adults and people with disabilities, it routinely defers to the research agencies. The missions of the sponsoring SBIR and STTR agencies, such as the large program within the NIH, are closely tied to agency priorities and awards related to biological products. NIH may use its SBIR and STTR funds to enable the development of, for example, biotechnology, but invest minimally in advanced technology for quality of life, creating a barrier to its development and commercialization. Challenges to innovation and commercialization are compounded by the complexities of regulation, especially regulation of medical devices (Stevens-Hawkins and Walker 2005).

3.5 Regulation

Product regulation requires significant expertise in order to implement highly complex supervisory and oversight tasks in safety and efficacy. Advanced technology products must adhere to international or national standards, guidelines, and requirements for technical performance and national policies, regulations, and standards on public health, safety, and efficacy (CIRCULAR NO. A-119 Revised | The White House 2011). Table 3.4 presents selected examples of nongovernmental international and domestic standards bodies and organizations and government regulatory agencies that play key roles in the development and commercialization of advanced technologies.

TABLE 3.4

Selected Government Agencies and Nongovernmental Organizations Involved in the Process of Regulation and Standards Setting

Agency/Organization	International	U.S. Govt.	Non–Govt.	Mission
International Organization for Standardization	X			Prepares international standards for all technologies other than electrical standardization
International Electrotechnical Commission	X			Prepares international standards for electrical, electronic, and related technologies
American National Standards Institute			X	Promotes and facilitates voluntary consensus standards
U.S. National Institute of Standards and Technology (NIST)		X		Promotes U.S. innovation and industrial competitiveness by advancing measurement science, standards, and technology in ways that enhance economic security and quality of life
U.S. Occupational Safety and Health Administration (OSHA)		X		Ensures safe and healthful working conditions by specifying safeguards for equipment
U.S. National Highway Safety Administration (NHSA)		X		Educates, supports research, develops, and implements safety standards and enforcement activity related to automobile and highway safety
U.S. Access Board		X		Develops and maintains design criteria for the built environment, transit vehicles, telecommunications equipment, and for electronic and information technology. Provides technical assistance and training on these requirements and on accessible design and continues to enforce accessibility standards that cover federally funded facilities
U.S. Food and Drug Administration		X		Promotes health by reviewing research and approving new products, ensures foods and drugs are safe and properly labeled, works with other nations to "reduce the burden of regulation," and cooperates with scientific experts and consumers to effectively carry out these obligations
Federal Trade Commission (FTC)		X		Plays a supporting role to FDA in enforcing advertising law for medical devices (restricted devices). FTC's primary jurisdiction relates to "unrestricted devices" rather than to device labeling. The commission is particularly intent on preventing marketers from misrepresenting their products to consumers

TABLE 3.4 (continued)

Selected Government Agencies and Nongovernmental Organizations Involved in the Process
of Regulation and Standards Setting

Agency/Organization	International	U.S. Govt.	Non–Govt.	Mission
Federal Communications Commission (FCC)		X		Regulates interstate and international communications by radio, television, wire, satellite, and cable in all 50 states, the District of Columbia, and U.S. territories. The FCC works with the FDA to harmonize regulation of remote devices which use communications

Technical standards organizations routinely establish, by research and consensus, standards which specify the materials to be used in making products as well as how they are to perform. Technical standards, adherence to which is often voluntary, are developed by consensus bodies, often from industry (CIRCULAR NO. A-119 Revised | The White House 2011). These standards must be consistent with U.S. law. The International Electrotechnical Commission (IEC), for example, prepares standards for particular types of technology such as electric and electronic products, while others such as the ISO prepares standards for most other technologies. Leaning edge software from Lean & Zoom and the PerMMA wheelchair referred to earlier, like most products, adhere to technical standards. Standards organizations establish standards which may eventually be adopted by regulatory agencies such as the FDA. In 2005, the American National Standards Institute (ANSI) approved a health level standard for capturing information to support the reporting of adverse events, product problems, or consumer-associated complaints. The FDA has piloted the standard in order to substantiate its use for electronic medical device reporting.

Government agencies have responsibilities for implementing safety, effectiveness, and health regulations and standards. The U.S. National Highway Traffic Safety Administration (NHTSA) develops and implements safety standards for motor vehicle and highway safety. DriveCAP which aims at improving driver safety is subject to NHTSA oversight as well as state regulation. Agencies such as the Occupational Safety and Health Administration in the U.S. Department of Labor have requirements for the safety of equipment in the workplace. The U.S. Access Board is responsible for the development of accessibility standards targeted for the population which is disabled. The mission of the FDA, an independent regulatory agency, includes protecting the public health by assuring the safety, effectiveness, and security of medical devices.

3.5.1 Standards and Regulatory Organizations

Standards organizations and regulatory agencies often work to positively impact U.S. competitiveness by addressing the interplay of standards with intellectual property, competition, and innovation (Insight 2011). These efforts may involve regulatory agencies working closely with industry to develop guidelines that put them at a competitive advantage while assuring the public interest (CIRCULAR NO. A-119 Revised | The White House 2011). However, the language of regulation may itself be a barrier to industry compliance. Regulatory language is not easily translated into the language of technical product requirements. Findings from an electronic information industry case study show that research on approaches to language alignment is beneficial to both industry and government agencies such as the Access Board. The study aimed at understanding and evaluating one company's attempt to align its product development language with legal disability accessibility requirements and to generalize this understanding into best practices (Breaux et al. 2008). Findings indicate that contextualizing legal requirements within a specific industry domain, such as electronics, and addressing specific products such as computers reduced ambiguity.

3.5.2 Medical Device Regulation

The purpose of regulation of medical devices, as with most regulation, is to protect the public. Medical devices, such as implantable pacemakers, may pose significant risk and also sustain and support human life. The Global Harmonization Task Force which works closely with WHO and the FDA are examples of international and federal government organizations that are responsible for achieving effective medical device regulation (U.S. Food and Drug Administration 2010a). These bodies have both the bureaucratic and scientific expertise to address complex scientific problems involving safety and effectiveness.

Medical devices became regulated in the United States in 1976 following a U.S. Senate finding that faulty medical devices had caused 10,000 injuries, including 731 deaths. The FDA's Center for Devices and Radiological Health (FDA CDRH) is responsible for carrying out laws and regulations that relate to the development, testing, manufacturing, labeling, marketing, and distribution of medical devices. The FDA definition of medical devices (Table 3.1) focuses on intended use such as the diagnosis of disease or other conditions; the cure, mitigation, treatment, or prevention of disease; and the means of affecting the structure or any function of the body. Medical devices include a wide range of products that vary in complexity and application. Tongue depressors, medical thermometers, total artificial hearts, stents, x-ray machines, hearing aids, wheelchairs, and iPhone medical apps are all examples of medical devices.

3.5.2.1 Basic Regulatory Requirements

The basic FDA regulatory requirements for which the medical device industry must comply are introduced in this section. In many cases, promotional claims determine the regulatory status of the product. Drive Cap, for example, may avoid using the term health in its promotional claims for the product to avoid being placed into an FDA regulatory category. However, if the Drive Cap system is put into cars as part of clinical practice in order to collect and use the data to assess or direct driver behavior, then Drive Cap may fall within FDA regulation. There are gray areas between wellness programs and disease programs where FDA guidance is unclear. Obesity, as a disease, is often difficult to distinguish from general physical conditioning. Coaching and monitoring devices, such as those developed at CAT, CREATE, and QoLT research centers, fall into these gray areas.

The FDA has established classifications for approximately 1700 different generic types of devices and grouped them into 16 medical specialties, referred to as panels (U.S. Food and Drug Administration). Each of these generic types of devices is assigned to one of three regulatory classes based on the level of control necessary to assure the safety and effectiveness of the device. These medical classes are defined in Table 3.5, with examples provided for each class.

Medical devices are classified according to safety and effectiveness risks posed by the device. Approximately 67% of device types, all from either Class I or Class II, were

TABLE 3.5

Definitions of Medical Device Classes with Examples

Class (U.S. Food and Drug Administration)	Example (U.S. Food and Drug Administration 2009)
Class I devices are subject to the least regulatory control. They present minimal potential for harm to the user and are often simpler in design than Class II or Class III devices	*Examples of Class I devices* include elastic bandages, examination gloves, and hand-held surgical instruments…
Class II devices are those for which general controls alone are insufficient to ensure safety and effectiveness and for which existing methods are available to provide such assurances	*Class II devices* include powered wheelchairs, infusion pumps, and surgical drapes
Class III devices are those for which insufficient information exists to ensure safety and effectiveness solely through general or special controls. Class III devices are usually those which support or sustain human life, are of substantial importance in preventing impairment of human health, or present a potential unreasonable risk of illness or injury	*Class III devices* include implantable pacemaker, pulse generators, HIV diagnostic tests, automated external defibrillators, and endosseous implants

exempt from premarket review (Institute of Medicine (U.S.), Committee on the Public Health Effectiveness of the FDA 510(k) Clearance Process 2011). Class I devices are defined as having the least harm, and therefore are subject to the least regulatory control while Class III pose the greatest risk. Postmarket surveillance studies are required under certain conditions such as when a device is reasonably likely to result in serious adverse health consequences for some users (Wizemann and Institute of Medicine (U.S.), Committee on the Public Health Effectiveness of the FDA 510(k) Clearance Process 2011). Policy criteria which FDA uses to make a determination of a postmarket surveillance study include new or expanded conditions of use for existing devices and significant changes in device characteristics. Applying a standard of least burdensome approach, the FDA requires a manufacturer to produce a scientifically sound answer to the question to be addressed in postmarket surveillance using methods ranging from nonclinical testing of the device to randomized control studies (Center for Devices and Radiological Health 2006). Nonetheless, some stakeholders, especially industry, view postmarket surveillance as an increased regulatory burden.

3.5.2.2 Regulatory Process

Medical devices may travel down two distinct FDA regulatory pathways on the way to the marketplace. These pathways are the 510(k) process and the premarket approval process. FDA exempts almost all Class I devices and some Class II devices from the 510(k) process.

3.5.2.2.1 510(k) and Premarket Approval

In 2003–2007, approximately 31% (15,472) of all devices entered the market through the 510(k) pathway (U.S. Government Accountability Office 2009). The 510(k) process begins with a premarketing submission made by a sponsor to FDA to demonstrate that the device to be marketed is as safe and effective, that is, substantially equivalent, to a legally marketed device that has already received FDA approval. A multiuser health kiosk, developed by QoLT (Research Projects—Quality of Life Technology Center 2011), for example, appears substantially equivalent to kiosks that have already undergone FDA review such as the Xeperex Health Care Kiosk (Thompson 2010). Therefore, the kiosk may receive a shorter and simpler review process than a new product without a substantially equivalent counterpart.

FDA reviews 510(k) submissions in a 90 day timeline. If there are unaddressed scientific issues, the review scientists can ask for additional information and put the submission temporarily on hold. If FDA determines that the information about a product provided by the sponsor meets the standard of substantial equivalence, therefore conforming to a product already cleared by FDA, the product is cleared for marketing in the United States (Office of Device Evaluation and Center for Devices and Radiological Health 2000). If FDA finds that there is no equivalent for the device, or that the new device does not have equivalent performance to the identified FDA-cleared device, the new device is deemed not substantially equivalent. It then may travel the premarket approval route.

Approximately 1% of all devices enter the market through the premarket approval process. A premarket approval requires a sponsor to submit an application to FDA requesting approval to market or to continue marketing a Class III (high risk) medical device. Approval is based on scientific evidence that provides reasonable assurance that the device is safe and effective for its intended use or uses. FDA reviews premarket approval submissions on a 180 day timeline. As with the 510(k) process, if there are unaddressed scientific issues, the review scientists can ask for additional information and put the submission temporarily on hold. If a product is a first of a kind, or if it presents unusual issues of safety and effectiveness, it is generally reviewed by an advisory panel of outside experts before being approved. If FDA finds that a product is safe and effective, it receives an official approval order for marketing in the United States. If the FDA finds that a product is not safe and effective, it will not be approved. Even under the investigational device exemption process, where a device is the object of an investigation, the study may not begin until FDA approves the study or provides a determination that the investigation is no significant risk (Investigation Device Exemption (IDE): IDE Approval Process 2011).

Premarket approval requires companies to demonstrate independently that a new medical device is safe and effective via the submission of clinical data to support claims made for the device. Demonstration of safety and effectiveness may involve clinical trials which can be expensive. Postmarket approval studies may be ordered for the highest-risk medical devices for which premarket approval is sought, similar to the requirement stipulated by the FDA for some devices undergoing consideration in the 510(k) clearance process (Wizemann and Institute of Medicine (U.S.), Committee on the Public Health Effectiveness of the FDA 510(k) Clearance Process 2011). All studies that are ordered for premarket approval are hypothesis-driven and have deadlines and deliverables. The PERMMA is an advanced assistive robotic device that may be viewed as similar to the iBOT, an FDA-approved advanced assistive robotic device from the Independent Technology Division of Johnson & Johnson that was classified as a Class III medical device. After submission of clinical data by its sponsor, the iBOT was successfully reviewed by the FDA which set down strict guidelines and limitations regarding the user population (Schultz 2010; Seelman 2010).

3.5.2.3 New Medical Devices

The FDA has initiated and proposed enhanced processes to move devices though the clearance process. The humanitarian use device (HUD) procedure offers a pathway to allow for commercialization of Class III (high-risk) devices and is designed to address commercialization in small markets (U.S. Food and Drug Administration 2010). This procedure is intended to benefit patients by treating or diagnosing a disease or condition that affects or is manifested in fewer than 4000 individuals in the United States per year.

A manufacturer's R&D costs could exceed its market returns for diseases or conditions affecting small patient populations. To obtain approval for a HUD, a humanitarian device exemption (HDE) application is submitted to FDA. An HDE application is similar in both form and content to a premarket approval application, but it is exempt from the effectiveness requirements of a premarket approval. As of January 25, 2010, the CDRH HDEs list was composed of highly medicalized devices such as a Transcatheter Pulmonary Valve designed to restore pulmonary valve function while delaying the need for open-heart surgery (U.S. Food and Drug Administration 2010c). Advanced Technology products are not usually highly medicalized devices, so the HDE may not apply.

The FDA has proposed two initiatives within what it refers to as an Innovation Pathway to facilitate development and evaluation of innovative medical devices. The initiatives will create a Priority Review Program for Pioneering Technologies and streamline the de novo Pathway (CDRH Innovation Initiative 2011). The Innovation Pathway would establish a priority review for pioneering medical devices, within the 510(k) process by front-loading critical aspects, such as identifying appropriate clinical endpoints and key scientific questions, and seeking advice from external experts in order to provide a more timely and efficient regulatory review process (CDRH Innovation Initiative 2011). The agency has identified the first submission for the Priority Review Program, a brain-controlled, upper extremity prosthetic developed by DARPA.

The FDA refers to its second initiative as the de novo market review classification process. De novo was created to provide a mechanism for the classification of certain lower-risk devices for which there is no predicate and, therefore, not appropriate for the 510(k) process. The de novo classification process is intended to apply to lower-risk devices that are classified into Class III through the 510(k) process. The de novo process is most applicable when the risks of a device are well understood and appropriate special controls can be established to mitigate those risks. Possibly because de novo is not part of the FDA 510(k) process, which the IOM views as needing replacement, IOM noted that de novo has the potential to provide a better premarket review of Class II devices and to provide the basis for a better regulatory model than 510(k).

In July 2011 the FDA issued draft guidance on Mobile Medical Applications (U.S. Food and Drug Administration, Center for Devices and Radiological Health, and Center for Biologics Evaluation and Research 2011). The mHealth (mobileHealth) system is composed of medical device technologies, communication technologies, network infrastructure, and software technologies. Industry has requested clarity from FDA on a number of topics and provided its own guidance to FDA (mHealth Regulatory Coalition 2011). Industry questions how FDA will distinguish between mHealth use for health and wellness and medical use? Within the complex mHealth system, what will be regulated and under which of the three FDA classifications of device regulation? *Institute of Medicine study of FDA 510(k) clearance process* (Institute of Medicine (U.S.), Committee on the Public Health Effectiveness of the FDA 510(k) Clearance Process 2011).

The FDA is under increasing external and internal scrutiny for performance of medical device software and other advanced technology (Institute of Medicine (U.S.), Committee on the Public Health Effectiveness of the FDA 510(k) Clearance Process 2011). An IOM workshop report revealed that malfunctioning software may cause death or serious injury, such as when an infusion pump controlled by malfunctioning software infuses a higher or lower level of medication than prescribed, with possible catastrophic results. IOM has recommended that the FDA should review and update its guidance on software validation. Many advanced technologies for quality of life use software so they may be subject to enhanced regulation in the near future. The FDA is actively monitoring medical and health care apps in mobile phone app stores. Applications where a smart phone is connected in any way to imaging are under scrutiny. Mobile devices may be regulated depending on who uses them (patients, medical personnel) and their intended use (Institute of Medicine (U.S.), Committee on the Public Health Effectiveness of the FDA 510(k) Clearance Process 2011). Both the General Accountability Office and the IOM have urged FDA to upgrade its personnel, resources, and regulatory process to meet the demands of advanced technology regulation. Even more dramatically the IOM struck at the core standard in the FDA regulatory 510(k) process, substantial equivalence, noting that it did not provide reasonable assurance of safety and effectiveness, especially for emerging technologies. The IOM recommended that FDA design a new medical device–integrated premarket and postmarket framework for Class II devices.

The FDA regulatory process for medical devices has been examined in this section. Stakeholders have been highly critical of the process. A robust, global medical device industry, driven by opportunities for commercialization of advanced technology, has criticized the regulatory burden and complexity of the process. The Government Accountability Office and the IOM have questioned the adequacy of the process to protect the safety of the public, especially the adequacy of FDA review of emerging new technology. The IOM has indicated that the FDA 510(k) process is flawed, especially the standard of substantial equivalence, and called for reforms. The FDA has responded by opposing the IOM recommendation for eliminating the 510(k) process. It has introduced initiatives to streamline the clearance process. Industry and the scientific community do not appear to have a common agenda which will create tension within the FDA (Walker 2011). In the short term, these internal and external forces will create uncertainty for the various stakeholders who have established assumptions and routines in their interactions with FDA.

The good news for many stakeholders is that 67% of Class I and II device types were exempt from premarket review. Depending on risk, many advanced technology products may meet the standard for exemption, thus enabling more rapid commercialization. The bad news, particularly for industry, is that the level of regulation in the medical device industries is heavy and increasing (IBIS World USA 2011). On the one hand, postmarket surveillance and postmarket studies increase the regulatory burden carried by industry. On the other, postmarket surveillance may serve the public interest in safety and effectiveness of medical devices.

The existing FDA regulatory process poses at least two major barriers to commercialization, especially for new products. The FDA substantial equivalence standard requires that the new product be substantially equivalent to a product legally marketed prior to May 28, 1976. This standard is a barrier to commercialization because it puts new technologies at a disadvantage. The science driving new technology such as the PerMMA, a robotic wheelchair, may not have been developed in 1976. If a new device cannot meet the standard of substantial equivalence, it must be reviewed in the FDA's premarket approval process which is longer and may add burdensome costs, such as those incurred in clinical trials and filing fees. Premarket applications filing fees to FDA for FY 2011 for regular business is $236,298 and for small business $59,075. For 510(k), the submission fee to FDA is $4348 for regular business and $2174 for small business (Institute of Medicine (U.S.), Committee on the Public Health Effectiveness of the FDA 510(k) Clearance Process 2011).

The 510(k) process also poses a major barrier to reimbursement of new products. Because a 510(k) order places a device in an existing payment category based on the substantial equivalence standard, this classification may preclude assignment of a new Healthcare

Common Procedure Code (HCPC) which is a necessary prerequisite to CMS payment decisions (Dobbins 2006). Nonetheless, the majority of new medical devices that go to market each year do not raise billing-code coverage or payment questions (Raab and Parr 2006). Most of these technologies fit into existing coding and payment categories or are similar to existing items for which coverage determinations have already been made. But when new devices or the procedures associated with their use do not fit into established insurance categories, their adoption may be markedly hindered by lack of reimbursement by third-party payers.

3.5.2.4 Stakeholders

The medical device literature transmits a strong message that enabling strategies to initiate approval of a medical device must begin early and engage multiple stakeholders, such as industry trade associations, consumer groups, researchers, and other members of the scientific community (Richner 2009; GHTF: Global Harmonization Task Force 2010). Researchers and industry should begin their investigations of the regulatory status of a device early in the product development stage. The success of each stakeholder group may be enhanced by support from a different stakeholder group. The medical device industry derives legitimacy for their product from support by the scientific community and patient and consumer groups with compelling medical and health needs. Consumers and researchers benefit from access to the regulatory expertise of the medical device industry. Consumers can be effective communicators of their needs and priorities to the research community, the medical device industry, and regulators.

3.5.2.5 Reimbursement of Medical Devices

Policies guiding medical device reimbursement are complex and contentious, in part because of the tension between those trying to speed the adoption of new medical technology and procedures and those concerned with controlling the costs of health insurance (Raab and Parr 2006c). This section will review various payment models and categories of payers, with a focus on CMS, its mission, procedures and processes, and Medicare. As Table 3.1 on medical device definitions indicates, CMS uses the term DME to refer to medical devices for which it may provide a benefit. CMS reimbursement policies will be examined with particular attention to coverage of advanced technologies for quality of life. Advanced technologies of interest include wheelchair seating coaches that use hardware, software, and intelligence to communicate with the user about the need for seating adjustments in order to prevent pressure ulcers. Other examples include wheelchair add-on items such as a robotic arm or a sit–stand option and tracking and monitoring devices.

3.5.2.6 Payers and Other Stakeholders

Industries involved with medical devices as defined by FDA and CMS are quick to point out that Medicare is the largest purchaser of health care services in the United States (Raab and Parr 2006). Private payers use Medicare prices as benchmarks in negotiating rates with health care providers. Commercial purchasers typically pay more than Medicare, and public purchasers such as Medicaid pay less than Medicare. Those involved in AT, such as wheeled mobility and adaptive seating and position systems, have a somewhat different perspective (Lipka 2009). Daniel Lipka, former president of the National Registry of Rehabilitation Suppliers, which is a trade association, has specified the following list of payers: commercial insurance, Medicare, Medicaid, state-supported workers compensation programs, and vocational rehabilitation services. He notes that there are literally thousands of different insurance carriers with several different types of health care plans. The Department of Veterans Affairs' (VA) Prosthetic and Sensory Aids Service (PSAS) is the largest and most comprehensive provider of prosthetic devices and sensory aids in the world (about PSAS—Prosthetics and Sensory Aids Services [PSAS] 2010), with eligibility for most VA benefits based on honorable discharge from active military service.

Spokespeople across the medical device industries are as one in indicating that medical device manufacturers must go beyond FDA clearance to achieve commercial success (Doughterty 2009). They must align product value, such as indications of improved clinical outcomes, with improved technology performance, cost-effective management of chronic conditions, and improved quality of life. Finally, they must communicate these values to a constellation of stakeholders, including CMS, health care providers, patients, and industry organizations, all of whom can exert pressure on CMS and in the U.S. Congress to make decisions about medical device policy which reflect various stakeholder positions.

3.6 Payment Models

The literature generates a clear message that successful commercialization increasingly requires developers and manufacturers to think early on about regulatory approval and reimbursement strategies for their new devices. On the one hand, advanced technologies have a broad range of applications that include medical use, health and wellness (prevention), and support for activities of daily living and social participation. On the other hand, the market is mostly structured by a third-party payment model highly influenced by restrictive Medicare regulation guidelines such as medical necessity and in-the-home use.

Reimbursement policy for monitoring devices provides a striking example of the medical use emphasis in Medicare reimbursement. In a study focused on monitoring devices, the authors laid out three different reimbursement models (Rao and Pietzsch 2009): third-party payment, out-of-pocket patient payment, and piggybacking onto in-hospital care payment and/or out-of-pocket patient payment only. When a monitoring device is used for a medical purpose and is highly invasive, such as a central line that continuously monitors a patient's circulatory status, the third-party payment model is most appropriate. Reimbursement is difficult to obtain for minimally invasive devices such as semi-invasive continuous glucose monitors, so the patient-pay business models may be the alternative. The study authors indicated that for noninvasive devices, such as coaches and sensors, hospital-pay and patient-pay business models are advised. In another recent study of remote health monitoring, the term "payment puzzle" was used to describe a major barrier to commercialization of monitoring technology (Sarasohn-Kahn and California HealthCare Foundation 2011). Medicare does not broadly support remote monitoring and barely half of Medicaid programs provide for some remote health monitoring applications. The study reports that it is uncertain that consumers will be willing to pay for remote health monitoring.

3.6.1 Centers for Medicare and Medicaid Services

The CMS and its predecessor agencies date back to 1965. On July 30, 1965, the President of the United States, Lyndon B. Johnson, signed into law legislation bills that created Medicare and Medicaid and helped extend access to medical services to the elderly and the poor. As a result, the American health care system was fundamentally transformed. Paying for the care of senior citizens and the poor changed from the local, state, and private realm to a federal responsibility. Since their initial implementation, these programs have absorbed an increasingly higher percentage of the national budget and have posed new problems for the wealthy, poor, young, and old.

With a budget of approximately $650 billion and serving approximately 90 million beneficiaries, the CMS plays a key role in the overall direction of the health care system. CMS aims to expend its resources in a way that both improves health care quality and lowers costs. CMS decisions are guided by its legislation, internal decision-making process, regulation, Medicare program manuals, and contractor policies (Dobbins 2006). Medicare reimbursement is based on an input–output, transactional model of care. Therapies and related procedures designed for cure or at least reduction of disease and impairments create value as found in providing direct measurable effects in patient outcomes (Rao and Pietzsch 2009; Munnecke and Ion 2010). This model is less effective in measuring outcomes from health and wellness, prevention, and rehabilitation devices. Stroke prevention, for example, may combine a number of prevention activities such as diet, monitoring blood pressure, and managing diabetes. These activities, whether measured individually or in combination, do not produce clear cause-and-effect evidence to substantiate outcomes such as fewer visits to the hospital. The transactional model is also less effective in measuring functional outcomes (ADLs and IADLS) and community reintegration. Again, advanced technology products including wheelchair seating coaches and monitoring devices are at a disadvantage. These advanced technologies also may combine a number of wellness and prevention, and rehabilitation activity supports, the outcomes for which whether measured individually or in combination do not produce clear cause and effect evidence of reduced readmissions.

The Medicare benefits policy process is composed of three components: coverage, coding, and payment. Devices must meet the requirements of each of these components in order to be reimbursed. These components are the subject of the next section. Examples are culled from each component to illustrate how Medicare attempts to incorporate new advanced technology into its policies.

3.6.2 Medicare Coverage

Medicare coverage serves as an important gateway for new medical technology and procedures. New medical procedures and technologies must fit within a covered benefit category set out in the Medicare statute, in this case, the DME benefit. DME includes home oxygen equipment, hospital beds, walkers, and wheelchairs (July 8, 2011 Federal Register (76 Fed. Reg. 40,498) 2011). Medicare defines DME as equipment that (a) can withstand repeated use, (b) is primarily and customarily used to serve a medical purpose, (c) generally is not useful to a person in the absence of an illness or injury, and (d) is appropriate for use in the home. CMS is proposing to add an additional 3 year requirement to the definition of durable for coverage of DME (Centers for Medicare & Medicaid Services 2011). Industry and consumer groups are opposing this requirement, arguing that since the proposed rule does not apply to existing devices, these devices will have a significant advantage

TABLE 3.6

Selected Sections of the Medicare Act Pertaining to Durable Medical Equipment

Medicare Benefit Categories
Section 1812 of Medicare Act, Medicare Part A: Items and services (e.g., supplies, equipment, diagnostic, or therapeutic services) provided during covered inpatient hospital stay: inpatient acute hospital, critical access hospital, and skilled nursing facility
Section 1832 of Medicare Act, Medicare Part B: Outpatient diagnostic and therapeutic services and supplies, items and services provided in physician offices (including "incident to" physician services), and DME used in the home

over new devices that enter the market (ITEM: Independence Through Enhancement of Medicare and Medicaid Coalition 2011).

CMS' national coverage determination for speech generating devices provides an informative example of the coverage challenges faced by advanced technologies (U.S. Centers for Medicare and Medicaid Services 2011). Speech-generating devices, as defined by CMS, provide individuals with severe speech impairments with the ability to meet functional speaking needs. Devices that do not meet this definition are characterized by their capability for running software for purposes other than (in addition to) speech generation. These devices include computers and PDAs (which may be programmed to perform the same function as a speech generating device) that may also be useful to someone without severe speech impairment. Single-purpose device requirements are very restrictive. Multiuse devices enhance multiple functionalities, including instrumental activities of daily living such as telephone communication. Table 3.6 shows Medicare benefit categories for medical devices such as speech generating devices.

These benefit categories specify the location of use for DME. Part A is insurance that helps to cover inpatient care in hospitals, skilled nursing facility, hospice, and home health care. Though Medicare will not cover speech generating devices under Part A, it will provide this coverage under Part B. The latter helps to cover medically necessary services like doctors' services, outpatient care, home health services, and other medical and preventive services. The Affordable Care Act of 2010 made important changes to Medicare-covered preventive services, including the removal of deductibles and co-pays for many services, as well as the addition of the new Annual Wellness Visit (AWV) benefit (Medicare Learning Network 2011).

Medicare's National Coverage Determination process also imposes a "Reasonable and Necessary" standard which can be interpreted to mean that the item or service should improve health outcomes overall for Medicare beneficiaries (Centers for Medicare & Medicaid Services 2007, 2010a). When making national coverage determinations, CMS evaluates relevant clinical evidence to determine whether the evidence is of sufficient quality to support a finding that an item or service that falls within a benefit category is reasonable and necessary for the diagnosis or treatment of illness or injury or to improve the functioning of a malformed body member.

Under certain limited conditions, Medicare will pay some nursing home costs for Medicare beneficiaries who require skilled nursing or rehabilitation services (Medicare. gov—Paying for Nursing Home Care 2010). When setting DME payment policy, Congress recognized the responsibility of institutions to meet patients' medical needs, regardless of the primary payer (Medicare and Medicaid) for the stays. Consequently, each nursing home must provide DME as an integral part of its basic daily rate unless it is not providing primarily skilled care or rehabilitation.

3.6.3 Coding

If CMS determines that a device meets coverage benefit requirements, then it moves on to the coding stage. Medicare coding is still another area of complexity, the understanding of which is a challenge to stakeholders. Nonetheless, codes are necessary for reimbursement of clinicians and devices and, thus, are of considerable interest to industry, practitioners, and end users. As indicated previously, most medical devices fit into existing codes. Codes identify medical technologies and procedures and serve as the basis for insurer coverage and payment determination for both. Codes are also needed to implement billing procedures for payment for both services and medical devices.

CMS developed its coding policies for services based on coding conventions defined in the American Medical Association's Current Procedural Terminology (CPT) manual (Centers for Medicare & Medicaid Services 2011). Coding for medical equipment is encompassed in the Healthcare Common Procedural Coding System (HCPCS) maintained by CMS. In order to receive Medicare reimbursement, advanced technology products must have a code. However, advanced technologies often require new codes. The process of establishing a new code is lengthy and the outcome is unpredictable. There are a number of strategies to influence CPT Code development (Hills; Hayes 2001). Emerging technologies should include a combined FDA and CPT strategy which includes obtaining specialist support. Stakeholders should identify CPT gatekeepers and decision makers and review their positions on coverage and benefits. Collaboration is encouraged and should be pursued with other groups with similar coding interests. Finally, stakeholders benefit from identifying individuals actually serving on the AMA code development committee and communicating with those who may be helpful while avoiding the appearance of lobbying.

3.6.4 Payment

If the device is determined to meet coverage policies and receives a code or is categorized under an existing code, then it moves on to the payment stage. The CMS administers Medicare through a defined administrative regulatory process where prices are set prospectively (Centers for Medicare & Medicaid Services 2010d), resulting in payment amounts for reimbursement that are predetermined and fixed according to the Prospective Payment System (PPS). The payment amount for a particular service is derived based on the classification system of that service, for example, diagnosis-related groups (DRGs) such as liver transplants (Averill et al. 2003) or DRGs for inpatient hospital services for liver transplants.

CMS uses separate PPSs for reimbursement to acute inpatient hospitals, home health agencies, hospice, hospital outpatient, inpatient psychiatric facilities, inpatient rehabilitation facilities, long-term care hospitals, and skilled nursing facilities. Medicare makes use of more than a dozen distinct major payment systems to reimburse more than 1 million providers and suppliers for care and services. These systems vary in how rates are set for new procedures and technologies. For instance, CMS may assign new technologies to existing payment groups such as DRGs or establish fee schedule rates. In either case, CMS has been criticized for not covering the costs of new items (Raab and Parr 2006). Industry analysts predict that new health care legislation, with its new payment methods, will support a trend of shifting the financial burden from insurers to care providers (Schneider 2010). Physicians and hospitals will pay even closer attention to clinical outcomes associated with technologies, especially with respect to its impact on costs.

3.6.5 Approaches to Enhancing Coverage of DME and Breakthrough Technologies

Medicare has a responsibility to pay enough for beneficial new technologies to ensure beneficiaries' access to care while simultaneously remaining a prudent purchaser. Medicare has instituted innovation initiatives, including the CMS Innovation (CMI) Center that was established in 2010. The CMI, which will begin full-scale operations as part of the CMS in 2011, will be responsible for developing at least 18 reform models specified in the new health care law adopted in 2010 that is entitled the Patient Protection and Affordable Care Act. The models include patient-centered medical homes, community-based health teams to support small-practice medical homes, and the use of health information technology to coordinate care for the chronically ill (Center for Medicare and Medicaid Innovation Must Implement Payment Reforms Rapidly 2011). While too early to know the impact of their implementation, these models may incorporate advanced technology such as monitoring devices that enhance individuals' ability to track their own health, functional status, or response to treatment or that enables others, particularly health care providers, to assess these parameters remotely.

Beginning in 2000, Congress took steps to ensure access by Medicare beneficiaries to new breakthrough technologies (Clyde et al. 2008). These technologies must meet the following three conditions: the technology must be new, which the CMS generally defines as within 2–3 years following FDA approval or market introduction, if later; the existing MS-DRG payment for the service involving the technology must be inadequate as demonstrated by meeting thresholds calculated annually by the CMS; and the technology must be a substantial clinical improvement over existing services. Through the use of CMS discretionary power and in conjunction with passage of the Medicare Prescription Drug Improvement and Modernization Act of 2003, Medicare's New Technology Add-On Payment Program evolved (U.S. Medicare Payment Advisory Commission 2003). While technologies that have qualified have shown value, they are highly medicalized such as rechargeable implantable spinal cord stimulators for chronic pain (Clyde et al. 2008).

Medicare has been conservative about extending the DME benefit to technology that traditionally have been used outside of what it determines to be medically necessary. In 2007, CMS made a coverage determination indicating what would be reimbursable for the iBOT 4000 Mobility System, an advanced robotic mobility system not unlike QoLT's PerMMA (Centers for Medicare & Medicaid Services 2007). These technologies combine emerging technologies such as robotics and ICT. They can provide additional function through add-ons and customization such as a robotic arm or stand and sit and coaching. Despite the FDA's positive review of the iBOT, described previously in this chapter, CMS determined that coverage would be limited to the standard function of this medical device. The iBOT meets the definition of DME as a wheelchair used in the patient's home that is reasonable and necessary for beneficiaries who have a personal mobility deficit which is sufficient to impair their participation in mobility-related activities of daily living in customary locations in the home. The CMS decided to reimburse the approximately $22,000 iBot like a regular wheelchair, at about $6,000. Coverage did not extend to the new technological functionality on the iBOT, such as a stair climber, four-wheel balancer, and remote functions which are associated with activities of daily living and participation in society.

Medicare has two approaches to help beneficiaries obtain DME such as sit and stand when they may fail to meet medical necessity criteria or when the beneficiary wishes to upgrade and obtain equipment that may not be covered based on medical need

(Crane and Minkel 2009). The two approaches are Advanced Beneficiary Notification (ABN) and Advanced Determination of Medical Coverage (ADMC). The first approach, ABN, is a written notice that a health care provider or his/her designee gives to a Medicare beneficiary before outpatient items or services are rendered, when the health care provider believes Medicare will not pay for some or all of the items or services (Advance beneficiary notice of noncoverage (ABN) Part A and Part B 2011). ABNs are restricted for provision to beneficiaries enrolled in Original (fee-for-service) Medicare. The Original Medicare Plan is a fee-for-service plan that covers many health care services and certain drugs, enabling a beneficiary to go to any doctor or hospital that accepts Medicare. The ABN allows the beneficiary to make an informed decision about whether to receive services that he/she may be financially responsible for paying. The ABN serves as proof that the beneficiary has knowledge that a service may not be covered by Medicare, prior to receiving that service. ADMC is an optional process by which CMS provides a DME provider and the beneficiary with a coverage decision prior to delivery of an item (Coverage and Medical Policy 2008). Not all DME items are eligible for the ADMC process, and the coverage determination provided does not guarantee payment for the device.

Medicare national coverage determinations have been the target of criticism from many different constituencies (Raab and Parr 2006). National coverage review times are much longer than the FDA's process for clearance or approval of new medical technologies (Medical Technology Leadership Forum 2002; U.S. Department of Health and Human Services 2003). An individual review for a coverage determination ranges from 280 to 811 days, and it takes an average of 219 days to implement these decisions once they have been made. CMS coding has also been the subject of considerable criticism (Raab and Parr 2006). Insurers are reluctant to reimburse for new technology HCPCS codes because they lack a track record of eligibility for reimbursement. Many researchers are unfamiliar with the process to pursue a new code.

DME providers, seeking redress for what they perceive as CMS' restrictive policies, have taken their arguments to Congress (NCART: National Coalition for Assistive and Rehab Technology 2010). They argue that the CMS DME benefit was created over 40 years ago to address the medical equipment needs of elderly individuals. However, technology has advanced and the Medicare population has expanded. In 1972, Medicare was extended to cover people under 65 with permanent disabilities who qualified for Social Security Disability Insurance (SDI) (Dale and Verdier 2003). In 2009, Medicare covered 45 million people, including 7 million persons with disabilities less than 65 years of age (Neuman 2009). This population that tends to qualify for Medicare based on their disability and not their age consists of individuals with diagnoses such as cerebral palsy, muscular dystrophy, multiple sclerosis, spinal cord injury, amyotrophic lateral sclerosis, and spina bifida. Nonetheless, the CMS proposal to add a 3 year requirement to the definition of durable for coverage of DME suggests that CMS may be more sensitive to cost and efficiency factors than to factors related to equipment upgrade or introduction of next generation equipment. Therefore, the outlook is not particularly positive for securing Medicare as a stable reimbursement source for rehabilitation and wellness and prevention equipment.

Medicare has reduced the length of reviews and adjusted its procedures in response to other criticisms, but it has not adjusted policies that impact noncovered disability groups who are under 65 years of age. In response to its responsibilities under the Patient Protection and Affordable Care Act, CMS has initiated activities related to telemedicine and the medical home. Therefore, depending on the successful implementation of Patient Protection and Affordable Care Act, opportunities for reimbursement for advanced technology may emerge.

3.7 Assistive Technology

The original AT legislation, Technology-Related Assistance for People with Disabilities Act of 1988 (Tech Act), and later amendments were introduced during a period of disability civil rights activism that peaked in 1990 with the passage of the Americans with Disabilities Act (Assistive Technology Training Online Project 2005). AT was seen as having the potential to provide opportunities for increased independence and participation in all of life's activities. Including any item, piece of equipment, software, or product system that is used to increase, maintain, or improve the functional capability of individuals with disabilities, AT addresses an individual's mobility, sensory, or cognitive needs at the functional level. The Tech Act as amended supports the development of training and delivery systems for AT devices and services for people of all ages. However, it does not provide reimbursement for the technologies themselves. The definition of AT migrated from the Tech Act to other legislation including the Individual with Disabilities Education Act (IDEA) and the OAA. While Congress has allocated funding for AT within IDEA, AT has been minimally funded within the OAA. Some government programs such as Social Security, Veteran's Benefits, Workmen's Compensation, and Medicaid pay for AT, with the U.S. Rehabilitation Services Administration an important source of funding for those with disabilities who want to work.

Estimates from the Survey of Income Program Participation showed that 54 million persons, or about 20% of the U.S. population, have activity limitations or disabilities (Carlson et al. 2005). About half of these individuals use assistive devices and technologies or special equipment such as canes, wheelchairs, special beds, or special telephones as well as medical devices and rely on home modifications or school or workplace accommodations or modified cars or vans to perform daily tasks and activities. A review of AT payment sources revealed that 48% of these individuals used devices paid for by themselves or their families; 75% of persons with home accessibility features reported that they or their families had borne the entire cost of such modifications.

While AT is widely regarded as an enabler of improved function among individuals with disabilities, the absence of reimbursement is a major barrier to their access to AT. The impact may fall most heavily on older adults who do not work and, therefore, cannot secure reimbursement from Vocational Rehabilitation or Workmen's Compensation. Older adults are also a key target market for advanced technologies which promote wellness and prevention. However, many older adults cannot afford to pay for AT.

3.8 Conclusions

The legal and regulatory policy framework for advanced technology and less formal forces such as activities of stakeholders have been explored in this chapter. Enablers and barriers to innovation and commercialization have been identified. Advanced technology has emerged as an important driver of change. The legal and regulatory framework is under pressure to change. But major stakeholders have not come to a consensus about the nature of reform, especially in the regulatory process, creating uncertainty for those involved in regulation. New policies are needed to balance the nation's need for medical cure with its needs to support wellness, prevention, and rehabilitation. Evidence to support the value of advanced technology to dampen the cost of health care and improve the health of U.S. citizens has not been sufficient to convincing policy makers in the Congress and the White House.

IOM's *Enabling America* reports on the weakness in the federal programs in disability and rehabilitation research and the general insufficiency in the magnitude of the programs (Brandt et al. 1997). The R&D, regulatory and reimbursement framework for today's advanced technology was developed during an earlier period when the promise of technology for quality of life was less obvious and lifespan was shorter. Policy was developed based on a medical model which, at the research stage, aimed at cure and in regulation and reimbursement at highly medicalized devices. Definitions of technology in public health insurance programs have a strong bias to medical use which limits the scope of coverage, as in the case of the CMS benefit for DME. In turn, restricted coverage creates a barrier to public reimbursement. CMS coverage criteria, especially in-the-home use restrictions, are in contrast to the objectives of the Americans with Disabilities Act which is supportive of broad social participation for people with disabilities. In the case of speech generating devices, benefit coverage actually limits the technical specifications of the device to single-purpose devices. Coverage does not extend to advanced technology, such as the iPAD, which provides a variety of supports for individual function and participation, including generation of speech. Public reimbursement coverage policy is particularly important because advanced technology for quality of life does not yet have integrated industrial structure and a stable out-of-pocket consumer revenue stream.

Pressure from agencies outside the U.S. advanced technology legal and regulatory framework may generate change in the framework. The IOM reports which recommends replacement of the FDA 510(k) clearance process and its substantial equivalence standard, if implemented, may lead to the development of a process more appropriate to review of robotics, software, and other advanced technologies. WHO and the International Standardization Organization (ISO) have adopted definitions of devices which distinguish between those devices which are for medical use such as pacemakers and those for quality of life such as motorized scooters and tilt and lift wheelchairs. WHO and ISO definitions could become models for the global marketplace. WHO's efforts in globalization of medical device regulation also may be an enabling factor in commercialization of advanced technology which enjoys an increasingly global marketplace.

Policy research on cost and benefits is needed to assist policy makers in decisions about resource allocation. However, the weakness of the CMS input–output model for measuring the impact of multiple activity rehab, wellness, or prevention interventions suggests the need to generate and legitimize other models to measure costs and benefits. Technology researchers would benefit from access to case studies of technology submissions as they move through the FDA and the CMS processes. While the CMS decision process is not transparent, the R&D community would also benefit from case studies of the process for development of new CMS product codes acquisition. Studies of the technology transfer process from the development to early commercialization stages would help academic researchers who may not be familiar with strategies to move their products to market. Disability accessibility regulation often applies to nonmedical products such as wheelchair bus ramps which are not subject to FDA regulation and CMS reimbursement policy. The cost of these products is usually absorbed by a particular industry such as companies in bus transportation. Industry would benefit from studies that crosswalk accessibility regulation with technical specifications for products. The development of new models for regulation of advanced technology is an obvious research priority. Research modeling regulatory frameworks appropriate to advanced technology would be a welcome outcome of the IOM's criticism of the FDA 510(k) medical device clearance process. Domestic and international studies of regulatory and nonregulatory approaches to protection of public safety in the adoption of complex advanced technology would be a valuable supplement to a focus on research on regulation.

Difficult questions persist about who wants, who needs, who benefits from, and who should pay for advanced technologies for quality of life. Forces external to the legal and regulatory framework for advanced technology, such as health care costs, are major issues in the broad public policy arena. Health care accounts for 16% of the country's gross domestic product, the highest among the world's industrialized nations. Over the past decade, the pace of total health care spending has grown faster than inflation and the growth in national income. The Patient Protection and Affordable Care Act enacted in March of 2010 by the U.S. Congress is but one example in a political arena highly polarized around health care provision and payment models ranging from privatization to socialized single payer government provider. If the new Act is implemented, most individuals will be able to purchase policies so that payers' pricing and risk management systems will need to be redesigned (Pawar and Pietraszek 2010). The Act proposes a tax on device companies which will affect profitability (Medical Device Manufacturing in the United States: Market Research Report, 33451b 2010). By expanding coverage to a broader range of patients through a significant loosening of the eligibility criteria for enrollment in Medicaid, the Act may also serve as an enabler to industry because medical device demand will increase. Under Title III of the Patient Protection and Affordable Care Act, CMS is required to improve the quality and efficiency of health care through its new Center for Medicare & Medicaid Innovation. The Center is charged with developing models, including medical homes and health information technology, which, if found to be cost effective, safe, and efficacious, may generate expanded benefits with positive impacts on advanced technology commercialization.

Advanced technology, health care costs, new legislation, and activities by IOM and the WHO all impact on the somewhat "crusty" regulatory and reimbursement framework. However, their impact on policy awaits political feasibility and consensus in the political arena. Therefore, researchers, developers, clinicians, consumers, and industry stakeholders in the advanced technology policy framework will pursue innovation and commercialization within a context characterized by uncertainty.

References

About PSAS—Prosthetics and Sensory Aids Services (PSAS). 2010. U.S. Department of Veterans Affairs, 2010 [cited September 2010]. Available from http://www.prosthetics.va.gov/About_PSAS.asp

Advance beneficiary notice of noncoverage (ABN) Part A and Part B. 2011. Accessed May 2012 at http://www.cms.gov/Outreach-and-Education/Medicare-Learning-Network-MLN/MLNProducts/downloads/ABN_Booklet_ICN006266.pdf

Assistive Technology Training Online Project. 2011. *Assistive Technology Laws: AT Legislation.* School of Public Health and Health Professions, University of Buffalo, The State University of New York 2005 [cited February 2011]. Available from http://atto.buffalo.edu/registered/ATBasics/Foundation/Laws/atlegislation.php

Averill, R. F., N. Goldfield, J. S. Hughes, J. Bonazelli, E. C. McCullough, B. A. Steinbeck, R. Mullin, A. M. Tang, J. Muldoon, L. Turner, and J. Gay. 2003. *All Patient Refined Diagnosis Related Groups (APR-DRGs): Methodology Review.* Wallingford, CT: Clinical Research and Documentation Departments.

Bauer, S. M. 2003. Demand pull technology transfer applied to the field of assistive technology. *The Journal of Technology Transfer* 28 (3–4): 285–303.

Bauer, S. M. and S. Arthanat. 2010. SBIR and STTR programs for assistive technology device development: Evaluation of impact using an ICF-based classification. *Assistive Technology Outcomes and Benefits* 6 (1): 39–72.

Beard, J. 2008. DARPA'S bio-revolution. In *DARPA: 50 Years of Bridging the Gap,* edited by United States Defense Advanced Research Projects Agency and United States Department of Defense, Office of the Secretary of Defense. Tampa, FL: Faircount LLC.

Björn, F. 2009. *Programme for Health Technologies: Call for Innovative Technologies Background and Process.* Geneva, Switzerland: World Health Organization.

Brandt, E. N., A. M. Pope, and Institute of Medicine (U.S.), Committee on Assessing Rehabilitation Science and Engineering. 1997. *Enabling America: Assessing the Role of Rehabilitation Science and Engineering.* Washington, DC: National Academy Press.

Breaux, T. D., A. I. Antón, K. Boucher, and M. Dorfman. 2008. Legal requirements, compliance and practice: An industry case study in accessibility. In *Proceedings of the16th IEEE International Requirements Engineering Conference,* September 8–12, 2008, Barcelona, Spain. Los Alamitos, CA: IEEE Computer Society.

Carlson, D., N. Ehrlich, and National Institute on Disability and Rehabilitation Research (U.S.). 2005. *Assistive Technology and Information Technology Use and Need by Persons with Disabilities in the United States, 2001.* Washington, DC: U.S. Department of Education, National Institute on Disability and Rehabilitation Research.

CDRH Innovation Initiative. 2011. Accessed May 2012 at http://www.fda.gov/MedicalDevices/NewsEvents/WorkshopsConferences/ucm241095.htm

Center for Devices and Radiological Health. 2006. Postmarket surveillance under section 522 of the Federal Food, Drug and Cosmetic Act. In *Guidance for Industry and FDA Staff.* Silver Spring, MS: U.S. Food and Drug Administration. Accessed September 2011 at http://www.fda.gov/MedicalDevices/DeviceRegulationandGuidance/GuidanceDocuments/ucm072517.htm

Center for Medicare and Medicaid Innovation Must Implement Payment Reforms Rapidly. 2011. PhysOrg.com 2010 [cited February 2011]. Available from http://www.physorg.com/news195195889.html

Centers for Medicare & Medicaid Services. 2007. *CMS Manual System: Pub 100-03 Medicare National Coverage Determinations—Transmittal 65.* U.S. Department of Health and Human Services. Accessed September 2011 at http://cms.gov/Regulations-and-Guidance/Guidance/Transmittals/downloads/R74NCD.pdf

Centers for Medicare & Medicaid Services. 2008. U.S. Department of Health and Human Services [Revised December 2008]. Available from http://www.medicare.gov/Publications/Pubs/pdf/11045.pdf

Centers for Medicare & Medicaid Services. 2010a. U.S. Department of Health and Human Services [cited September 2010]. Available from www.cms.gov

Centers for Medicare & Medicaid Services. 2010b. Overview durable medical equipment, prosthetics/orthotics and supplies fee schedules. U.S. Department of Health and Human Services, September 13, 2011 [cited September 2010]. Available from www.cms.gov/DMEPOSFeeSched

Centers for Medicare & Medicaid Services. 2010c. Medicare coverage database. U.S. Department of Health and Human Services, 2010 [cited September 2010]. Available from https://www.cms.gov/medicare-coverage-database/overview-and-quick-search.aspx?id=8

Centers for Medicare & Medicaid Services. 2010d. Overview prospective payment systems—General information. Department of Health and Human Services 2010 [cited September 2010]. Available from https://www.cms.gov/ProspMedicareFeeSvcPmtGen/01_overview.asp

Centers for Medicare & Medicaid Services. 2010e. Overview national correct coding initiatives edits. U.S. Department of Health and Human Services 2011 [cited September 2010]. Available from www.cms.gov/national/correctcodinited

Centers for Medicare & Medicaid Services. 2011. Overview end stage renal disease (ESRD) payment. U.S. Department of Health and Human Services, 2011 [cited September 2011]. Available from https://www.cms.gov/esrdpayment/

Cheng, M. 2003. *Medical Device Regulations: Global Overview and Guiding Principles.* Geneva, Switzerland: World Health Organization.

CIRCULAR NO. A-119 Revised | The White House. 2011. Office of Management and Budget 2011 [cited January 2011]. Available from http://www.whitehouse.gov/omb/circulars_a119

Clyde, A. T., L. Bockstedt, J. A. Farkas, and C. Jackson. 2008. Experience with Medicare's new technology add-on payment program. *Health Affairs (Millwood)* 27 (6): 1632–1641.

Coverage and Medical Policy. 2008. *DME MAC Jurisdiction C Supplier Manual.* Nashville, TN: CIGNA Government Services.

Crane, B. and J. Minkel. 2009. Legislation and funding. In *The Industry Profile on Wheeled Mobility,* edited by S. Bauer and M. E. Buning. Buffalo, NY: Rehabilitation Engineering Research Center on Technology Transfer.

CREATE. 2011. Center for Research and Education on Aging and Technology Enhancement 2010 [cited August 2011]. Available from http://www.create-center.org/

Dale, S. B. and J. M. Verdier. 2003. Elimination of medicare's waiting period for seriously disabled adults: Impact on coverage and costs. In *Issue Brief (Commonwealth Fund); Variation: Issue Brief (Commonwealth Fund).* Place Published: Commonwealth Fund, Task Force on the Future of Health Insurance. http://www.cmwf.org/programs/medfutur/dale-waitingperiod-ib-660.pdf

Dobbins, K. L. 2006. Getting CMS reimbursement for medical technology products: Reimbursement for medical technology, overview of CMS coverage. FDLI & Clinical Device Group.

Doughterty, E. J. 2009. Reimbursement advocacy: Multiple avenues to success. Paper read at *12th Annual Coverage, Reimbursement and Health Policy Conference,* November 10, Washington, DC.

Engineering Research Centers Association. 2010. About the ERCs. National Science Foundation [cited September 2010]. Available from http://www.erc-assoc.org/

Field, M. J., A. M. Jette, and Institute of Medicine (U.S.), Committee on Disability in America: A New Look. 2007. *The Future of Disability in America.* Washington, DC: National Academies Press.

Foster, R. W. 1982. Cost-based reimbursement and prospective payment: Reassessing the incentives. *Journal of Health Politics, Policy and Law* 7 (2): 407–420.

GHTF: Global Harmonization Task Force. 2010. [cited September 2010]. Available from www.ghtf.org

Hayes, M. G. 2001. *Reports on CPT Codes and Assistive Technology.* Arlington, VA.

Heerkens, Y. F., T. Bougie, and M. W. de Kleijn-de Vrankrijker. 2000. Classification and terminology of assistive products. In *International Encyclopedia of Rehabilitation,* edited by M. Blouin and J. Stone. New York: CIRRIE.

Hills B. J. CPT codes: Tips and Strategies change to: Medical Device Manufacturers Association. Reimbursement Reform: M. Beebe, The coding process and the impact on innovation. [Accessed September 2011] Available from http://www.medicaldevices.org/node/832

IBIS World USA. 2011. [cited November 2011]. Available from http://clients.ibisworld.com/launch.aspx?show=1

Independence Technology—A Johnson & Johnson Co. Ibot (Power Wheelchairs)—USA Techguide. 2011. United Spinal Association 2011 [cited August 2011]. Available from http://www.usatechguide.org/itemreview.php?itemid=903

Independence Technology, L.L.C. 2011. [cited August 2011]. Available from http://www.ibotnow.com/

Insight. 2011. http://www.gtwassociates.com/answers/insight-v13-n01.html

Institute of Medicine (U.S.), Committee on the Public Health Effectiveness of the FDA 510(k) Clearance Process. 2011. Medical devices and the public's health the FDA 510(k) clearance process at 35 years. Place Published: National Academies Press. http://www.nap.edu/openbook.php?record_id=13150

Investigation Device Exemption (IDE): IDE approval process. 2011. U.S. Food and Drug Administration.

ITEM: Independence through Enhancement of Medicare and Medicaid Coalition. 2011. [cited September 2011]. Available from http://www.itemcoalition.org/

Item Coalition letter to Donald M. Berwick, MD, MPP Administrator Centers for Medicare & Medicaid Services. 76 Fed. Reg. 40,498, July 8, 2011 Federal Register. 2011. U.S. Government Printing Office. [Accessed September 2011] Available from http://www.christopherreeve.org/atf/cf/%7B3d83418f-b967-4c18-8ada-adc2e5355071%7D/ESRDREGULATION0811.PDF

Jordan, J. F. 2010. Innovation, commercialization and the successful start-up (working paper). http://www.heinz.cmu.edu/research/407full.pdf

July 8, 2011 Federal Register (76 Fed. Reg. 40,498). 2011. U.S. Government Printing Office.

Lane, J. P. 1997. Technology evaluation and transfer in the assistive technology marketplace: Terms, process and roles. *Technology and Disability* 7 (1–2): 5–24.

Lane, J. P. 2003. The state of the science in technology transfer: Implications for the field of assistive technology. *Journal of Technology Transfer* 28 (3–4): 333–354.

LeadingAge: Aging Services Technologies. 2011. LeadingAge [cited August 2011]. Available from www.leadingage.org/SubSection.aspx?id=533

LeadingAge: Center for Aging Services Technologies. 2011. LeadingAge [cited August 2011]. Available from www.leadingage.org/cast.aspx

Lipka, D. 2009. Supplier perspectives. In *The Industry Profile on Wheeled Mobility*, edited by S. Bauer and M. E. Buning. Buffalo, NY: Rehabilitation Engineering Rese288-ach Center on Technology Transfer.

Market Research Reports & Analysis | IBISWorld US. 2010. IBISWorld 2010 [cited September 2010]. Available from www.ibisworld.com

Medical Device Manufacturing in the US: Market research report, 33451b. 2010. [Accessed May 23, 2012]. Available from http://www.pr-inside.com/medical-device-manufacturing-in-the-r2431944.htm

Medical Technology Leadership Forum. 2002. MTLF FORUM Medicare Coverage Policy: The balance between local and national decision making. Washington, DC.

Medicare Learning Network. 2011. MedicarePREVENTIVE. SERVICES. In *Quick Reference Information: Preventive Services*, edited by C. F. M. M. Services. Washington, DC: U.S. Department of Health and Human Services.

Medicare.gov—Paying for Nursing Home Care. 2010. U.S. Department of Health and Human Services [cited September 2010]. Available from http://www.medicare.gov/nursing/payment.asp

mHealth Regulatory Coalition. 2011. [cited November 2011]. Available from http://mhealthregulatorycoalition.org/

Munnecke, T. and H. W. Ion. 2010. A transformational notion of health 2000 [cited September 2010]. Available from http://www.munnecke.com/papers/D20.doc

National Institute for Public Health and the Environment. 2010. WHO—FIC homepage. WHO Collaborating Centre for the FIC in the Netherlands 2010 [cited September 2010]. Available from http://www.rivm.nl/who-fic/ISO-9999eng.htm

NCART: National Coalition for Assistive and Rehab Technology. 2010. National Coalition for Assistive and Rehab Technology 2009 [cited May 2010]. Available from http://www.ncart.us/

Neuman, T. 2009. Medicare 101: The Basics. The Henry J. Kaiser Family Foundation. Available from http://www.kaiseredu.org/Tutorials-and-Presentations/Medicare-the-Basics.aspx

Office of Device Evaluation and Center for Devices and Radiological Health. 2000. Use of standards in substantial equivalence determinations. In *Guidance for Industry and for FDA Staff*. Silver Spring, MD: U.S. Food and Drug Administration.

Pawar, M., and W. E. Pietraszek. 2010. The new IT landscape for health insurers. McKinsey on Business Technology, http://execseries.mgt.ncsu.edu/files/2010/08/IT_Landscape_for_health_insurers.pdf

Quality of Life Technology Center. 2011. [cited August 2011]. Available from www.cmu.edu/qolt

Raab, G. G. and D. H. Parr. 2006a. From medical invention to clinical practice: The reimbursement challenge facing new device procedures and technology—Part 1: Issues in medical device assessment. *Journal of American College of Radiology* 3 (9): 694–702.

Raab, G. G., and D. H. Parr. 2006b. From medical invention to clinical practice: The reimbursement challenge facing new device procedures and technology—Part 2: Coverage. *Journal of American College of Radiology* 3 (10): 772–777.

Raab, G. G., and D. H. Parr. 2006c. From medical invention to clinical practice: The reimbursement challenge facing new device procedures and technology—Part 3: Payment. *Journal of American College of Radiology* 3 (11): 842–850.

Rao, S. K. and J. B. Pietzsch. 2009. Policy-induced constraints in the design and commercialization of monitoring devices: An assessment of three technologies' reimbursement models. *Journal of Medical Devices, Transactions of the ASME* 3:2.

Research Projects—Quality of Life Technology Center. 2011. [cited August 2011]. Available from http://www.cmu.edu/qolt/Research/projects/index.html

Richner, R. 2009. Medical Affairs & Markets: Reimbursement 101 Developing Strategies for Product Cycle Planning. [Accessed May 23, 2012] Available from http://www.medicaldevices.org/issues/Reimbursement

Sarasohn-Kahn, J. 2011. The connected patient: Charting the vital signs of remote health monitoring. Oakland, CA: California HealthCare Foundation. http://www.chcf.org/~/media/MEDIA%20LIBRARY%20Files/PDF/T/PDF%20TheConnectedPatient.pdf

SBIR (Small Business Innovation Research). 2011. U.S. Government [cited August 2011]. Available from www.sbir.gov/about/about-sbir

Schneider, C. E. 2010. Tracking reimbursement and payment trends. MD+DI: Medical Device and Diagnostic Industry. www.mddionline.com/article/tracking-reimbursement-and-payment-trends

Schultz, D. G. 2010. FDA Letter granting premarket approval for iBOT 3000 mobility system. U.S. Department of Health and Human Services 2003 [cited September 2010]. Available from http://www.accessdata.fda.gov/cdrh_docs/pdf2/P020033a.pdf

Schwartzel, E. 2011. 'Leaning' edge software from Lean & Zoom, a CMU spinoff, creates national buzz. *Pittsburgh Post-Gazette*, January 21, 2011.

Seelman, K. D. 2010. Social enablers and barriers to adoption of assistive robots: Case studies of the iBOT and PerMMA. Paper read at *Second International Symposium on Quality of Life Technology*, Las Vegas, NV.

Silverstein, S. M. 2011. Common examples of healthcare IT failure. Drexel University 2010 [cited August 2011]. Available from http://www.ischool.drexel.edu/faculty/ssilverstein/cases/?loc=cases&sloc=negligent_homicide

Sirat, Z. 2011. LeadingAge CAST mission and vision. LeadingAge, April 29, 2011 [cited August 2011]. Available from www.leadingage.org/CAST_Mission_and_Vision.aspx

Stevens-Hawkins, L. and M. Walker. 2005. HL7 Individual Case Safety Report Release 1: Implementation Guide for FDA Medical Device Reporting. U.S. Food and Drug Administration. Accessed September 2011 at http://www.fda.gov/downloads/ForIndustry/DataStandards/IndividualCaseSafetyReports/UCM161178.pdf

The WHO Family of International Classifications. 2011. World Health Organization 2011 [cited August 2011]. Available from http://www.who.int/classifications/en/

Thompson, B. M. 2010. *FDA Regulation of Mobile Health: Mobihealthnews 2010 Report*, edited by B. Dolan.

Thompson 2010. Investigation device exemption (IDE): IDE approval process (2011). http://www.thompson.com/images/tpg/pdfsamples/XRAY_TOC.pdf

Timmers, P. 2011. ICT addressing societal challenges. In *European "Fp8" Workshop—Innovation for Society*, Bruxelles, Belgium.

U.S. Centers for Medicare and Medicaid Services. 2011. National Coverage Determination (NCD) for Speech Generating Devices (50.1) 2001 [cited November 2011]. Available from http://www.cms.gov/medicare-coverage-database/details/ncd-details.aspx?NCDId=274&ncdver=1&NCAId=8&ver=6&NcaName=Augmentative+and+Alternative+Communication+(AAC)+Devices+for+Speech+Impairment&MCDId=6&McdName=Factors+CMS+Considers+in+Opening+a+National+Coverage+Determination&bc=BEAAAAAAEAAA&

U.S. Department of Health and Human Services. 2003. Report to Congress on national coverage determinations for fiscal year 2002. Washington, DC: U.S. Department of Health and Human Services.

U.S. Food and Drug Administration. 2010a. Device classification. U.S. Department of Health and Human Services [cited February 2010]. Available from http://www.fda.gov/MedicalDevices/DeviceRegulationandGuidance/Overview/ClassifyYourDevice/default.htm

U.S. Food and Drug Administration. 2010b. Device advice: Comprehensive regulatory assistance. U.S. Department of Health and Human Services 2010 [cited September 2010]. Available from http://www.fda.gov/medicaldevices/deviceregulationandguidance/default.htm

U.S. Food and Drug Administration. 2010c. Humanitarian device exemption. U.S. Department of Health and Human Services 2010 [cited May 2010]. Available from http://www.fda.gov/MedicalDevices/DeviceRegulationandGuidance/HowtoMarketYourDevice/PremarketSubmissions/HumanitarianDeviceExemption/default.htm

U.S. Food and Drug Administration. 2010d. Listing of CDRH humanitarian device exemptions. U.S. Department of Health and Human Services, 2010 [cited May 2010]. Available from http://www.fda.gov/MedicalDevices/ProductsandMedicalProcedures/DeviceApprovalsandClearances/HDEApprovals/ucm161827.htm

U.S. Food and Drug Administration. 2011. U.S. Department of Health and Human Services 2011 [cited November 2011]. Available from http://www.fda.gov/MedicalDevices/default.htm

U.S. Food and Drug Administration, Center for Devices and Radiological Health, and Center for Biologics Evaluation and Research. 2011. Mobile medical applications (DRAFT). In *Guidance for Industry and FDA Staff*. Silver Spring, MD: U.S. Food and Drug Administration.

U.S. Government Accountability Office. 2009. Medical devices FDA should take steps to ensure that high-risk device types are approved through the most stringent premarket review process: Report to Congressional Addressees. Washington, DC: U.S. Government Accountability Office.

U.S. Medicare Payment Advisory Commission. 2003. Payment for new technologies in Medicare's prospective payment systems. In Report to the Congress. Medicare payment policy. Washington, DC: Medicare Payment Advisory Commission.

United States Congress Senate Special Committee on Aging. 2008. Recognition of excellence in Aging Research Committee Report. Washington, DC: U.S. Senate Special Committee on Aging.

Unofficial Compilation of the Older American Act of 1965 as amended in 2006 (Public Law 109–365). Available from http://www.aoa.gov/aoaroot/aoa_programs/oaa/oaa_full.asp#_Toc153957648

Walker, E. P. 2011. Medical news: IOM device report gets strong response. *MegPage Today*, LLC 2011 [cited September 2011]. Available from http://www.medpagetoday.com/PublicHealthPolicy/FDAGeneral/27806

Wizemann, T. M. and Institute of Medicine (U.S.), Committee on the Public Health Effectiveness of the FDA 510(k) Clearance Process. 2011. Public health effectiveness of the FDA 510(k) clearance process: Measuring postmarket performance and other select topics: Workshop Report. Washington, DC: National Academies Press.

Part II

Design, Development, and Evaluation

4

Assessing Needs, Preferences, and Attitudes Using Survey Methods

Scott R. Beach

CONTENTS

4.1 Introduction

The first three chapters of the book set the broad context for the remainder of the book by providing working definitions of quality of life and quality of life technologies (QoLTs), describing who might benefit from such technology, and presenting a general model of the facilitators and barriers of technology uptake. The goal of this chapter is to describe the use of survey methods for understanding broad user attitudes and preferences for QoLT. These surveys would typically be conducted in the early phases of QoLT design, prior to the development of specific technology system prototypes (although they could also be used in later phases of the iterative design, development, and evaluation process to be described in Chapters 5 and 6).

The focus of this chapter is on the use of survey methods to assess potential end-user attitudes and preferences in a broad, general sense in order to better define and understand the potential market for QoLT. The types of data that might be collected in this phase include *general attitudes and preferences about potential QoLT design parameters* such as basic form factor (e.g., anthropomorphic or "human-like" qualities in assistive robots); interface modality; preferences for passive or active systems; how "smart" or intelligent the system should be; the type, frequency, and specificity of feedback the system should provide; how the system affects social connectedness; privacy issues like the use of video cameras versus sensors to gather behavioral data; and preferences for who should have access to such data. Surveys might also collect data on *general attitudes toward proposed or imagined QoLT systems*, including, for example, perceptions of willingness to use, safety, functionality, likelihood of improving quality of life, ease of use and learning to use, anxiety about use, embarrassment or stigma of use, privacy impacts, and willingness to pay for the technology. Note that these parameters are derived from the model of technology uptake presented in Chapter 2. Survey methods should be used to collect data both from potential direct users of QoLT (i.e., the older or disabled adult) and other stakeholders such as family/professional caregivers, healthcare providers, and industry. While the specific issues addressed for the various stakeholders may differ, any systematic attitudes/preferences analysis should target multiple stakeholder perspectives.

This chapter begins with a brief overview of survey methodology with a focus on issues that are particularly relevant to the conduct of surveys to inform QoLT design. The next section provides a focused review of work being done by other researchers involving survey methods that is relevant to broad preferences for QoLT and illustrative of the survey design issues raised in the first section. The chapter concludes with an overview of surveys conducted by the CMU/Pitt QoLT Engineering Research Center (ERC). The description of our own and others' work is meant to provide examples of the issues and challenges that QoLT design teams encounter when conducting surveys with potential QoLT stakeholders. They also illustrate the range of potentially valuable data that can be obtained from surveys to help inform the design of QoLT.

4.2 Survey Methodology and QoLT

Surveys involve the collection of standardized data (i.e., measurement) from samples of clearly defined populations (i.e., sampling) (Groves et al. 2009). One of the distinguishing features of surveys is that sample sizes should be relatively large to provide enough cases for quantitative statistical analyses that allow general conclusions about the population of interest. This contrasts with smaller-sample qualitative methods like focus groups, which are used primarily to get rich and detailed perspectives on needs and preferences for QoLT or in-depth reactions to actual system prototypes (see Helal et al. 2008 for examples). The "representativeness" of the samples for qualitative studies is generally of less concern than ensuring that the participants are members of the target stakeholder population and that at least some range of background characteristics and views are included. Both sampling and measurement pose unique challenges in the context of conducting QoLT preference surveys. These challenges are discussed briefly here.

4.2.1 Sampling

In terms of sampling, the target populations for QoLT preference surveys should be defined to include "potential users of QoLT"—potential because the systems are generally still in development at this stage. This population includes older adults and baby boomers (generally defined as 45–64 years old)—both currently disabled and nondisabled—current users of assistive technology (who are often also disabled), and other stakeholders such as informal family caregivers, healthcare providers, and industry representatives. One of the challenges in sampling these populations—particularly disabled, AT users, and caregivers—is their relatively low prevalence in the general population. This makes drawing representative probability samples labor intensive and costly due to extensive screening requirements. Recall that the population-based epidemiological surveys reviewed in Chapter 1 are large-scale, primarily government-funded efforts. It is possible to obtain representative population-based samples of potential QoLT users, and we describe a few examples in the following.

However, QoLT design teams and researchers may have to make sampling design compromises in order to get large enough samples and remain within budget constraints. Some of these compromises include the use of online web panels that allow targeting of specific disability and health groups, the use of readily available mailing lists or clinic populations, and the development and the use of research registries of special populations. The main limitation of these approaches is that they are not pure probability samples, and most online panels have the additional problem of only including individuals with access to computers. Finally, surveys of healthcare professionals and industry representatives come with their own challenges, the main ones being difficulty gaining access and the lack of comprehensive lists (sampling frames) from which to draw true probability samples. Again, QoLT design teams will need to make design trade-offs such as the use of readily available providers and incomplete lists, to sample these important potential QoLT stakeholders.

4.2.2 Measurement

Turning to the measurement of QoLT preferences, the fundamental challenge is the fact that many systems in question do not yet fully exist. Thus, either more general issues–related preferences for technology need to be addressed (e.g., general attitudes toward and the use of technology, general privacy concerns related to technology) or respondents must be presented with hypothetical descriptions of QoLT systems and function and be asked to imagine themselves needing the technology. More specific questions about hypothetical QoLT design parameters can then be asked. Questions can always be raised about the validity of such survey responses to imagined, hypothetical systems, but there are approaches to addressing this problem. For one, by surveying those who are most likely to need and use QoLT in the future, and can perhaps better imagine needing and using such systems—disabled older adults, baby boomers, current users of AT, and caregivers—we hope to obtain more valid responses.

Another key survey design parameter is the mode of administration. To date, we have used two general approaches. First, we have employed traditional self-administered surveys (via the web and paper and pencil) with text-based hypothetical descriptions of QoLT systems as stimuli. More recently, we have incorporated visual stimuli (videos) of prototype systems and related behaviors that hopefully increase realism and the vividness of the experience and result in more valid survey responding. Of particular interest are comparisons between responses to text-based versus visual stimuli depicting similar QoLT systems. Examples of this work from the QoLT ERC are presented as follows.

4.3 Illustrative Surveys Targeting Attitudes and Preferences for QoLT

Much of the current work on preferences for QoLT-related systems is being done with small samples using qualitative methods like focus groups (Helal et al. 2008). However, there a few sources of survey data on broad attitudes, usage, and preferences for assistive and other technologies that deserve mention. Note that these examples involve both currently existing technology (i.e., computers, the Internet, and home safety devices) as well as systems that are just on the horizon. We will see in the following when we discuss our QoLT ERC work that more futuristic, longer-term horizon technologies can also be the focus of surveys.

One major source of population-based data on the use of existing computer-based technology in the United States—specifically the Internet—is the Pew Research Center's Internet & American Life Project, which has involved repeated random digit dialing (RDD) telephone surveys of U.S. adults (Pew Research Center 2011). RDD involves the random selection of telephone numbers (both listed and unlisted) from the set of all potential phone numbers covering the target geography of interest (in the case of the Pew surveys, the United States), and is the standard method for generating representative probability samples of telephone households. Current state-of-the-art RDD surveys like the Pew Center's include both landline and cell phone interviews to account for the fact that approximately 25% of U.S. households are cell-phone only (Blumberg et al. 2011). The current survey conducted in May 2011 (n = 2277) shows that 78% of Americans are currently online (up from 46% from the first survey in 2000). Internet usage is related to age, with adults 18–29 (95%), 30–49 (87%), and 50–64 (74%) being much more likely to be online than those 65 and older (42%; Pew Research Center 2011).

These data show fairly high penetration of computer use through baby boomer age (64), and increasing usage among older adults (the online rate for 65+ was 12% in 2000), providing evidence for an increasingly technology-savvy population of potential QoLT users. This is a good example of the use of a probability sample survey to obtain data on the usage of existing technology from a nationally representative sample. Also, the measurement issues raised earlier about hypothetical systems are not relevant here as the focus is on computers and the Internet. The Pew surveys provide the best estimates of the current size of the populations with and without access to the Internet and computers.

Another group doing work in this area and using large sample surveys is the Center for Research and Education on Aging and Technology Enhancement (CREATE) based at the University of Miami. Czaja et al. (2006) examined predictors of the use of various existing technologies in a comprehensive study of 1204 adults age 18–91 recruited via advertisements, newspapers, flyers, etc., from the Miami, FL, Tallahassee, FL, and Atlanta, GA, areas. The study included questionnaires, which were administered both in person and self-administered; tapping attitudes toward and the use of computers and other technologies; and a detailed battery of cognitive tests (plus other psychosocial variables). The researchers categorized the sample into younger (18–39), middle-aged (40–59), and older (60–91) age groups for analyses. Czaja et al. (2006) found that older adults reported less use of technology and less experience with the World Wide Web, confirming the Pew findings reported earlier. The study also found that lower use of technology among older adults was partially mediated or explained by higher levels of computer anxiety, lower levels of computer efficacy, and lower levels of "fluid intelligence" (analytical reasoning), despite higher levels of "crystallized intelligence" (world knowledge).

The authors stressed the importance of developing effective anxiety reduction training techniques to increase the likelihood of successful adoption and use of technology by older adults. These results reinforce the need for QoLT system designers to strive for simple, intuitive user interfaces and to develop effective training strategies for end users and other stakeholders. This work also illustrates a large-scale effort that, while not relying on population-based probability sampling (i.e., the study relied on volunteers recruited from ads), did have a large sample and, most importantly, a comprehensive assessment battery that allows for detailed examination of the correlates and predictors of technology attitudes and use.

Another survey effort that directly relates to preferences for QoLT called *Healthy@ Home* was conducted in December 2007 by the American Association for Retired Persons (Barrett 2008a). This survey used nationally representative online/web panels of 907 older adults (age 65+) and 1023 caregivers (reporting that they are "currently or in past 12 months providing unpaid help to a relative or friend 50 years or older"), using Knowledge Network's (KN) *Knowledge Panel*®. This panel is recruited using RDD telephone and address-based probability sampling methods, with noninternet households provided with Web TV/laptop computers in order to include participants without access to computers.

The *Healthy@Home* survey focused on older adults' and caregivers' awareness of, willingness to use, and perceived benefits and barriers for three classes of technology: (a) personal computers; (b) home safety devices (alarms, appliance regulation devices, activity monitors, sensors to detect falls, and cooking aids); and (c) personal health and wellness devices (personal emergency response systems, telephone-based monitoring, TV-based monitoring with provider communication, electronic pillbox, Internet monitoring with provider communication, and electronic pillbox with provider monitoring). Thus, the survey explored attitudes and preferences for already existing QoLTs. The survey provided *still photographs* of various technologies for respondents to react to in order to aid responding.

Some of the main findings for *older adults* (65+) included the following:

- The vast majority would prefer to receive help in their own home if they need help caring for themselves.
- While older adults have a limited awareness of new technology, they would be willing to use a variety of systems to maintain social contact, gather information, be safe at home, and promote their personal health and wellness.
- For home safety devices, willingness to use exceeded awareness for all systems.
- While older adults perceived physical safety and emotional peace of mind as potential benefits of home safety technology, many expressed concerns about costs.
- Seven in ten older adults say these devices may not be something they need.
- Results for personal health and wellness devices parallel those for home safety devices—willingness exceeds awareness; despite safety, peace of mind, and comfort as potential benefits, there was great concern over costs, and 70% thought they may not need these technologies.

Some of the main findings for *informal caregivers* included the following:

- While awareness of the various technologies for help in caring for their loved one varied greatly, willingness to use the devices was generally high.
- Willingness to use the various technologies generally exceeded awareness of the technology.
- Caregivers providing higher levels of care were generally more willing to use the various technologies.
- More than 8 in 10 caregivers thought they would have some or a great deal of difficulty persuading the people they help to use the technology.
- While perceiving many potential benefits of the various technologies, caregivers were also quite concerned about costs.

The survey report recommended increasing older adult and caregiver awareness of the range of technology either available (or on the horizon) that could provide increased safety, peace of mind, and social connectedness (Barrett 2008a). The issues of cost and the reluctance of older adults' to think they need such technology must be addressed before widespread adoption can occur. The *Healthy@Home* survey raises many fundamental issues for QoLT design teams to consider. It also illustrates the use of large, probability samples of older adults and caregivers to conduct surveys about existing technology. However, as the survey results showed, many of the respondents were not aware of the existence of such technology. From a measurement perspective, the survey was interesting in its use of still photographs to help respondents better understand the technologies being discussed and perhaps lead to more valid responding. This is a "middle ground" approach between written descriptions and video stimuli, and has the advantage of not requiring special software in order to actually view a video.

Another set of surveys focused on caregivers of older and disabled adults, and their use of technology has been conducted by the National Alliance for Caregiving (NAC) and American Association of Retired Persons (AARP 2009). The 2009 *Caregiving in the U.S.* survey (also conducted in 1997 and 2004) included questions on caregiver use of technology for the first time. The survey used primarily RDD telephone sampling (with some oversampling of minorities using more targeted methods) to gather data from 1480 caregivers. Some of the highlights from the 2009 *Caregiving in the U.S.* survey include the following:

- A population prevalence rate of 28.5% of adults in the United States providing informal care (65.7 million caregivers).
- The new questions on the use of technology showed that almost half (45%) of the caregivers reported using some form of technology to help care for the recipient.
- The most commonly used device was an electronic organizer/calendar (24%).

The following technologies were also used by a small but significant portion of caregivers:

- Emergency response system such as Lifeline (12%)
- A device that electronically sends information to a doctor or care manager to help manage care recipient health care (11%)
- An electronic sensor that can detect safety problems in the home and take steps to help (falls, leave stove on, etc.) (9%)
- A website or computer software to keep track of care recipient personal records (7%)

In sum, the survey reveals that a small but significant minority of informal caregivers (7%–12%) is using technology like emergency response systems, electronic communication of recipient health data to providers, electronic sensors for safety, and websites/software for tracking personal records. These data show a substantial potential market for QoLT among informal caregivers and provide general guidance for the design of such systems. The survey is also an example of using the telephone to provide verbal descriptions of existing technologies to a representative national sample of caregivers of older and disabled adults and children with disability.

Another NAC-sponsored survey conducted in 2011 was the *e-connected family caregiver survey* (United Healthcare and the National Alliance for Caregiving 2011). This was a web-based survey of 1000 members of a national voluntary, opt-in online survey panel who met the following criteria: (1) age 18 and over; (2) provided at least 5h/week of unpaid care to a friend or relative who needs help due to illness, disability, or frailty; and (3) had already used some sort of technology to help them with caregiving (Internet, blogs, electronic calendar/organizer, etc.). The survey obtained feedback on receptivity to 12 technologies, including 4 caregiver support technologies (caregiver mentor matching service, decision support tool, training simulations, and coaching software), and 8 technologies to facilitate caregiving (video phone system; caregiving coordination system; passive movement monitoring system; symptom monitor and transmitter; medication support system; interactive system for physical, mental, and leisure activities; transportation display; and personal health record tracking). The technologies were presented using text-based descriptions. Respondents were asked how likely they would be to use the technology (or if they already used it), how helpful they think it would be, and about various perceived barriers to use and adoption of the technology. To reduce burden, each respondent rated only 6 of the 12 technologies (2 caregiver support and 4 caregiving facilitation, randomly chosen).

Results were summarized with a matrix showing helpfulness versus barriers for each technology, which were categorized into those with the "greatest potential" (helpful, low barriers), those with "moderate potential" (helpful, high barriers), and those with the "least potential" (less helpful, high barriers). Technologies showing the "greatest potential" included

- Personal health record tracking (which had the highest perceived helpfulness and lowest perceived barriers)
- Caregiving coordination system
- Medication support system

Caregiver training simulations and the caregiver decision support tool were also in the "greatest potential" category, but were rated less positively. Technologies rated as having "moderate potential" included symptom monitor and transmitter; the interactive system for physical, mental, and leisure activities; the video phone system; and the passive movement monitoring system. Finally, caregiving coaching software, transportation display, and caregiver mentor matching service were rated as having the "least potential."

In sum, the survey shows that potential adoption of new technologies by caregivers involves consideration of both costs and benefits, and that those with the greatest current potential may be the most practical (i.e., health record tracking, medication support, and caregiver coordination). Other technologies like symptom monitor and transmitters, video phones, and passive movement monitoring may be helpful but various barriers to use—primarily cost and resistance to use by care recipients—must be overcome before they are adopted. The survey is also interesting from a methodological point of view in two ways. First, the sampling strategy was unique in that the survey targeted caregivers who were already using technology to assist with caregiving. This ensured that the respondents would be more likely to be able to imagine using the technologies described and hopefully provide more valid responses. However, in order to attain this, a nonprobability, opt-in volunteer web survey panel had to be accessed. The cost of using a random sampling approach with screening for not only caregivers but those also using technology to aid in caregiving would have been prohibitive. Second, the techniques of having the respondents react to only 6 of the 12 technologies to reduce burden is notable. While the benefits of the approach are obvious, the disadvantage is the reduced sample sizes (and different, but partially overlapping mix of respondents) responding to each specific technology. Both of the methodological issues illustrate the trade-offs that designers of QoLT surveys often need to make.

There is other work involving surveys of attitudes toward and the use of technology that is relevant to the identification of broad QoLT preferences (see Barrett 2008b for a review). The purpose of this brief review was to point to some of the most relevant recent work in this area that illustrates the issues involved with conducting surveys of QoLT attitudes and preferences. We now turn to a description of surveys being conducted by the QoLT ERC.

4.4 Surveys Conducted by the QoLT ERC

Our survey work in the QoLT ERC has focused on many of the broad attitudes and preferences for QoLT systems that have been discussed in this chapter. We have focused our surveys on general attitudes about potential QoLT design parameters and general attitudes toward proposed or imagined QoLT systems. The surveys we have conducted to date are summarized in Table 4.1, which includes detailed descriptions of the samples, target populations, mode of survey administration, target measurement domains, and major findings. The surveys highlight the sampling and measurement issues discussed at the beginning of the chapter. This section of the chapter will provide brief summaries of the survey methods and key findings, and the chapter concludes with a summary discussion of recommendations for sampling and measurement when conducting QoLT surveys. The main difference between our work in the QoLT ERC and the work just reviewed is that we have attempted to get feedback on technology *that generally does not yet fully exist* rather than existing technology. Since our goal was to inform the technology design and development process, we felt it important to assess attitudes about hypothetical as opposed to real systems.

The first survey was conducted with a national opt-in volunteer web panel that targeted disabled and nondisabled baby boomers (age 45–64) and older adults (65+). Though not a representative probability sample and comprised of only Internet users, the panel offered the opportunity to collect data from a large sample (n = 1610), and more importantly, to target specific disability groups—physical disability, rheumatoid arthritis, stroke, emphysema, and multiple sclerosis—as respondents (see Table 4.1). We reasoned that these groups would be more likely to be able to imagine needing the QoLT systems we presented. For this survey, we used traditional written scenarios to describe hypothetical QoLT technologies being developed by the ERC. We were also interested in informational privacy concerns relating to the sharing and recording of sensitive health and functional behavior information by QoLT systems. This survey also contained items from standard batteries we developed measuring general attitudes toward technology and the release of private information, health and disability status, assistive technology use, health-related quality of life, and demographic variables. This standard battery was used in most of the surveys reported here.

The key findings were that respondents were least accepting of sharing information about toileting and driving behavior, sharing it with the government or insurance companies, and having the information be recorded via video (versus sensors; see Table 4.1 for detailed findings). Figure 4.1 presents results on acceptability of having private health and functional information recorded by video with sound, video without sound, and sensors. There was a clear preference for sensors over video, and respondents were

TABLE 4.1

QoLT ERC Surveys of Attitudes and Preferences for QoLT

Sample/Source/Sample Size (References)	Target Population(s)	Mode of Administration	Target Measurement Domains	Major Findings
Survey 1				
National opt-in volunteer web panel (Survey Sampling International; SSI) (n = 1610) (Beach et al. 2009a; Matthews et al. 2010)	Nondisabled baby boomers (age 45–64) (303) Nondisabled older adults (age 65+) (610) (specifically targeted disability groups of any age): Physical disability (348) Rheumatoid arthritis (103) Stroke (101) Emphysema (74) Multiple sclerosis (71)	Web-based text only	General technology attitudes Factors in choices to use technology General privacy concerns about release of personal information *Evaluations of hypothetical QoLT systems—safe driving, active home (robots), virtual coach, and Personal Mobility and Manipulation Appliance (PerMMA)* (including perceived applicability of system to respondent) Willingness to pay for system *QoLT informational privacy concerns around target behavior:* • Toileting • Taking meds • Moving about the home • Cognitive ability • Driving behavior • Vital signs/health status Recipient of information: • Family • Healthcare providers • Insurance co. • Researchers • Government	Respondents least accepting of sharing personal health information: • About toileting and driving behavior • With government and insurance companies • And recording PHI using video (versus sensors) More disabled respondents more accepting of sharing, recording PHI Older slightly more accepting than younger Respondents with more positive attitudes toward technology in general were more accepting Those with more general privacy concerns were less accepting Current AT use was not related to acceptance of recording and sharing of PHI Respondents who thought the QoLT systems applied to them were more positive in their evaluations of the systems

(continued)

TABLE 4.1 (continued)

QoLT ERC Surveys of Attitudes and Preferences for QoLT

Sample/Source/Sample Size (References)	Target Population(s)	Mode of Administration	Target Measurement Domains	Major Findings
			Method of recording: • Video with sound • Video without sound • Sensors Technologies to improve QOL to develop in near future (open-ended) Health/disability/AT use/QOL Demographics	Themes from open-ended: • Develop technology that enhances independence at home, delay LTC placement • QoLT should assist with both physical and cognitive deficits • Safe driving technology would be useful • Privacy concerns and trade-offs between reduced privacy and independence • Cost is a major concern • QoLT that reduces human contact should be avoided
Survey 2 Local (Pittsburgh, PA) Gerontology Research Registry (n = 350) (Beach et al. 2009b)	Disabled and nondisabled older adults (60+)	Mailed paper and pencil	General technology attitudes Factors in choice to use technology General privacy concerns about personal information *QoLT informational privacy concerns* (replication—same as earlier) Explicit QoLT *trade-offs* and *"tipping points"* focused on: • Reduced privacy versus independence (avoidance of nursing home) • Reduced privacy versus enhanced function (IADL, ADL, Transfers) • Reduced efficiency versus enhanced function	Replication of informational privacy findings from Survey 1 Respondents less willing to make trade-offs for independence or function when QoLT involves: • Video cameras throughout the home • System takes twice as long as human to perform tasks • 5–10 h of required training • About 1 h/day of maintenance • Reduced opportunities for social interaction Respondents least willing to trade-off reduced social interaction More educated respondents were generally more willing to make trade-offs than less educated

		• Heavy training requirements versus enhanced function • Heavy maintenance versus enhanced function Recued social interaction versus enhanced function Health/disability/AT use/QOL Demographics	Respondents with higher levels of disability more willing to make trade-offs than nondisabled (replication of Survey 1)
Survey 3 National Wheelchair user Registry (n = 277) (Beach et al. 2010)	Current manual or power wheelchair users age 18 and older (mean age 54.5)	Mailed paper and pencil	Same as that given earlier (Gerontology Research Registry)—surveys identical	Replication of informational privacy findings from Surveys 1 and 2 Respondents less willing make trade-offs for enhanced ADL function when QoLT involves video cameras throughout the home Were slightly more willing to accept full video coverage of home for prevention of LTC placement Respondents less willing make trade-offs for enhanced ADL function when QoLT involves: • System takes twice as long as human to perform tasks • 5–10 h of required training • About 1 h/day of maintenance • Reduced opportunities for social interaction Respondents least willing to trade-off reduced social interaction More educated respondents were generally more willing to make trade-offs than less educated

(continued)

TABLE 4.1 (continued)

QoLT ERC Surveys of Attitudes and Preferences for QoLT

Sample/Source/Sample Size (References)	Target Population(s)	Mode of Administration	Target Measurement Domains	Major Findings
				Respondents with mobility problems and spinal cord injury more willing to make trade-offs than nondisabled (replication of Survey 1)
				Respondents with more positive general attitudes toward technology were more willing to trade-off reduced privacy for prevention of LTC placement
Survey 4				
Health care providers at the University of Pittsburgh Medical Center (UPMC) System Conference attendees e-mail distribution lists (n=107) (unpublished data)	Health care providers (physicians, RN, nurse practitioner, physician assistant)	Paper and pencil (at conference)	Perceived trustworthiness of data generated by various sources including nontechnical: • PCP • Specialists • Home health facilities • Nursing homes/assisted living facilities • Community health screenings • Patients and family members And technology: • Telehealth monitors • Wearable monitors • Environmental monitors • Other monitors (type of data—e.g., vital signs, diagnoses, psychological assessment, behavior, and activity—varied by source) Perceived usefulness of data from the source for clinical decision making	Providers generally perceive technology sources as trustworthy
				Wearable monitors are seen as most trustworthy, followed by environmental and telehealth monitors
				Technology sources seen as more trustworthy than home health and nursing homes, community health screenings, and patients and family
				Technology sources (as a whole) seen as less trustworthy than PCPs and specialists, except for wearable monitors (no difference)
				Actual experience with receiving data from the technology did not affect perceived trustworthiness
				PCPs and specialists are seen as most trustworthy among the nontechnology sources
				Community health screenings seen as least trustworthy

Survey 5	Baby boomers and older adults	Web-based with the following:	(For technology) ever received data from this source? Discipline, specialty, length of practice	
National web panel (representative)		Written scenarios		
Knowledge Networks (KN) (*Knowledge Panel®*) (n = 500) (unpublished data)		Video stimuli	*Written scenarios:* Acceptability of *kitchen, personal care, and safe driving* technology performing varying levels of assistance:	*Written scenarios:* Less comfort with driving technology actually helping with tasks
			• Monitor performance and share info. with family / doctor	More safety concerns for all three types of technology when it actually helps with tasks than when simply providing coaching and advice
			• Monitor and provide evaluative feedback	Privacy was a concern for all three types of technology
			• Monitor and coach, give advice	Respondents generally preferred human assistance to technology assistance
			• Monitor and help complete task	Respondents strongly preferred human control to technology control
			Outcomes:	Perceived likelihood of ever needing help with all three tasks was somewhat low
			• Comfort with technology	
			• Safety concerns	Respondents would be willing to pay fairly small amounts out of pocket each month for all three types of technology
			• Perceived invasion of privacy of technology	
			• Preference for technology versus human assistance with task	
			• Preference for technology versus human control in operation of technology	
			• Perceived likelihood of needing help with task in the future	
			• Willingness to pay out of pocket for technology	

(*continued*)

TABLE 4.1 (continued)

QoLT ERC Surveys of Attitudes and Preferences for QoLT

Sample/Source/Sample Size (References)	Target Population(s)	Mode of Administration	Target Measurement Domains	Major Findings
			Video stimuli:	*Video stimuli:*
			• *Bathing Robot* ("hard" versus "soft" systems) (same outcomes as those given earlier) "Virtual valet" car parking system	Fairly low comfort levels and high safety concerns for both "hard" and "soft" bathing robots (no differences in ratings) After viewing robot bathing videos, respondents strongly favored human versus technology assistance and human control of technology (these ratings were more extreme than for the written personal care scenario)
			• Outcomes: Trust in system accuracy and safety (absolute and versus human valet)	Low to moderate levels of trust in the "virtual valet" to park their car accurately and safely
			• *General* attitudes toward system (learning to use, make life easier, embarrassing to use)	Perceptions that the "virtual valet" would be easy to learn to use and not embarrassing to be seen using; but less clear about whether it would make life easier
Survey 6				
National web panel (representative)	Disabled and nondisabled baby boomers and older adults	Web-based with video stimuli	Acceptability of varying levels of privacy masking for video data of a fall (full video, masking, stick figure, text only/sensors)	"Context-free" stick figure and text only/sensors are seen as less invasive than either full motion or "blurry" videos
Knowledge Networks (KN) (*Knowledge Panel*)		Randomized experiment	Randomized between-subjects experiment embedded within population-based survey	The majority of respondents were willing to share all types of fall data if it would prevent nursing home placement
Time-Sharing Experiments for the Social Sciences (TESS) project (n = 1800) (unpublished data)			Perceived invasion of privacy of this type of monitoring in bedroom, bathroom, kitchen Trade-offs of sharing video info. to remain in home, avoid LTC placement	Most willingness to share context-free data The approximately 8% who were current caregivers were more accepting of sharing fall data than noncaregivers

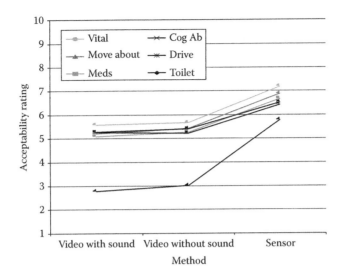

FIGURE 4.1
Acceptability of having different types of personal health information recorded with videos versus sensors among middle-aged and older adults.

particularly concerned with having toileting behavior recorded via video. In addition, those reporting higher levels of disability were more accepting of sharing the information (Beach et al. 2009a). This implies that those most in need may be most willing to trade reduced privacy for increased function provided by QoLT. Consistent with this argument, we also found that respondents who thought the QoLT systems applied to them personally were more positive toward the systems than those who did not (Matthews et al. 2010).

Our next surveys (Surveys 2 and 3, Table 4.1) were conducted using traditional paper and pencil methodology and utilized existing research registries of older adults and wheelchair users (the survey instruments were identical). This sampling methodology was chosen for several reasons. First, we wanted to continue targeting groups that would be more likely to be currently disabled, or to become disabled in the future, and thus be more likely to relate to the QoLT scenarios (Gerontology Registry). In the case of the wheelchair users, disabled adults currently using a "lower technology" assistive device are a potential market for future QoLT systems and are more likely to identify with the presented scenarios. We also wanted to use mailed paper surveys to insure that we captured individuals without access to the Internet, which we had not done with the first national web survey panel. Thus, we wanted to replicate the findings on informational privacy concerns from the national web survey with samples that included noncomputer users. The 350 older adults who completed the survey were members of a local Gerontology Research Registry at the University of Pittsburgh who had agreed to be contacted for studies relating to aging, family caregiving, coping with illness and disability, and other topics. The 277 wheelchair users were participants in a national research registry who had agreed to participate in studies on issues related to living with a disability and the use of assistive technology. The primary goal of the registry surveys was to follow up more explicitly on the idea of trade-offs (e.g., less privacy for increased function and independence) suggested by the prior results showing that more disability was related to more acceptance of sharing private health information (Beach et al 2009a). We used a measurement strategy where we

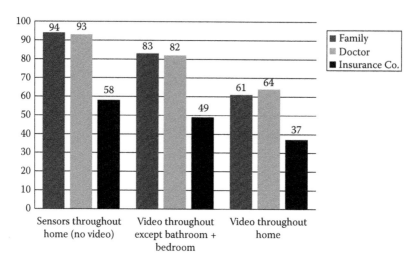

FIGURE 4.2

Percent of middle-aged and older respondents agreeing with different levels of home monitoring and sharing data with varying targets to prevent going to a nursing home.

posed explicit trade-offs (e.g., video cameras throughout your home, but it will prevent you from having to go to a nursing home; takes 5–10 h to learn to use the technology, but will increase ADL/IADL function) and asked in a yes/no format whether they would be willing to accept the technology given the conditions. This trade-off approach was also an attempt to directly measure perceived costs and benefits that may be potentially related to user uptake (see Figure 2.1, Chapter 2).

Key findings included respondents being less willing to make trade-offs for independence (prevention of nursing home placement) or function (help with IADL/ADL tasks) when the QoLT systems involve video cameras throughout the home; the system takes twice as long as a human to perform tasks; the system takes 5–10 h to learn how to use; and 1 h/day to maintain. The findings were generally consistent between the older adults from the Gerontology Registry and the wheelchair users, and the specific findings presented next are for the combined samples (Beach et al. 2009b, 2010). Figure 4.2 shows acceptance of differing levels of home monitoring and data sharing with family, doctors, and insurance companies assuming the technology would prevent nursing home placement. Older adults and wheelchair users were least accepting of video monitoring throughout their home— particularly if the data were to be shared with their insurance company—even if such monitoring would prevent nursing home placement. Video monitoring except for the bedroom and bathroom was more acceptable. Respondents were generally unreceptive to sharing any type of data with insurance companies regardless of the potential benefits, while they were more accepting of sharing with their doctor and family. Figure 4.3 shows acceptance of 2–3 and 5–10 h of training required for the use of technology that would provide ADL, IADL, and transfer assistance. Only slightly more than one-third would accept technology requiring 5–10 h of training, and there were significant minorities who would not accept 2–3 h to learn to use technology, even if it would enhance daily function. These findings reinforce the points made earlier about the requirements for technology that is intuitive and simple to use. Another dramatic finding was that respondents were generally unwilling to trade off reduced opportunities for social interaction, even if it meant enhanced function. Only about 30% of the sample was willing to make such a trade-off. Lastly, Respondents

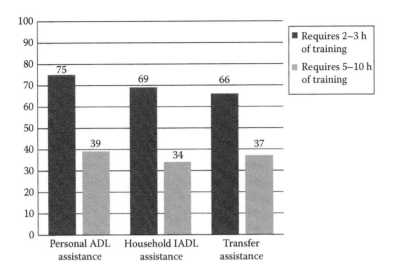

FIGURE 4.3
Percent of middle-aged and older respondents willing to accept 2–3 and 5–10 h of training to use technology that will provide assistance with activities of daily living, instrumental activities of daily living, and transfers.

with higher levels of disability (Beach et al. 2009b) and wheelchair users with more severe mobility problems or spinal cord injury (Beach et al. 2010) were more willing to make QoLT trade-offs, consistent with findings from the national web panel survey discussed earlier (Beach et al. 2009a).

The next survey (Survey 4, Table 4.1) shifted the focus to another key stakeholder group in QoLT—healthcare providers. For practical and cost-related reasons, a convenience sample of 107 University of Pittsburgh Medical Center providers who were attending a conference on technology and aging in Pittsburgh completed the paper and pencil survey. This was clearly not a representative sample and, in fact, by attending the conference these healthcare providers showed an interest in technology. However, given the exploratory nature of the topic—perceived trustworthiness and usefulness of data from nontechnology and technology sources—we thought it would still provide valuable preliminary information. Many of the QoLT systems under development at the ERC will ultimately involve the provision of data (e.g., vital signs, behavior patterns, and sleep patterns) to healthcare providers. A key question is whether providers will actually find the data generated by technology to be trustworthy and ultimately useful to clinical practice. The survey items asked about trustworthiness of data generated from both nontechnology (PCP, specialists, home health facilities, patients and families, etc.) and technology (telehealth monitors, wearable monitors, environmental monitors, and other monitors) sources.

The major finding of the survey was that the providers reported high levels of trustworthiness of data from technology, particularly wearable monitors. In fact, data from the technology sources were seen as more trustworthy than data from home health agencies, nursing homes, patients and family, and community health screenings, which were seen as least trustworthy. While technology sources as a whole were seen as less trustworthy than PCP's and specialists, wearable monitors were seen to be as trustworthy as these expert sources. Finally, actual experience with the various types of technology was not related to perceived trustworthiness. While the results need to be viewed with some caution given the potentially technology-savvy convenience sample of providers, they are encouraging for QoLT designers.

More recently, we have begun to incorporate a combination of rich visual stimuli and nationally representative web panels to assess attitudes and preferences for QoLT. The first of these surveys (Survey 5, Table 4.1) used a combination of traditional written scenarios and video stimuli to depict QoLT systems for 400 baby boomers and 100 older adults. We used the Knowledge Networks *Knowledge Panel*, a web panel recruited using probability sampling that provides noncomputer households with laptops and an Internet connection to complete surveys (also used in the *Healthy@Home* survey described earlier). The written scenarios described kitchen, personal care, and safe driving QoLT applications that would perform varying levels of assistance (monitor behavior and share with doctor, provide individual feedback, provide coaching and advice, and help perform tasks; see Table 4.1). The videos depicted (1) robots providing bathing assistance (comparing "hard" mechanical versus "soft, balloon" skin robots showed in random order), and (2) a "virtual valet" system which allows the human driver to get out of the vehicle and guide the technology with a hand-held device to park the car in "tight spots." The written scenarios were presented first, the robot bathing videos second, and the "virtual valet" video last. Outcome measures included general comfort with the technology, safety and privacy concerns, preferences for human versus technology assistance and control, perceived likelihood of needing help with the task in the future, and willingness to pay out of pocket for the technology. One of our key hypotheses driving this work is that rich visual depictions of QoLT should result in more valid survey responding than hypothetical written scenarios. Thus, we were particularly interested in comparing responses to written versus video stimuli.

Some of the key findings included moderate levels of comfort with the technologies, but also moderate to high safety and privacy concerns. These perceptions varied by type of technology (kitchen, personal care, and driving) and intensity of help provided by the technology. There were also moderately strong preferences for human assistance and individual control over technology, and generally low willingness to pay out of pocket for QoLT. Respondents were also likely to perceive a fairly low likelihood of ever needing assistance with the various tasks. The "virtual valet" self-parking system video raised challenges regarding trust, accuracy, and safety relative to a human valet. Reactions to the robot bathing videos were generally quite negative, and this did not vary by the "hard" mechanical versus "soft, balloon" skin. In fact, the responses to these videos were more negative than those to the written scenarios depicting personal care technology across all outcome measurement domains. For example, Figure 4.4 shows preference for human assistance versus technology assistance in response to the written scenario depicting personal care technology and the two robot bathing videos. Whereas nearly half of the sample showed either preference for technology (21%) or "no preference" (26%) in response to the written scenario, only 11% and 9% showed a preference for technology and 13% had no preference after viewing the robot bathing videos. After viewing the robot bathing videos, over three-fourths of the sample preferred human assistance versus only slightly more than half in response to the written scenario. It should be noted that the written and video depictions were by no means directly comparable—the written scenario about personal care mentioned "things like getting in and out of bed, dressing, and toileting" and not bathing per se. Nonetheless, the results are interesting, and the survey shows the potential value of using rich stimuli to depict QoLT systems to large, representative samples.

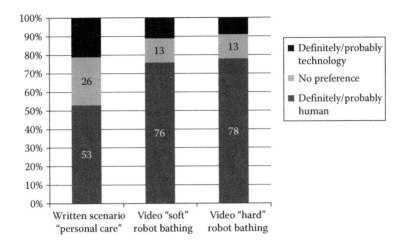

FIGURE 4.4
Percent middle-aged and older respondents preferring human versus technology assistance with personal care and bathing for written scenario and video depictions of technology.

The last survey shown in Table 4.1 also involved the use of video stimuli in a large, representative sample, again using the Knowledge Networks *Knowledge Panel*. The survey made use of the Time Sharing Experiments for the Social Sciences (TESS) program which allows researchers—selected via peer review—to add survey items to large, ongoing panel surveys at no cost. This survey illustrates another potentially useful method for gauging attitudes and preferences for QoLT—the use of a combination of randomized experiments and large probability sample surveys. The survey was designed to assess the acceptability of varying levels of video "masking" or "anonymization" in the context of falls monitoring. In this survey, 1800 baby boomers and older adults were randomly assigned to see one of four videos capturing an older adult reaching for something in a cupboard and falling in a kitchen setting: (1) a full video version, (2) a "blurred" video version that preserved some context, (3) a context-free "stick figure" version, and (4) a "text-only/sensor" version (no picture, but text alerting to the fall). The key outcome was perceived invasion of privacy if this type of video data were to be shared, and we hypothesized that respondents would be more concerned with privacy invasion in the full motion condition than in the other three conditions. The privacy invasion question was asked relative to the video being taken in the bedroom, bathroom, and living room. Preliminary results suggest that in fact the full motion video is seen as more invasive than the context-free "stick figure" or the text-only/sensor versions. However, somewhat surprisingly, the "blurry" video that preserved context was seen as *more invasive* than the full video version. The data have only recently been collected, and follow-up analyses are being conducted to explore this finding in more depth.

In sum, the surveys conducted thus far by the QoLT ERC have utilized a variety of sampling and measurement strategies, each with their own strengths and weaknesses. Our primary challenge has been to obtain attitude and preference data for QoLT systems that do not yet fully exist. Our experiences, along with the surveys by other groups reviewed in Section 4.3 focusing on existing technologies, lead to some general recommendations for sampling and measurement when conducting QoLT surveys. These are presented in the last section of this chapter.

4.5 Summary Recommendations for QoLT Survey Methods

This chapter has reviewed issues and considerations for using survey methods to measure broad attitudes and preferences for QoLT. We provide an overview of survey methodology with a focus on sampling and measurement issues of particular relevance to QoLT, and reviews of other work as well as our own using surveys focused on technology and QoLT. We draw on this discussion to propose a few broad recommendations for conducting QoLT surveys.

First, QoLT design teams need to think carefully about the type(s) of technology that are the focus of the survey and use this to help define the both the target population and measurement strategy. For *technology that already exists* (e.g., computers and the Internet, home safety devices, and electronic medication reminders), a variety of populations (e.g., general population, older adults, disabled adults, and caregivers) are relevant. Existing technology also allows for a variety of measurement approaches, including verbal descriptions by telephone, written descriptions via paper or web, and visual presentation (e.g., pictures and video). *Hypothetical or futuristic technologies that do not yet fully exist* require more targeted sampling strategies—for example, baby boomers, disabled and/or older adults, assistive technology users, caregivers, and healthcare providers—to increase the likelihood that the respondent can imagine actually needing and using the technology. Measurement is also more challenging for nonexistent, futuristic QoLT. There are questions as to whether traditional written, text-based scenarios about hypothetical QoLT systems produce valid data. Thus, the use of rich visual stimuli in these surveys is encouraged where possible, as one of our recent surveys found fairly large differences in responses to video versus written scenarios for personal care technology.

With regard to sampling in QoLT surveys, while large probability samples are recommended, and have been used in numerous surveys as described in this chapter, they are not always feasible. Designers of QoLT surveys often need to make trade-offs between gaining access to the most relevant populations—for example, adults who have suffered a stroke, wheelchair users, and healthcare providers—and not having the resources or the opportunity to use pure probability sampling methods. The surveys described in this chapter have used such techniques as opt-in web panels, registries, and convenience samples. While these methods are reasonable and can certainly produce valuable data for QoLT design, researchers should be cautious in generalizing results from such samples.

On the measurement side, we have documented the challenges involved in collecting survey data on technology that does yet exist. Researchers conducting QoLT surveys must think very carefully about mode of administration (telephone, paper, web, and in-person) and, more importantly, how the technology is conveyed to the respondent. Written scenarios may work well with existing technology that is familiar to respondents, but visual stimuli may be required to obtain valid survey data for less familiar or nonexisting technology. Again, trade-offs may need to be made when attempting to access special populations who may only be contactable by certain modes (mail and telephone), thus requiring written or verbal descriptions of technology. We should note that pictures/photographs can be included in traditional paper surveys, and this should be considered.

In sum, when possible, designers of QoLT surveys should attempt to combine probability methods to obtain representative samples with measurement strategies complemented by rich visual stimuli such as pictures and video. We have begun to conduct such surveys using the Knowledge Networks *Knowledge Panel*. When such optimal designs are not feasible, QoLT survey designers should think carefully about the potential sampling and measurement trade-offs involved when interpreting their data. This will increase the likelihood that survey methods will be valuable in helping to inform the ultimate design of QoLT systems that are likely to positively impact quality of life.

References

Barrett, L.L. 2008a. Healthy@Home research report. AARP Foundation, Washington, DC.

Barrett, L.L. 2008b. *Older Adults' and Family Caregivers' Perceptions and Use of Technology to Maintain Independence: A Literature Review*. Washington, DC: AARP Foundation.

Beach, S.R., Schulz, R., Downs, J., Matthews, J., Barron, B., and Seelman, K. 2009a. Disability, age, and informational privacy attitudes in quality of life technology applications: Results from a national web survey. *ACM Transactions on Accessible Computing* 2, Article 5, 5:1–5:21.

Beach, S., Schulz, R., Downs, J. et al. 2009b. End-user perspectives on privacy and other trade-offs in acceptance of quality of life technologies. Paper presented at the *First International Symposium on Quality of Life Technology*, Pittsburgh, PA.

Beach, S., Schulz, R., Seelman, K., Cooper, R., and Teodorski, E. 2010. Trade-offs and tipping points in the acceptance of quality of life technologies: Results from a survey of manual and power wheelchair users. Paper presented at the *Second International Symposium on Quality of Life Technology*, Las Vegas, NV.

Blumberg, S.J. and Luke, J.V. 2011. Wireless substitution: Early release of estimates from the National Health Interview Survey, July–December 2010. National Center for Health Statistics. http://www.cdc.gov/nchs/nhis.htm (accessed October 15, 2011).

Czaja, S.J., Charness, N., Fisk, A.D. et al. 2006. Factors predicting the use of technology: Findings from the Center for Research on Aging and Technology Enhancement (CREATE). *Psychology and Aging* 21:333–352.

Groves, R.M., Fowler, Jr., F.J., Couper, M.P., Lepkowski, J.M., Singer, E., and Tourangeau, R. 2009. *Survey Methodology* (2nd edn.). Hoboken, NJ: John Wiley & Sons.

Helal, S., Mokhtari, M., and Abdulrazak, B. (eds.). 2008. *The Engineering Handbook of Smart Technology for Aging, Disability, and Independence*. Hoboken, NJ: John Wiley & Sons.

Matthews, J.T., Beach, S.R., Downs, J., Bruine de Bruin, W., Person-Mecca, L., and Schulz, R. 2010. Preferences and concerns for quality of life technology among older adults and persons with disabilities; National Survey results. *Technology and Disability* 22: 5–15.

National Alliance for Caregiving (NAC) and American Association of Retired Persons (AARP). 2009. *Caregiving in the U.S.* Bethesda, MD: NAC.

Pew Research Center. 2011. Who's online: Internet user demographics. http://pewinternet.org/Static-Pages/Trend-Data/Whos-Online.aspx (accessed on October 18, 2011).

United Healthcare and the National Alliance for Caregiving (NAC). January 2011. *e-Connected Family Caregiver: Bringing Caregiving into the 21st Century*. Bethesda, MD: NAC.

5

Design and Development Process*

Judith T. Matthews, Karen L. Courtney, and Annette DeVito Dabbs

CONTENTS

5.1 Introduction

Quality of life (QoL) technologies that meet the day-to-day needs of older adults and persons with disabilities must address complex challenges posed by aging, impairment, and the environmental context in which they are used. Potential beneficiaries vary widely in their capabilities, resources, and desire for novel devices and systems that may extend their capabilities, prevent or detect disease and disability, or enable remote or self-monitoring of health and function. Market forces and public policy undoubtedly

---

* Portions of this chapter appear in *Proceedings of the IEEE* (Schulz et al., in press).

influence the availability and adoption of QoL technologies, but perceptions of usability and usefulness are at least as important in light of the qualitative difference such innovation could make in daily life.

As noted in Chapter 2 on facilitators and barriers to uptake, QoL technologies that are unresponsive to a real-world need or considered too complex, intrusive, or stigmatizing are apt to be rejected or abandoned. While some technologies may be universally appealing and beneficial regardless of age or ability, people with chronic disorders stand to gain the most from these technologies. They are also the most vulnerable to injury or worsening of their conditions, should errors or failures occur. Indeed, poor design may not only decrease acceptance, it may also compromise safety and ultimately add to rather than reduce daily stress among users across the age and ability spectrum. Addressing these high stakes issues during the design and development process increases the likelihood that the resulting features and functions of QoL technologies will be safe, acceptable, and helpful.

Creativity and inspiration can lead to technological solutions independent of an identified need. However, a scientifically sound, needs-driven approach to the design and development of QoL technologies is essential to their success. Likewise, success depends upon developers understanding the unique capabilities and preferences of target users and the nature of tasks to be performed. From the initial needs assessment to the final evaluation of effectiveness, developers in multidisciplinary teams should repeatedly elicit input from the constellation of persons who are likely to be affected by the technology being developed.

In this chapter, we discuss various practical approaches to the design and development of QoL technologies, emphasizing involvement of potential end users (henceforth also referred to as users) early and often throughout the process. The concepts and methods presented are not geared to any particular technology, although exemplars are provided for clarity. Instead we provide background and describe strategies for developing any technological application intended to improve QoL by affecting health or functional ability. In addition to this emphasis on the user-centered design process, we offer an overview of important design guidelines to be considered during development of QoL technologies for older adults and persons with disabilities.

5.2 Moving from Need to Solution

The findings from the needs assessment process described in Chapter 4 provide the basis for design and development of QoL technologies. Users often suggest functionalities that would be advantageous and features that would be desirable. Conceptually, this information helps to identify the design space where innovation would be beneficial. The identified needs can further be used to identify the design space attributes described in the Preface, including (1) the functional domain targeted (physical, psychological, cognitive, sensory); (2) the type of support needed (compensatory, preventive and maintenance, or enhancing); (3) the extent of user involvement required (passive or interactive); and (4) the amount of system intelligence needed to be responsive to the user's abilities, needs, preferences, and environment. By employing the same framework to locate both needs and solutions, we can design technology to fit the target user, and later assess the fit between person and technology at both the individual and aggregate levels.

5.2.1 Example 1: Virtual Coaching for Home-Based Therapeutic Exercise

A virtual coach system that we are developing provides a case in point. Despite ample evidence that adherence to a home-based exercise program significantly reduces the pain, stiffness, and functional impairment associated with knee osteoarthritis, adherence to such regimens remains low. The result may be significant loss of gains achieved during a time-limited course of physical therapy. Though some individuals diligently engage in therapeutic exercise as prescribed at home, others perform their exercises incorrectly or not at all, with adherence waning over time (Pisters et al. 2010; Rejesky et al. 1997; Thomas et al. 2002). Physical therapists and other clinicians currently rely on self-report to learn whether and how well the exercises are being done. Individuals may refer to printed instructions when exercising at home, but they typically receive neither performance guidance nor real-time feedback in that setting.

To address these issues of mobility disability (functional domain), we are devising a virtual coach system for home use (maintenance or enhancement support). The system will rely on accelerometers applied to strategic locations on the body to detect the quality and quantity of therapeutic exercise as it is performed (Taylor et al. 2010). Based on its interpretation of this sensor information (system intelligence), the virtual coach system will offer real-time instruction, encouragement, and feedback to the user through visual and auditory prompts (interactive involvement) issued by an avatar displayed on a monitor screen.

5.2.2 Direct and Indirect Users

QoL technology users are more than just the individuals with identified health or functional needs. Users may also include stakeholders such as family caregivers, clinicians and other service providers, and third-party payers who interact directly or indirectly with the QoL system or device. For our virtual coach system, the person with knee osteoarthritis is the primary direct user. However, physical therapists and other health professionals who prescribe exercise or access electronic progress reports from remote locations are also considered users. So too are family members who encourage the person with knee osteoarthritis to use the system or help to set it up, apply the accelerometers, or interpret the instructions and feedback provided by the avatar. Agency administrators overseeing service delivery may be users as well. Though not interacting with the system for personal benefit, these latter stakeholders may aggregate health or functional outcome data at the institutional level to inform decisions regarding resource allocation for their clients.

5.3 Establishing Requirements

In the initial design of a QoL technology, it is important to establish the requirements that must be met by the solution. In a requirements analysis, both the designers and the users take an active role in a process of identification, refinement, modeling, and specification. That is, they engage in a process of recognizing the issue, evaluating and synthesizing the options, modeling a possible solution, and developing technical specifications. Involving an array of users at various points along the technology development trajectory strengthens the end-product.

The designers initiate this process by translating a user need into a requirement description of the desired capabilities of the QoL technology. At this point, the focus is on what the technology should provide, not on how the technology will do it. The influence of designers at this stage is critical, as users alone may gravitate toward descriptions of how a technology solution should perform rather than describe what it needs to accomplish. An overemphasis on how the solution is to be achieved will often unnecessarily limit generation of alternative solutions.

5.3.1 Example 2: Developing a Space Pen

While development of a "zero-gravity pen" in the early days of the space program may be an urban legend, it nicely illustrates the importance of distinguishing the *what* from the *how* in a requirements description. In this example, a description of a *what* requirement would be "an instrument that writes in a low- or no-gravity environment," whereas a *how* requirement description would be "a pen that writes on paper in a low- or no-gravity environment." The how requirement description would have eliminated an existing technology such as the pencil as a potential solution, as well as other solutions such as a wax slate with a clear plastic sheet and stylus (a common children's toy). While these alternative solutions might later prove to be undesirable for other reasons, it would be important not to discard potential solutions unintentionally through inadequate requirement descriptions at the outset.

5.3.2 Refining the Requirements

Once the basic requirements have been identified, they need to be further refined in terms of functional versus nonfunctional requirements. Functional requirements include the essential functions of the technology and the capacity to map real-world relationships between input and output as well as to define how to handle exceptional situations. In the aforementioned example, writing, or the making of a mark on a display, would be a functional requirement of the system. Nonfunctional requirements define the constraints within which the technology solution must work. For example, the technology may need to interface with legacy systems or use a particular communication protocol. For the writing instrument in space, an obvious constraint would be the low- or no-gravity environment in which it must function. Efforts to refine the requirements at this stage should be driven by what task the technology needs to perform rather than a desire to begin to limit alternative solutions.

5.4 Weighing Alternatives

After the requirements of the solution have been identified and refined, the design team must evaluate potential solutions for their adequacy in meeting the need. At this juncture, existing technologies may be identified and, if deemed inadequate, the feasibility of developing new QoL technology solutions must be considered. Existing technologies may suffice. Or they may meet the need with some modification, and thus provide an interim, if not permanent, solution. After reviewing potential solutions and assessing their feasibility, the design team will choose a solution to pursue.

Refinement of requirements for the writing instrument for the space program could have stipulated that it be capable of creating a permanent record, or it could have resulted in a further constraint that no instruments with sharp points or flammable materials be used. With these additional requirements, the alternative solutions of pencils or wax slates would no longer have been appropriate alternatives. In this case, the design team might conclude that development of a pen that would write in a low- or no-gravity environment is the ideal solution.

5.5 Modeling the Solution

Once a solution pathway has been determined, modeling is the next step in transforming the user need into a QoL technology design. Modeling is used to represent the various aspects of the QoL technology, including user interactions, data flow, and contextual function. Like the user-centered design process described later in this chapter, modeling is an interactive, iterative process between designers and users. In this stage, designers must ascertain what data or components are needed for the prescribed function. The flow of information and control between the user and the technology must be clearly described. Finally, the behavior of the system, or how it is expected to perform, needs to be described in detail using one of several different modeling conventions such as unified modeling language, or UML.

5.6 Documenting Specifications

The last step in moving from an identified user need to a testable QoL technology is specification of the technology solution, which consists of detailing function and performance, the interfaces and interactions among various elements of the technology, and the identified solution constraints. Because technology design and development are iterative processes, maintaining and updating this documentation is crucial for developing the project management plan and keeping the project within scope. These specifications provide the roadmap for the project. Transforming this specification roadmap to the final product requires careful consideration of the users throughout the development process. The principles of user-centered design can guide developers of QOL technologies through the development phase.

5.7 User-Centered Design

Human factors are critically important in the design of QoL technologies, as they influence how people interact with the systems and devices that result. The focus of human factors is on the physical, cognitive, sensory/perceptual, emotional, and communication capabilities of individuals in relation to specific tasks they need to perform in particular environments (Stanton et al. 2005). Knowledge of human factors should inform interface design for all QoL technologies, with the aim of improving their safety, efficacy, and effectiveness.

The basic tenet of user-centered design is that intended users are the final arbiters of what works and what does not. Understanding users and their tasks, ascertaining the acceptability and usefulness of a novel technology during its design and development, and testing the technology with various stakeholders in a variety of environments are central principles of user-centered design. Application of these principles serves to improve ease of use, performance, reliability, and user satisfaction. By involving individuals who are directly or indirectly affected by a technology, designers and developers are more likely to produce a system or device that fits both the user and the task (Gould and Lewis 1985).

5.7.1 Principle 1: Focus Early on Users and Their Tasks

Assessing the characteristics of users, analyzing their tasks, and determining how they think a technology solution could assist them with task performance are key to ensuring correspondence among the users' abilities, the task requirements, and the features and functionalities of the technology (Goodhue and Thompson 1995). This knowledge helps to determine whether a technology is likely to modify or promote task performance. It also enables designers to be reasonably certain that the technology and user interface will be appropriate for the intended users.

Developers of QoL technologies have at their disposal a variety of established techniques to assess the characteristics and needs of intended users and stakeholders (see Table 5.1). Though a few of these techniques require accrual of large samples, many rely on small samples. Some characteristics such as age bracket, gender, and primary language are easy to ascertain by observation. Less obvious are characteristics such as health literacy, cognitive and physical ability, amount of experience with existing technologies, and idiosyncratic traits of the population of interest, which merit systematic investigation. As described in detail in Chapter 8, *epidemiologic studies* that estimate the prevalence of unique characteristics in the target population and *large-sample surveys* of intended direct users and other stakeholders, whether conducted in person, by phone, or via the web,

TABLE 5.1

Sample Techniques for Assessing Users and Tasks

Technique	Description
Epidemiologic studies and surveys	Data collection of user characteristics from larger samples, enabling generalization of the findings to the population of potential end users
Interviews	Individual interviews conducted with an actual or potential user, either in person or by phone to ascertain user characteristics (demographics, health and functional status, experience with computers and other technology, attitudes, preferences, and concerns about tasks or technologies)
Contextual inquiry	Observation of users performing tasks where they are usually performed (e.g., home, school, work) to reveal user characteristics, the nature of the task, and performance difficulties, and to identify ways that technology may support or enhance performance or permit evaluation of design features over time
Focus groups	Structured series of group discussions between a facilitator and actual or potential users in a nonthreatening environment to elicit their preferences and perceptions of needs and barriers to performing certain tasks or using technologies; interaction and exchange of ideas among group participants encourages richer data about tasks that are shared or performed jointly
Group-individual synthesis	To elicit user response to description or demonstration of a technology in development, based on one-on-one interviews, quick conferencing among interviewers, and final group discussion
Storyboarding	Presentation of initial concepts, rules, and assumptions about task performance and proposed technologies, using pictures and graphs to elicit reaction among potential users
Task analysis	Decomposition of a task in terms of the actions, processes, and capabilities required for safe performance, conducted to inform the design and functionality for a novel technology or to assess the person-technology fit for task performance
Think aloud	Process by which a user provides running commentary, giving voice to thoughts about processes, preferences, and barriers that come to mind while performing usual tasks prior to introduction of a novel technology
Workflow modeling	Synthesis of user task pattern and process data

are valuable sources of relevant information. *Market analyses* of adaptive products and services for older adults or persons with disabilities typically profile the pool of potential customers and examine trends that may influence market share. *Interviews* enable developers to learn what users think and feel about topics ranging from the difficult challenges of everyday life to the pros and cons of available solutions and what would motivate people to embrace QoL technologies.

These assessment techniques elucidate the diversity of attitudes, beliefs, and capabilities that should be taken into account in the design and development process. Such knowledge can also guide selection of potential users for consultation or periodic testing of the design solution. For instance, understanding potential users' hearing ability, visual acuity, cognitive function, and psychomotor skills would be important when designing a technology that relies on adequate hearing and vision, the ability to comprehend and retrieve information, manual dexterity, and eye–hand coordination to meet users' needs. The virtual coach system described earlier illustrates this point. During the design phase, we specified that the avatar providing auditory and visual feedback to the user and offering instruction about moving differently or adjusting the placement of sensors would have to accommodate the wide variation in hearing, vision, cognition, sensation, and dexterity prevalent among the largely middle-aged and older population affected by osteoarthritis of the knee.

An array of techniques also exists for assessing tasks (see Table 5.1). These are broadly defined in terms of the work or functions that a system or device is intended to support. Observing potential users actually performing a task enables designers to understand how their goals, interests, and learning styles may affect the use and effectiveness of a particular technology solution.

Contextual inquiry is one such method for understanding the nature and difficulty of tasks for given user groups. This ethnographic technique involves field observation and interviews with users as they perform tasks in their usual environment, offering insight into how people actually perform and structure the tasks and the capabilities required to perform them safely and efficiently. A useful example is provided by Forlizzi et al. (2004) whose contextual inquiry informed development of design guidelines for assistive robotic technologies in support of aging in place. By interviewing and observing 17 older adults in their own residences as they carried out selected daily activities, the investigators learned how these individuals—some well and others in declining health—experienced aging in relation to products (i.e., artifacts, services, environments) that were available in their own homes. The meaning (e.g., status, stigma) ascribed to various products and the extent to which aging had affected how accessible and useful they were revealed that older adults want and use products that support their personal identity, dignity, and independence, but they abandon those that do not.

Conducting *focus groups* with 6–12 participants is another way to explore the relevant needs, preferences, experiences, and opinions of a relatively homogeneous assembly of individuals who are familiar with the issues or tasks that a QoL technology might address. When a series of focus groups is conducted for a given project, it is possible to examine trends and patterns among the ideas and recommendations expressed. Focus groups, however, are not intended as consensus-building sessions, because attempts to build consensus can discourage expression of contrary views. Rather, focus groups are meant to elucidate the meanings and understandings participants attribute to health and illness (Basch 1987; O'Brien 1993; Wilkinson 1998) as well as their range of experiences and their opinions, including concordant and divergent views (Krueger and Casey 2000).

For instance, Courtney et al. (2008a) conducted focus groups to inform the design of smart home technologies that would support older adults' desire to remain safe and independent at home for as long as possible and receive assistance only as necessary. Eleven residents of two continuing care retirement communities participated in a series of four sessions during which their preferences and willingness to adopt these QoL technologies were explored. The investigators initially described how a suite of sensors embedded throughout the home could passively collect data that would permit inferences to be made about a resident's safety and activity. They discussed various types of sensors that could be used to detect, for example, the use of kitchen appliances or meal preparation, falls, nighttime wandering, and excessive trips to the bathroom. The investigators suggested that this type of passive monitoring could benefit residents by enabling earlier detection of accidents or declining functional abilities and thus facilitate timely intervention to prevent problems or summon assistance when needed.

Recurring themes among the older adults' responses included the perception that *others* (not *oneself*, regardless of serious health conditions or functional limitations) may benefit from smart home technologies, that family members' concerns are likely to positively influence willingness to accept smart home technologies, and that choice about which particular technologies to adopt is essential to preserving older adults' sense of autonomy. These findings were validated in individual semi-structured interviews with three additional residents, and they provided valuable insights that should inform product design, business models, and marketing plans.

Downs et al. (2010) suggest another technique, the *group-individual synthesis* approach, which blends interview and focus group techniques, to elicit input regarding users and their tasks during development of novel QoL technologies. We used this approach to explore stakeholders' views about the four families of engineered systems (Active Home, Virtual Coach, Safe Driving, and Mobility and Manipulation) comprising the applied foci of our Quality of Life Technology (QoLT) Center. The details of our findings are less relevant here than the technique used to achieve them.

For each family of engineered systems, we convened a diverse mix of stakeholders including persons with the potential to be direct beneficiaries of the technology presented, family caregivers, clinicians and social service providers, researchers, and industry partners, all of whom had a vested interest in preventing or mitigating pertinent physical or cognitive challenges posed by aging and disability. After the lead engineer presented a brief overview and illustrated or demonstrated one or two novel technologies in the conceptual or proof-of-concept stage of research and development, stakeholders were interviewed individually to learn their concerns and suggestions. To preserve the anonymity of individuals who might have been reticent about sharing their impressions and reactions in an open discussion with the group, we rapidly culled the responses for recurring themes, then summarized and shared them with the stakeholder group for clarification and validation of our interpretation. These sessions often reinforced what the developers had assumed about users' needs and capabilities. They also provoked helpful discussion of contrary views that challenged the developers' preconceived notions about who might accept, if not embrace, their inventions and what constituted a workable solution.

Storyboarding is yet another effective tool for introducing preliminary design concepts, eliciting potential end users' reactions to a proposed QoL system or device, and validating the concept. This technique can be used in conjunction with all of the preceding techniques, except for interviews administered by phone. Many people find it difficult to grasp in the abstract a proposed technological solution that does not yet exist, whether intended for themselves or others. Indeed, words are often of limited value for conveying what a technology might look like, how it would work, when it could be used, and where it might be stored. Showing images of what the developers have in mind, including alternative designs and scenarios, can help

Friend finder

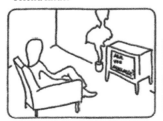 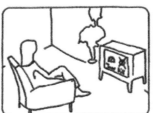 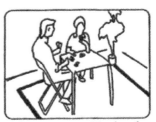

Mary's chair senses that she might be available for visitors and helps her post a message that she would like to play cards

Jane feels like socializing and notices that Mary is available to play cards

Jane goes over to Mary's and they play several games of cards

FIGURE 5.1
Sample storyboard sketches used to validate the SenseChair concept. (Used with permission courtesy of AIGA, www.aiga.org)

individuals to form a mental picture of the technology they are being asked to consider. This is the approach incorporated into "rich stimuli" survey research described in Chapter 4.

Illustrations including hand-drawn sketches, photos, and video animations can be presented to suggest how a QoL technology could be used by different people in different situations and environments (e.g., home, work, recreational or social settings). Beyond obtaining concept validation, designers often use storyboarding to identify additional requirements and constraints or correct flawed assumptions in their designs. Forlizzi et al. (2005) provide a sample illustration (see Figure 5.1) from a series of cartoon storyboards they presented to 10 older adults early in the design process for SenseChair, a robotic chair capable of sensing its occupant's position and movement and interacting with other household appliances to promote physical, social, and emotional health.

Task analysis, a technique from human factors engineering, entails deconstructing tasks into component subtasks and identifying the capabilities required to perform the components that the technology is intended to support (Crandall et al. 2006). Methods for *workflow modeling* and interpreting data derived from task analysis include hierarchical task analysis and affinity diagram building. The latter consists of sorting activities derived through task analysis into logical groups or categories, to guide decisions about how to support designated tasks. Hierarchical task analysis uses graphical flowcharts to depict the steps and sequence of required actions or behaviors involved in task performance. Designers and developers will find *Health Care Comes Home: The Human Factors* (National Research Council 2011) to be particularly instructive regarding application of these techniques to QoL technologies that facilitate completion of activities of daily living.

5.7.2 Principle 2: Measure Performance and Acceptability Empirically

Novel technology should be measured in terms of its performance and acceptability, that is, whether the technology supports tasks as intended and how useful users find it to be. Such usability testing requires evaluators to identify a priori the indicators and criteria that will be accepted as credible evidence of success for each stage of development. In addition to ascertaining users' views about the effectiveness and usefulness of a technology, designers typically assess several other factors. These include how easy or intuitive the system or device is to use initially or after a period of nonuse, how quickly tasks can be accomplished when using it, and how flexible it is to being used in various ways (see Table 5.2).

TABLE 5.2

Usability Factors and Empirical Measures

Factors	Definition	Objective Measures	Subjective Measures
Learnability	Ease with which use of device is learned so users can rapidly accomplish intended tasks	Clock time for new users to learn to accomplish the intended tasks	Users' ratings of the ease and time to learn the system
Effectiveness	Usefulness for supporting intended tasks	Successful performance of the intended tasks; measures of productivity	Users' ratings of the system's ability to promote their performance and productivity
Efficiency	Productivity once users have learned the system	Clock time to accomplish the tasks once users have learned the system	Users' ratings of the system's ability to improve the speed at which they perform
Errors	Frequency and severity of errors and ease of recovery from errors	Error rates trying to use system; severity of errors; recovery time for errors	Users' ratings of the impact of errors on using system and their ability to recover from errors
Flexibility	Variety of ways to achieve intended tasks	Number of different commands or routes to achieve the same goal	Users' ratings of system's ability to provide different commands or routes to achieve the same goal
Memorability	Ease with which casual users can return to the system without having to relearn	Memory failure rate on how to use system the next time; time to relearn the system after periods of nonuse	Users' ratings of the ability to remember how to use the system the next time and their ability to relearn the system after periods of nonuse
Satisfaction	Judgments about usability, aesthetics, acceptability, and pleasure derived from use	Frequency and duration of interaction with the system	Users' ratings of satisfaction with systems, user interfaces, and user interaction

Source: Nielsen, J., *Usability Engineering*, Academic Press, San Diego, CA, 1993; Guillemette, R.A., *The Evaluation of Usability in Interactive Information Systems*, Ablex Publishing, Norwood, NJ, 1995; Lindgaard, G., *Usability Testing and System Evaluation: A Guide for Designing Useful Computer Systems*, Chapman and Hall, London, U.K., 1994; Reed, S., *PC Comput.*, 5, 220, 1992; adapted from DeVito Dabbs et al., *Clin. Transplant.*, 23, 537, 2009.

Designers may also elicit users' assessments of how safe and secure they feel when using a system or device, how confident they are in its capacity to function as intended, and how concerned they are about attractiveness, obtrusiveness, and cost.

Conducting empirical testing at every stage involves using measures and techniques that are appropriate to the features and functionalities of interest. Typically, multiple sources of data are collected including observations, audio and/or video recordings, screen capture, and "think aloud" narratives that reflect test users' running commentary of their thoughts as they interact with a novel technology. Data from these various sources are then triangulated to determine usability successes and failures, which then inform modification of the technology over time. Decisions about future refinement are further influenced by practical considerations such as resource availability and feasibility.

Though initial usability testing may be conducted as a simulation or in a laboratory setting, the ultimate test of usability occurs under actual conditions or in settings in which users typically perform their tasks. It is noteworthy that indicators and criteria may differ among team members at the same stage. For instance, engineers may consider a technology to be performing adequately when its hardware and software perform flawlessly during usability testing in a laboratory environment. In contrast, clinicians may consider the technology successful only after it functions without errors when deployed in far less predictable residential and clinical environments.

5.7.3 Principle 3: Design and Test the Technology in an Iterative and Integrative Manner

Usability engineering refers to activities that are performed early and continued throughout development to ensure that all aspects of a technology work optimally to meet their users' needs. Iterative design is consistently rated as the most important determinant of design usability (Nielsen 1992). Considerable improvements can be achieved after the first iteration; additional usability issues appear in repeated tests after early, blatant problems have been resolved. The benefits of iteration and integration, in which all aspects of the user-centered design process are performed in a concurrent and coordinated manner, are indisputable. It should be noted, however, that particular attributes of usability will vary depending on the degree of user interaction possible at a given stage in the design and development process. In general, QoL technologies should be easy to learn to use, efficient with a low error or crash rate, and considered useful for accomplishing tasks.

5.8 Designing for Older Adults and Persons with Disabilities

Attention to human factors is particularly important when designing for aging and disabled individuals who stand to reap the most benefit from technologies that enhance their safety, independence, and QoL. Considerable variation exists in the manifestation of age-related changes and functional disability across these populations, as described in Chapter 3. Nevertheless, adherence to guidelines that address the most common age-related changes and prevalent impairments, regardless of age, provides reasonable assurance of usability for a large proportion of intended users.

Universal design, with its essential focus on products and environments that are usable regardless of whether or not people have limitations (Ostroff 2001), is a paradigm applicable to the design of QoL technologies in general, as discussed at length in Chapter 6. Fisk et al. (2009) provide excellent guidance for designing technology for older adults in particular. For people with functional limitations, Vanderheiden (2006, 2007, 2008) offers excellent recommendations as well. Detailed discussion of these guidelines and recommendations is beyond the scope of this book, though key elements warrant brief mention here. Whether a QoL system or device has a visual, audible, or haptic interface or is invisibly embedded in the environment, consideration must be given to the form and features of the technology itself as well as its effect on the user's surroundings.

5.8.1 Visual Presentation

As noted in Chapter 2, declining visual ability is a fundamental marker of aging. To accommodate changes in visual perception that accompany aging, illumination should be increased, glare and glossy surfaces should be avoided, and light sources should be adjustable. Using several light sources that are low in intensity is preferable to having a single, high-intensity light source. Text presented on paper or electronically should contrast well with the background color; white on black or black on white is best. Fonts that are 12 points in height or higher and unembellished (serif or san serif) are easier to read. Older adults find two-dimensional displays easier to view than three-dimensional ones, suggesting that novel virtual reality applications may be problematic for this population.

For persons of any age who are blind or have limited vision, cues to enable independent functioning should be as unobtrusive as possible and issued through portable, wearable, or permanently installed QoL technologies that signal hazards (e.g., dangerous terrain, traffic, intruders) or describe other important features of their surroundings. These technologies should use enhanced images, sound, or vibration, among other sensory indicators, to help individuals understand, interpret, and interact with their personal environments. Doing so would permit them to accomplish practical, everyday tasks such as locating and using household tools and appliances, thermostats, and security systems; accessing printed materials including instructions; and administering injectable medications or complex treatments. Among the unobtrusive designs in development are on-demand assistants that can project enlarged images onto walls or other surfaces or deliver verbal messages via ear bud.

5.8.2 Auditory and Haptic Presentation

Age-related changes in hearing point to the need for auditory interfaces that permit adjustment of sound levels. Frequencies above 4000 Hz are difficult for many to hear, and auditory alerts for warnings should reside within the 500–2000 Hz range and have a minimum intensity of 60 dB. Since hearing capability varies widely among older adults, auditory information should ideally be provided through other sensory channels such as visual images or vibration. Background noise and reverberation from conversation, music, or video should be kept to a minimum, with headphones and sound-dampening materials used to mitigate these environmental distractions. Lengthening natural pauses and slowing the rate of speech or other sounds (e.g., to signal a warning) facilitates comprehension. For vocal utterances, older adults prefer male voices when announcements are made and female voices to capture attention. When interfaces rely on users' tactile sensation, vibration should be issued at low frequencies (e.g., 25 Hz) to the upper rather than the lower body (e.g., to the face, lips, and fingers rather than the back, trunk, and feet), since sensitivity differs by site.

As with visual impairment, persons who are deaf or hearing impaired benefit from signals provided by QoL technologies through alternate or amplified sensory inputs. Unobtrusiveness is important to minimize the stigma that may be attached to the impairment or the technology associated with it, and to the emotional distress and social isolation that may result. Technologies that can isolate and interpret desired sounds (e.g., conversation with an individual, alarms) by separating them from background noise generated by other people or objects are very important. So too are technologies for omnidirectional detection and translation of sounds from sources beyond face-to-face earshot (e.g., when supervising children or for enhanced safety at work and while driving).

5.8.3 Input and Output

There are many ways for people to indicate their intentions or specify what they want a QoL technology to do (input). On/off buttons, point-and-click devices, and voice-activation or motion detection are among the most common mechanisms for entering input. Older adults who are novice computer users find a trackball easier than a mouse for double-clicking; using a stylus or touch screen tends to be even easier. Experienced older adults, on the other hand, are more likely to be adept at using a mouse and keyboard, particularly with larger monitors (20+ in.). Novice or experienced, older adults prefer CRT screens to LCD displays.

Speech recognition software and voice activated technologies are particularly helpful for individuals with severely limited manual dexterity who struggle to use a mouse, joystick, or touch screen. For some, large, clearly marked keypads work well, and redundant signals (e.g., text and sounds issued when a button is pressed on a remote control device) help to provide confirmation that an input message has been received by the system or device. When tremor results in unintentional delivery of multiple inputs on a touch screen, using the keypad arrows or a stylus with a built-up handle may work better.

An array of methods also exists for users to receive feedback (output) from a system or device. As with all visual display, contrast between characters and background should be high, and glare should be kept to a minimum. Changing settings for brightness, contrast, and color should be intuitive and easy. Visual warning signals should flash rather than be static, and vibration can be used to provide alerts in noisy settings.

The types of disabilities that affect people of all ages are essentially limitless, and in some situations design of input and output mechanisms may need to be tailored to individuals' unique capabilities. In addition to designing for simplicity and intuitive use to accommodate sensoriperceptual and motor deficits, designers should keep in mind the cognitive capabilities that typify their intended users. Cognitive impairment may take many forms, from lapses in memory and computational skill to spatial disorientation and wayfinding difficulty. Many assistive technologies are, in effect, ignorant of their users and thus cannot anticipate needs or modify their response in terms of functionality. QoL technologies, on the other hand, increasingly rely on intelligent interpretation of their users' behaviors, and therefore hold promise for being able to operate in a context-aware and context-responsive manner. This suggests that designers need to develop options for multiple, often redundant, input and output features to permit "on the fly" presentation of alternatives when a user has difficulty interacting with the default input or output features.

5.8.4 Interface Design

Several general guidelines figure prominently when designing interfaces through which older adults and persons with disabilities interact with QoL technologies. Simplicity and logical organization are of paramount importance, which means that the visual, auditory, and haptic input and output should be uncluttered, cognitive overload should be avoided, and the sequence of required actions should be intuitive. Permitting users to tailor various features (e.g., text size, sound quality, intensity of vibration) to their capabilities is essential, as is making sure that settings can be modified to allow ample time for inputting information and receiving or responding to feedback. Consistent formats for display of information such as step-by-step instructions, error messages, and confirmations indicating successful task completion are likewise important.

5.8.5 Training and Instruction

Helping older adults learn how to use QoL technologies involves strategies often employed across the age spectrum, regardless of level of ability. These include building skill and confidence by capitalizing on the user's prior knowledge or experience with similar features or functionalities, showing how the system or device works, and providing the opportunity to practice actual tasks in a setting that affords minimal distraction. The focus at the outset should be on essential information and tasks, so that learning is not impeded by extraneous explanations or noncritical features which can be presented after the basics have been mastered. Errors should be permitted, if it is safe to do so, but they should be corrected immediately with helpful feedback. Training sessions that are longer than 30–45 min should include 5–10 min breaks. Training materials, like training sessions, should be well organized, clearly labeled, and briefly presented without technical jargon.

5.8.6 Example 3: Designing a Multiuser Health Kiosk

We incorporated many of these design elements into a multiuser health kiosk developed through our QoLT Center specifically for the subpopulation of community-residing older adults with little or no Internet access and typically limited income. This project was prompted by evidence that timely self-monitoring of various health parameters can improve personal habits and yield better outcomes in terms of symptom management and disease control (see Chapter 11). It was also motivated by the lack of viable commercial products that met our design requirements and constraints. An earlier preliminary study that we conducted with a commercially available, multiuser health kiosk, one of few on the market, revealed this product to be very costly and unreliable, difficult for some older adults to use, and not customizable (Courtney et al. 2008b). Table 5.3 illustrates the sometimes overlapping sequence of activities and major milestones for the series of studies subsumed under our Health Kiosk Project. The timeline begins with efforts to identify the need for the kiosk and ends with our current community-based usability testing.

During initial prototype development for our health kiosk, a description of the *what* requirement was "an extensible system to provide health maintenance support for both body and mind." A *how* requirement description might have been "a tablet computer with USB ports for peripheral measurement devices." This latter description would have eliminated other solutions such as a standard desktop computer with a standard monitor, a desktop computer with a touch screen monitor, or even a smartphone.

We had many functional requirements for this multiuser health kiosk, which had to (1) be usable by persons who were mobile with or without an assistive device such as a cane, walker, scooter, or wheelchair; (2) be portable for use and storage within a congregate residential setting or senior center; (3) operate where wireless Internet access was not always available; (4) measure and track parameters of physical, psychological, and cognitive function; (5) display longitudinal data capture and print reports; (6) limit users' access only to their own information; (7) allow for easy addition of different types of peripheral measurement devices; and (8) facilitate communication among users, health care providers, and a kiosk administrator. Nonfunctional requirements included the kiosk being capable of interfacing with legacy systems and using a particular communication protocol.

Further refinement of our requirements stipulated that the hardware components of the kiosk had to be commercially available (for easy replication), and no keyboard or mouse interface could be used due to concerns about computer-naïve users. With these additional requirements, the alternative solutions of phones or desktop computers with standard monitors were no longer appropriate alternatives. Given the requirements and design constraints, our team concluded that development of a kiosk based on a desktop computer with a touch screen interface with cellular network internet access was the ideal solution.

The resulting multiuser health kiosk, now in its third iteration (see Figure 5.2), has been built to be Americans with Disabilities Act (ADA)-compliant. It consists of a desk-sized platform that can be used from either of two sides. Below the desktop is a locked cabinet for a computer and an unlocked cabinet that contains a printer and supply of paper.

TABLE 5.3

Timeline of Health Kiosk Activities: Conceptualization through Usability Testing

Activity	2006	2007	2008	2009	2010	2011	2012
Need identified for multiuser kiosk for older adults to measure, track, and share health and functional information	■	■					
Input regarding system design and study methods obtained from clinicians and community agency administrators serving community-residing older adults		■	■			■	
Institutional Review Board approval obtained for human subjects research			■		■		
Pilot Study #1: Feasibility of wellness intervention using commercial telehealth kiosk; focus groups with staff and older adults pre/post-implementation		■	■				
Novel multiuser health kiosk conceptualized by clinicians, technology developers, and community partners				■			
Proof-of-concept by students in rapid prototyping course—Health Kiosk v1.0				■			
GUI and cabinet redesign by students—Health Kiosk v2.0				■	■		
Construction of kiosk by cabinet maker and integration of software and medical devices by staff programmer—Health Kiosk v3.0					■		
Pilot Study #2: Laboratory usability testing of Health Kiosk v3.0 with older adults						■	
Modification of kiosk based on findings of Pilot Study #2						■	
Pilot study #3: Community-based usability testing with older adults							■

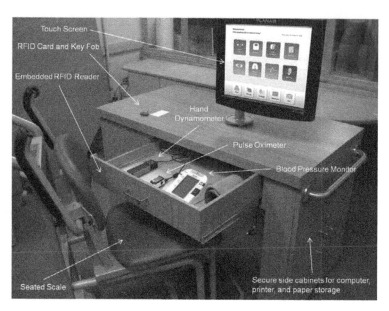

FIGURE 5.2
(See color insert.) Multiuser health kiosk.

A touch screen monitor mounted on the desk surface has a swivel base and hinged arm that make adjustment easy from either side. The desktop also has embedded speakers, and individual users are identified by passing an radio frequency identification (RFID) card or key fob over an RFID reader.

The two-way drawer, accessible from either side of the kiosk, contains various commercially available devices (e.g., pulse oximeter, blood pressure cuff, hand dynamometer) that enable automated measurement of physiologic and physical parameters such as peripheral oxygen saturation, pulse, blood pressure, and grip strength. The drawer also contains headphones that can be used to screen for hearing impairment or to limit exposure of the kiosk's audio output to the user alone, thus enhancing privacy or reducing distraction from ambient noise. A seated scale is situated on one side of the kiosk, and the opposite side provides access to the two-way drawer (and automated devices within) for individuals who use scooters or wheelchairs. All devices including the seated scale are integrated with the computer, and all measurements taken are automatically entered into a secure database.

The graphical user interface on the touch screen monitor provides guidance for obtaining physiologic and physical measurements (e.g., blood pressure, grip strength) as well as text-based, self-report measures pertaining to health and functional ability (e.g., symptoms, mood, appetite, energy level, preventive health practices, exercise, physical and functional status). Users can view and print summary reports of their measurements as well as graphs that depict secular trends. Another feature is the kiosk's messaging function which permits communication between the user and the kiosk administrator or designated primary health care providers with whom threshold values (e.g., within normal range versus out of normal range) can be set, brief reports may be shared, and queries and responses can be exchanged. Several standard psychosocial measures have been adapted for display and delivery on the kiosk, including the Falls Efficacy Scale

(Tinetti et al. 1990), Pittsburgh Sleep Quality Index (Buysse et al. 1989), the Morisky 4-Item Self-Report Measure of Medication-Taking Behavior (MMAS-4) (Morisky et al. 1986), and Cost-Related Nonadherence items (CRN-2) (Soumerai et al. 2006), among others.

The health kiosk targets multiple domains (physical, psychological, cognitive, sensory) in support of older adults' health and functional needs by providing support that may be compensatory, disease preventing, or health maintaining or enhancing. It is a decidedly interactive QoL technology that at present records the various measurements obtained, but it has been developed with the capacity to learn patterns of use, monitor trends across parameters, suggest changes in threshold values or measurement frequencies, and provide instruction and feedback, all directed toward improving self-management.

Initial usability testing conducted in a laboratory setting with seven older adults recruited from two community partners affiliated with our QoLT Center—an in-home service provider for frail older adults and a retirees' service organization—revealed fixable shortcomings of the kiosk's hardware and software. These included an overly sensitive touch screen, visual displays that were difficult for some individuals to read or not intuitive to use, and verbal instructions that were either ambiguous or inadequately illustrated. Based on these findings, we revised the health kiosk's design to address the identified shortcomings.

Community-based usability testing is currently underway with 40 adults age 65 and older who live independently and are being recruited from four sites that offer socioeconomic and racial diversity: a senior center, a suburban continuing care retirement community, and two congregate housing communities in an urban and rural setting, respectively. Our field observations during usability testing with the first 19 study participants enrolled to date suggest that older adults find the kiosk fairly intuitive to use. They value its capacity to help measure and track information about their day-to-day health and functioning between medical encounters, for sharing with health care providers, and they think that older adults would use the kiosk.

To eliminate errors that occur when people either do not realize they have advanced to a new screen or skip past a screen due to tapping a "Next" button more than once, we continue to make adjustments to the sensitivity of the touch screen and to modify the screen display by varying the background color so that users can more easily discern when they have advanced from one screen to the next. We are in the process of adding audio instructions, relocating the chair scale to the right side of kiosk, and replacing it with a wheeled, adjustable height chair that faces the drawer and touch screen. This latter change is being made to accommodate very tall or overweight individuals whose legs do not fit comfortably under the desk kneehole, especially when they rest their feet on the foot platform while weighing themselves.

During upcoming usability testing sessions, we plan to evaluate whether drawer access is still needed from both sides of the kiosk, since wheelchair users may be able to use the kiosk on the same side as nonwheelchair users if the adjustable chair can be rolled out of the way. We anticipate that systematic analysis of the complete set of qualitative and quantitative data will yield more nuanced evidence of the usability of this QoL technology among the total sample as well as the subsamples from each of the four sites. Our next step will be a pilot feasibility intervention study aimed at learning whether older adults will use the health kiosk over time to set personal health and functional goals, enhance health and functional behaviors, and improve health care utilization or health and functional outcomes.

5.9 Conclusion

Successful design and development of QOL technologies require a clear understanding of the challenges posed by aging and disability. The enterprise also calls for careful consideration of the varied environments in which these challenges occur and the ability to anticipate the impact that resulting systems and devices may have on the people, services, and organizations involved. Willingness of designers and developers to engage potential users in meaningful collaboration throughout the process is as essential as this knowledge in combination with creativity and technical know-how.

Moving from an identified need to one or more viable solutions that can actually enhance independence and QoL among intended users should proceed in deliberate fashion. Though there is room for serendipitous discovery along the way, the path to solution should be carefully mapped, not haphazard, to ensure firm grounding in the nature of the challenge and contextual aspects of the design problem. This is especially important because designers and developers often dwell in very different life spaces from those whose needs they are addressing. With little or no experience in the realms of aging and disability—a fact for some, not a fault—engineers and computer scientists, among others, may be unrealistic in the assumptions they make and the solutions they propose. Perhaps most difficult is the frequent stipulation that QoL technologies be inexpensive, easy-to-use, and customizable in order to accommodate the heterogeneity that exists among people whose circumstances vary so widely in terms of capabilities and infirmities, living arrangements, social support, and financial resources.

Ensuring extensive user involvement throughout the design and development process is crucial because it affords the opportunity to see and hear firsthand what matters to the intended users, what would be considered useful and helpful, and what might actually work in relevant settings. The first step is identification of both direct and indirect potential users. As users' needs are understood and documented, the solution can be tailored by incorporating design elements that take into account their characteristics and capabilities as well as their preferences and concerns. This user-centered—rather than designer-centered—approach serves to strengthen the fit between tasks and QoL technologies for the people who will use them and the environments in which they will be used, and it provides a strong foundation for subsequent rigorous evaluation.

References

Basch, C. E. 1987. Focus group interview: An underutilized research technique for improving theory and practice in health education. *Health Educ Behav* 14:411–448.

Buysse, D. J., C. F. Reynolds III, T. H. Monk, S. R. Berman, and D. J. Kupfer. 1989. The Pittsburgh Sleep Quality Index: A new instrument for psychiatric practice and research. *J Psychiatr Res* 28:193–213.

Courtney, K. L., G. Demiris, M. Rantz, and M. Skubic. 2008a. Needing smart home technologies: The perspectives of older adults in continuing care retirement communities. *Inform Prim Care* 16:195–201.

Courtney, K. L., J. H. Lingler, E. Olshansky, and L. A. Garlock. 2008b. Community-based telehealth kiosks: First impressions. *AMIA Annu Symp Proc* :916.

Crandall, B., G. Klein, and R. R. Hoffman. 2006. *Working Minds: A Practitioner's Guide to Cognitive Task Analysis*. Cambridge, MA: MIT Press.

DeVito Dabbs, A. J., M. A. Dew, B. Myers et al. 2009. Evaluation of a hand-held, computer-based intervention to promote early self-care behaviors after lung transplant. *Clin Transplant* 23:537–545.

Downs, J. S., R. Schulz, S. Beach et al. 2010. Group-individual synthesis: A novel approach to garnering stakeholder input for engineered systems. Unpublished manuscript.

Fisk, A. D., W. A. Rogers, N. Charness, S. J. Czaja, and J. Sharit. 2009. *Designing for Older Adults: Principles and Creative Human Factors Approaches*, 2nd edn. Boca Raton, FL: Taylor & Francis Group.

Forlizzi, J., C. DiSalvo, and F. Gemperle. 2004. Assistive robotics and an ecology of elders living independently in their homes. *Hum Comput Interact* 19:25–59.

Forlizzi, J., C. DiSalvo, J. Zimmerman, B. Mutlu, and A. Hurst. 2005. The SenseChair: The lounge chair as an intelligent assistive device for elders. *Proc Conf Design User Experiences*, San Francisco, CA.

Goodhue, D. L. and R. L. Thompson. 1995. Task-technology fit and individual performance. *MIS Quart* 19:213–236.

Gould, J. D. and C. Lewis. 1985. Designing for usability: Key principles and what designers think. *Commun ACM* 2:300–311.

Guillemette, R. A. 1995. *The Evaluation of Usability in Interactive Information Systems*. Norwood, NJ: Ablex Publishing.

Krueger, R. A. and M. A. Casey. 2000. *Focus Groups: A Practical Guide for Applied Research*, 3rd edn. Thousand Oaks, CA: Sage Publications, Inc.

Lindgaard, G. 1994. *Usability Testing and System Evaluation: A Guide for Designing Useful Computer Systems*. London, U.K.: Chapman and Hall.

Morisky, D. E., L. W. Green, and D. M. Levine. 1986. Concurrent and predictive validity of a self-reported measure of medication adherence. *Med Care* 24:67–74.

National Research Council. 2011. *Health Care Comes Home: The Human Factors*. Committee on the Role of Human Factors in Home Health Care, Board on Human-Systems Integration. Division of Behavioral and Social Sciences and Education. Washington, DC: The National Academies Press.

Nielsen, J. 1992. The usability engineering life cycle. *IEEE Comput* 25:12–22.

Nielsen, J. 1993. *Usability Engineering*. San Diego, CA: Academic Press.

O'Brien, K. 1993. Using focus groups to develop health surveys: An example from research on social relationships and AIDS-preventive behavior. *Health Educ Q* 20:361–372.

Ostroff, E. 2001. Universal design: An evolving paradigm. In *Universal Design Handbook*, Eds. W. Preiser and E. Ostroff, pp. 1.3–1.11. New York: McGraw-Hill.

Pisters, M. F., C. Veenhof, F. G. Schellevis, J. W. R. Twisk, J. Dekker, and D. H. DeBakker. 2010. Exercise adherence improving long-term patient outcome in patients with osteoarthritis of the hip and/or knee. *Arthritis Care Res* 62:1087–1094.

Reed, S. 1992. Who defines usability? You do! *PC Comput* 5:220–232.

Rejesky, W. J., R. B. Lawrence, W. Ettinger et al. 1997. Compliance to exercise therapy in older participants with knee osteoarthritis: Implications for treating disability. *Med Sci Sports Exerc* 29:977–986.

Schulz, R., S. R. Beach, J. T. Matthews et al. In press. Designing and evaluating quality of life technologies: An interdisciplinary approach. *Proc IEEE*.

Soumerai, S. B., M. Pierre-Jacques, F. Zhang et al. 2006. Cost-related medication nonadherence among elderly and disabled Medicare beneficiaries: A national survey 1 year before the Medicare drug benefit. *Arch Intern Med* 166:1829–1835.

Stanton, N., P. Salmon, G. Walker, C. Baber, and D. Jenkins. 2005. *Human Factors Methods: A Practical Guide for Engineering and Design*. Aldershot, U.K.: Ashgate Publishing.

Taylor, P. E., G. J. M. Almeida, T. Kanade, and J. K. Hodgins. 2010. Classifying human motion quality for knee osteoarthritis using accelerometers. *Conf Proc IEEE Eng Med Biol Soc* 2010:339–343.

Thomas, K. S., K. R. Muir, M. Doherty, A. C. Jones, S. C. O'Reilly, and E. J. Bassey. 2002. Home based exercise programme for knee pain and knee osteoarthritis: Randomised controlled trial. *Br Med J* 325:752–756.

Tinetti, M. E., D. Richman, and L. Powell. 1990. Falls efficacy as a measure of fear of falling. *J Gerontol* 45:P239–P243.

Vanderheiden, G. C. 2006. Design for people with functional limitations. In *Handbook of Human Factors and Ergonomics*, 3rd edn., Ed. G. Salvendy, pp. 1387–1417. New York: John Wiley & Sons.

Vanderheiden, G. C. 2007. Redefining assistive technology, accessibility and disability based on recent technical advances. *J Technol Hum Serv* 25:147–158.

Vanderheiden, G. C. 2008. Ubiquitous accessibility, common technology core, and micro assistive technology. *ACM Trans Access Comput* 1, Article 10. http://dl.acm.org/citation.cfm?doid=1408760.1408764 (accessed October 27, 2011).

Wilkinson, S. 1998. Focus groups in health research: Exploring meanings of health and illness. *J Health Psychol* 3:329–348.

6

Universal Design for Quality of Life Technologies

Edward Steinfeld and Roger O. Smith

CONTENTS

6.1 What Is Universal Design?

Universal design is a set of practices that can help ensure development of effective quality of life technologies (QoLTs). The most common definition of universal design is "The design of products and environments to be usable by all people, to the greatest extent possible, without the need for adaptation or specialized design" [1]. This definition emerged from experience with barrier-free or accessible design. It became obvious that many accessibility features, like curb cuts or lever-handled door openers, benefit a much wider group of people than only people with disabilities. Early advocates argue that, in a diverse society, a broader understanding of end user populations is needed to reduce the need for specialized products, environments, and services. It should be noted that terminology such as "inclusive design," "design for all," or "transgenerational design" are sometimes used to address the same goals.

Despite the wide adoption of the aforementioned definition, concepts are maturing and new definitions are evolving. Over the past decade, a host of expanded universal design applications have emerged. Social participation, in particular, is being addressed more explicitly as a design outcome. This acknowledges that designing products to be usable by a broader population is not sufficient to ensure an improved quality of life for those who use them. If a product makes an individual feel or look awkward when using it, a consumer will avoid it, even if it is free of barriers to usability. Thus, the emotional response to a product, including the perception of stigma, is very important as well as usability.

Health and wellness goals, including safety, health promotion, and protection from exposure to environmental threats like toxic chemicals or pollution, are also being identified as part of universal design practice. Design for health and wellness leads to reduction in disability and, thus, has become an essential part of universal design. This has been recently acknowledged in health care legislation with new efforts in the Food and Drug Administration (FDA) around accessible medical devices.

Universal design is also being expanded beyond products and environments in applications related to policy, services, and business practices. For example, universal design has become a major force in K-12 education and the concept is embedded in the federal legislative mandate for inclusive education. Communication systems like voicemail have included universal design attributes such as providing multilingual options. And some supermarkets provide electric shopping carts with seats for its customers who have difficulty walking.

As currently conceived, universal design is perceived to be an unrealistic immediate objective for some applications. Some argue that the current lack of design expertise, the need for affordability and fiscal planning and other constraints require a longer-term plan for implementation. In these cases, universal design can be implemented as a continuous quality improvement process, including the establishment of benchmarks and measurement of progress. The incorporation of design strategies that are not possible today can be anticipated in the future [2].

In 2011 and 2012, Steinfeld and Maisel [3] and Steinfeld and Seelman [4] offer a definition that explicitly addresses all these issues: "Universal design is a process that increases usability, safety, health, and social participation, through design and services that respond to the diversity of people and abilities."

Clearly, universal design is not the same as "accessible design" or "assistive technology (AT)." Although accessibility is definitely a part of universal design, meeting the needs of people with disabilities and eliminating discrimination against this group is not the only focus. Universal design both treats accessibility in a broader way, and also provides benefits for people with disabilities that exceed minimum legally mandated levels of accessibility wherever possible. Like accessibility, AT is focused on the needs of people with disabilities, providing special aids and equipment to compensate for limitations in function. Universal design, on the other hand, produces products that can be used by a wide range of end users and, whenever possible, reduces the need for AT. Thus, the broader idea of providing "enabling technologies" for everyone is incorporated in universal design practice.

The most widely known tool for the application of universal design that helped define its parameters is a document called the Principles of Universal Design [1]. Since their publication, the principles defined in this document have been tested while putting them into practice, resulting in some discovery about their limitations. To many, they do not adequately reflect the contemporary understanding of the concept, as embodied in the revised 2011–2012 definition mentioned earlier [5]. To address these limitations, Steinfeld and Maisel [3] propose eight "goals of universal design" that more effectively address the intent of the concept:

1. Body fit—accommodating a wide range of body sizes and abilities
2. Comfort—keeping demands within desirable limits of body function and perception
3. Awareness—insuring that critical information for use is easily perceived
4. Understanding—making methods of operation and use intuitive, clear, and unambiguous
5. Wellness—contributing to health promotion, avoidance of disease, and prevention of injury
6. Social integration—treating all groups with dignity and respect
7. Personalization—incorporating opportunities for choice and the expression of individual preferences
8. Appropriateness—respecting and reinforcing cultural values and the social and environmental context of any design project

While these goals use more general terms than the initial universal design principles, they are more useful for broader applications and with fewer restrictions. They are intended to establish and organize information for universal design practice because they correspond to specific bodies of knowledge, and provide a more effective framework for measuring the achievement of universal design goals because they explicitly address the social participation and wellness issues. As Steinfeld and Maisel illustrate, they are compatible with the principles and can be mapped on them easily [3].

Since the 1990s, when universal design was formally defined, it has become a pervasive interdisciplinary design methodology. Since then, the concepts, definition, and terminology have matured. However, the fundamental concepts of universal design still elude most of the engineering and design fields. Universal design has not manifested strongly in engineering design education or in practice. A more in-depth introduction to universal design is needed to understand its implications and contributions to the design of QoLT. Although product designers desire guidelines and criteria for practicing universal design, the rest of this article focuses on the process of universal design. Universal design is not a "rule-based" activity. The criteria used in any project are a function of the economic, cultural, and technological context in which a product may be used, which makes the development of guidelines much more complex than when defining minimum accessibility criteria. In fact, new methods for developing guidelines and standards must be devised to implement universal design in a manner true to its ideals. Thus, we focus here on the business case for universal design and the process of implementing it rather than on guidelines, although we will address the needs for improving the knowledge base for practice and identify current efforts to develop guidelines and standards.

6.2 Overall Importance

Why is universal design important? The most general answer is that, in a global culture, the need to address diversity is more significant than in the past. Three trends have contributed this need: the increasing cultural diversity of societies, the increasing obesity rate, and the aging of the population [3]. Intersecting these trends, the growth of civil rights movements, a greater understanding of the relationship between design and health, and advances in technology have increased awareness of universal design goals and opportunities for implementing them. In particular, information technology has increased the potential for the use of design to respond to diverse needs, even to the point of individual customization within the context of mass production (i.e., "mass customization").

A review of some beneficiaries of universal design helps to demonstrate the trends that are leading to increasing demand for universal design. The following list demonstrates that the target population is much broader than only people with disabilities and elders [3]:

1. People who have temporary and permanent limitations in function due to body shape or stature like pregnant women, children, and "outliers" (e.g., very short, very tall, very light, or very heavy people)

2. Caregivers who have people dependent on them including families with small children, families with disabled members, spouses of older individuals serving as informal caregivers, and professional caregivers like personal care attendants and even nannies

3. People with psychosocial conditions like autism, Alzheimer's, and chronic depression who encounter social barriers but also may have limitations in motor activities, perception, and cognition

4. People with behavioral and/or functional limitations due to alcohol and/or drug dependency (both legal or illegal) or medications that alter perception or cognition

5. Minority ethnic groups or foreign visitors with culturally based traditions, preferences, and expectations, including differences in language, diet, social interaction norms, and related spatial behaviors

6. Low- and even middle-income populations who often experience lack of access to services and resources due to economic restrictions in residential location and mobility

7. People who are displaced from culturally normal living environments and find themselves in temporary living situations or in vulnerable or exposed conditions due to extreme events such as political unrest, war, or natural disasters

8. Abused spouses, children, or homeless people who need secure environments with specialized services

To put the size of the beneficiary population into perspective, data from the U.S. Census for some of the beneficiary populations show that over 50 million people have some type of disability; about 90 million Americans are considered obese; almost 20 million people have very tall or very short stature and are pregnant at any time; about 85 million families have a member with a disability; and over 130 million people have a chronic disease and, therefore, are at risk of disability [3].

6.2.1 Need for Universal Design in the Development of Quality of Life Systems

The term "QoLT systems" implies that individuals need products that will resolve current or future challenges in their quality of life. A wide range of potential challenging life activities can be addressed by QoLT systems. The World Health Organization's International Classification of Function (ICF) [6] delineates hundreds of areas of life activity and role participation. These activities and roles require successful functional performance ranging from personal care activities such as brushing ones teeth, to social and community gatherings like going out to a movie, to recreational activities like playing baseball, to work activities like using a computer, and to social role activities like taking care of an infant. In the aggregate, experiences in these activities and roles define our quality of life.

Conversely, substantial challenges to any one of these life activities and roles detracts from our quality of life. Therefore, all products that people use and environments they live in have the potential to facilitate quality of life for any person. QoLT systems, however, do not presuppose certain types of impairments, health, or social conditions that define the challenge of one's quality of life. For example, being blind, having a reading disability, being a nonnative language speaker, dealing with schizophrenia, or having a chronic respiratory disorder can all severely erode a person's functional performance in activities, thus decreasing their quality of life. Income, educational level, race, ethnicity, and gender are also important considerations. Steinfeld and Maisel illustrate how social characteristics intersect with disability and health conditions to amplify the challenges caused by physical, sensory, and cognitive limitations [3].

Overall, the intent of universal design for QoLT systems is to ensure that anyone is able to benefit from a QoLT system regardless of their functional challenges. This inclusive design approach has a good fit with QoLT system research and development goals. Designing to meet the needs of people with a very wide range of challenges is clearly daunting. The complete listing of functional impairments related to disablement ranges from the hundreds in the ICF. To help manage the design objective attempts to categorize have condensed the set to 42 [7], to 13, or in its basic simplicity 6 [8] or 3 [9]. For simplicity, designs can accommodate three basic types of challenges, sensory, motor, and cognitive. Every product should be tested with populations of people who represent each of the three basic types of challenges, but the actual groups involved may vary, depending on the target population for a design.

For example, in a recent project to create a health kiosk for retirement living residences, a team assembled a convenient set of health measures in a single system. These included a blood pressure cuff, an oxygen sensor, a weight scale, and a computer monitor displaying the health-related data to the individual. When testing the design, it quickly became apparent that many users who lived in retirement centers had poor hearing and poor vision, wore bifocals, might use the kiosk in a wheelchair or use walkers or canes for balance, etc. A new design was required to increase the size of the screen font displayed, simplify the display information, provide audio output for visual information and visual information for audio output, include a seated weight scale, and redesign the entire system so that it was more aesthetically appealing and less medical in appearance. Essentially, this design iteration of a QoLT system was a call back to universal design. Universal design is an upfront strategy that evaluates and predicts individual differences. In this case, a costly round of iteration would have been avoided by using an a priori universal design approach. Note that many communities have senior residences that serve large concentrations of older people who emigrated to the United States late in life to join their immigrant children. They come from different cultural groups and speak languages like Spanish,

Russian, or Chinese rather than English. Thus, not only should differences related to cognitive challenges cause by stroke and dementia be addressed but also those related to culture and language.

6.2.2 Benefits of Universal Design

The lifespan perspective is a good shorthand approach to summarize the benefits of universal design for everyone. Universal design provides tangible benefits at every stage of the lifespan: support for safety, security, and developmental progress for children; enhancing social integration and independence for young adults; reducing stress for working-aged adults; and maintaining independence for elders. Universal design has significant economic benefits to society. It can support health-promoting behaviors, reducing the cost of health care and rehabilitation for society as a whole. It can reduce the risks of work-related injury; support employment of people with disabilities and continued employment of key older workers, which all have significant economic benefits for employers; and improve environmental quality in the community by attracting riders to public transportation, improving walkability and enhancing recreation opportunities. Participation benefits include enhancing friendship formation, reducing stigma and social isolation, and continued civic engagement for elders. Finally, at the highest level of human development, universal design provides support for realizing individual potential throughout the lifespan. Three examples of universal design demonstrate these benefits.

Example 1: A business improvement district (BID) in New York City determined that much of the street furniture in the city was poorly designed. They hired an industrial designer and did research with visitors and businesses to identify the unmet needs in their district (mid-Manhattan). Then they developed new designs and worked with the city to develop and install new street furniture that would solve the most critical they identified. One product they developed was an improved street sign. Their research identified that reading the conventional street signs was difficult and led to orientation and wayfinding problems. They developed a new sign with much larger street names, easier to read fonts, and integral illumination (Figure 6.1). The signs were large enough that they could be mounted much higher, making them visible from further away. Not only were the signs easier to read by people with limited vision, they also were much more visible in the confusing and overstimulated environment of midtown Manhattan, benefiting the entire population, including tourists, business visitors, public safety professionals, delivery staff, and others. Moreover, they are particularly beneficial at night, when all people have limitations in vision.

Example 2: Computer access for people with disabilities initially was originally achieved through AT. An array of special software was developed to enlarge screen fonts and windows, enhance contrast, convert text to speech, enable the use of special input devices like sip n'puff systems, adjust key input to accommodate poor coordination and reduced range of motion, etc. The add-in software programs were difficult to find, limited in compatibility, and required expert assistance to install and maintain. So, experts in adaptive computing, led by the Trace Center at the University of Wisconsin, worked with Apple, IBM, and Microsoft to develop out of the box accessibility solutions that could be incorporated into operating systems. Today, all major computer operating systems have a suite of universal accessibility options that allows individual users to adjust the computer input and output to accommodate their needs (Figure 6.2). Moreover, everyone now has access to these features. They prove very helpful in improving usability,

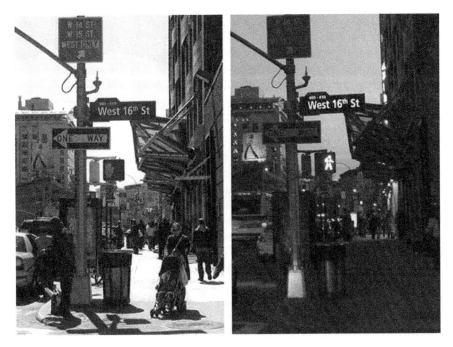

FIGURE 6.1
Enhanced street signs in Manhattan. (Courtesy of Marco Castro/Chelsea Improvement Company, New York.)

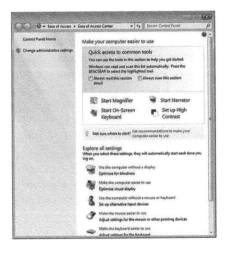

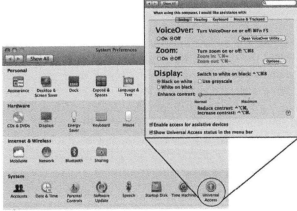

FIGURE 6.2
Accessibility options in Windows and Macintosh operating systems.

especially in situations where the work environment may put unusual demands on input and output tasks. But, most importantly, the integration of such systems increases the availability of adaptations to people with disabilities, reduces dependence on experts for assistance, improves integration into the workforce, and helps to improve productivity of older workers. All of these benefits are delivered at a lower cost as they are built in as a component of computer operating systems. And, they are updated continuously as the operating systems are updated.

Example 3: The mobile phone is an important enabling technology, especially the smartphone. Smartphones demonstrate the value of universal design on two levels. First, consider the general implications of a mobile telephone technology on human civilization. Professionals in the field of vision impairments estimate that more than 95% of people with visual impairments carry mobile phones. To this group, they can be compared to a "lifeline" due to the added security and connection they provide when they need assistance. People with mobility disabilities also obtain more security and safety by carrying mobile phones. Due to the availability of mobile phones, they can travel more independently and take more risks than in the past, knowing that if a car breaks down, an entrance is blocked, or they fall in a bathroom, they can summon assistance. People with hearing impairments are also heavy users of mobile phones because they can send text messages with them.

At one time, deaf people used text telephone (TTYs) to communicate but they only could communicate with other people who had TTYs. Today, the TTY is headed for extinction because mobile phones are so much cheaper, can be used to send anyone a message, and can be carried in a pocket or purse. Some deaf people even use texting to communicate in person with people who hear without the need of an interpreter, particularly for short transactions like making purchases in stores. But, mobile phones clearly provide universal benefits. For example, parents and children with mobile phones can always be in reach of one another; mobile phones enhance productivity by allowing members of work teams to communicate with each other wherever they are; and smartphones with real-time video improve social engagement of elders by allowing grandparents to watch their grandchildren do things in real time, like riding a bicycle for the first time. Low-income people can even benefit from the use of mobile phone technology. Purchasing a mobile phone eliminates activation fees whenever they move to a new residence, reduces monthly service charges through pay as you go plans, facilitates searching for employment and managing family affairs, and reduces dependency on unreliable public phones.

If the mobile phone has redundant visual, tactile, and voice interfaces, its usability is enhanced for everyone. Once, we needed separate systems for each of these interface types. Today, the smartphone is becoming a universal platform for all three interfaces. Furthermore, to insure that people who are blind, deaf, or have motor impairments can access a smartphone easily, simplified interface design is a key design goal. Thus, individuals with moderate cognitive impairments can use the phone. Of course, this also enables people without disabilities to use the phone in more situations and environments. When a driver of an automobile is watching the road and is effectively functionally blind in doing other tasks, audio can be used; a patron in a noisy environment like a bar or restaurant is functionally hearing impaired and benefits from visual or tactile equivalent information. Smartphone hardware provides the needed transducers, the operating systems can offer the consistent and necessary framework, and the software interface design can offer the end user a universal design… all to create a more highly portable, flexible, accessible, and safer product to accomplish a wider range of tasks and achieve a more equitable and higher quality of life.

6.3 Cost of Not Adopting UD

Lifetime costs increase without adoption of universal design (UD). The example used most often is the curb cut. When the curb cut is constructed at a corner, it provides access for baby strollers, delivery carts, hand trucks, bicycles, and wheelchairs. The cost increase for installing a curb ramp is usually only marginally more than the cost of a traditional curb. On the other hand, the expense of removing and replacing a curb later is very expensive. This is, in fact, one reason why the designers of new housing subdivisions try to guess where driveways will be needed. Estimating correctly, even once, saves the expense of breaking up curbs and repouring driveway entries.

Neglecting to incorporate UD features in products can lead to increased needs for after-market support or loss of market share. For the consumer this can result in much greater costs, for example, paying a premium to purchase special accessibility adaptations. For the manufacturer, it can result in the need to ramp up product development earlier than planned if competitors introduce improved usability, safety, or wellness features. The failure to initially adopt UD design is often an opportunity lost and revenue untapped. For example, if a cable television provider has an interface that it is too complicated for older users, they are essentially writing off the opportunity to attract a large segment of the population, one that has, as a group, the highest disposable income [3].

6.4 Models of Practice

In this section we discuss three complementary models of practice that can be adopted to implement universal design and have well-established methodologies: (1) enhanced ergonomic design, (2) AT as a design motivation and testing ground, and (3) participatory action research (PAR).

6.4.1 Enhanced Ergonomic Design

Ergonomic design is a field in which knowledge bases about human performance are applied to design problems. This field has a long history of evidence-based practice to solve real-world design problems. Ergonomics researchers place great value on consulting with end users in development projects through usability testing and focus groups. However, the application of best practices in ergonomic design will not necessarily achieve universal design. As an example, one of the most well-known of all general ergonomic principles, design for the largest part of the "bell curve" of characteristics and abilities (from the 5th through 95th percentile), excludes many people [10]. Rarely does an individual fit within this range for every characteristic or ability. A person with a long trunk may have short arms, or a person with short stature may have large hands. More significantly, circumstances of everyday life reduce human abilities all the time. We all are unfamiliar with a product or place, distracted by personal troubles, fatigued from too little sleep, or victim of a sudden storm or power blackout. Every person could find themselves "disabled," and functioning outside the 5th–95th percentile range, particularly with respect to mental processes. Universal design requires a readjustment of typical human factors and ergonomics (HFE) priorities.

Nevertheless, many basic principles of HFE can be applied to UD [3]. Rather than using older design strategies that only target 90% of the population, the UD goal is to include 100% of the population, or as close as possible to that ideal. Fortunately, the field of ergonomics has recognized the need to collect information on extremes of the population [11]. Both traditional human factors researchers and rehabilitation science researchers are developing an ever-expanding knowledge base on the characteristics and capabilities of groups like people with disabilities and elders. This knowledge should be tapped for universal design practice.

Contemporary ergonomics research puts emphasis on the emotional response to a product, environment or service, as well as the direct performance issues. The foundations of ergonomics lie in high performance settings like airplane cockpits, dangerous activities like assembly line work, and critical settings like nuclear power plant control rooms. Unlike these settings, ordinary consumers usually have the flexibility to avoid or abandon products and environments they do not like. Likewise, their emotional response will determine how much effort they invest in learning how to use new products and technologies. Research on "Kansei/Affective Engineering" and "Emotional Design" demonstrates how we can design products and environments to be appealing to people [12–14]. Nagamachi [13] cites the value of Kansei/Affective Engineering to the practice of universal design. He argues that by focusing on the affective aspects of product design, the designers take more of a human-centered approach to design, addressing the end users' needs, wants, and desires.

The process of ergonomic design may require other adjustments when applied to universal design. In universal design, the influence of personal factors and cultural context should receive more attention than it usually receives in traditional ergonomic design initiatives. The scientific literature tends to focus on generalizations that apply to large populations. In universal design we seek to address particulars and provide more choices and flexibility. Thus, more emphasis should be placed on direct involvement of end users in developing user requirements and user testing of prototypes prior to final design and even after product launch. Through this involvement, a deeper understanding of individual differences and contextual issues can be obtained.

Audible navigational instructions provide an example of the importance of emotions, individual differences, and context. The voice and language used for navigation affects the level of attention and acceptance of the end user. For example, to some groups and in some situations such as in s telephone voice mail menu, people may be more responsive to a soothing female voice than a commanding male voice. On the other hand, when avoiding mistakes is critical and a voice must cut through a noisy environment like at the end of a moving walkway, it may be better to use a startling voice and commanding language. And again, such directive language may be annoying when used to help people find the shortest route to the grocery store. Recently, Garmin [15] introduced character options for their navigational devices. One can now chose to use the voice and language of Darth Vader, Yoda, or Dora the Explorer to guide you through a maze of unfamiliar city streets instead of the ubiquitous friendly female voice (Figure 6.3). This option not only introduces entertainment value to the mundane task of following directions, but also allows an individual to customize their system to their preferences. Taking this approach one step further, individuals with hearing impairments may find certain voices difficult to hear. Now they have the opportunity to choose a different voice, for example, Darth Vader over Dora to improve perception. From a marketing perspective, it is likely that the entertainment value of the characters will actually increase sales to those who have heretofore done without a navigational device.

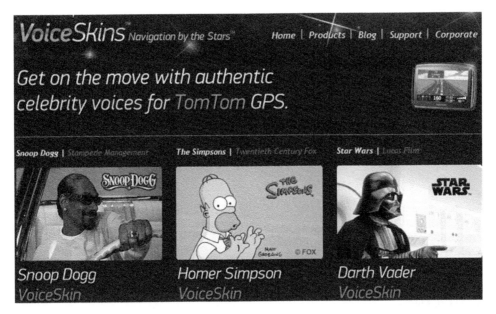

FIGURE 6.3
(See color insert.) Garmin navigation device with personalized voice.

6.4.2 Assistive Technology as a Design Motivation and Testing Ground

Throughout the history of industrial design, innovative AT and products conceived for special populations have evolved into mainstream consumer products due to the general value of their features. One example is the typewriter, originally conceived as a device to help a blind person write [16]. Another is the phonograph, which was developed because Alexander Graham Bell, a teacher of the deaf and hard of hearing, sought a way to amplify speech for people with hearing impairments. A third, text to speech, was originally developed by Ray Kurzweil to help blind people read the printed word.

Often, when first designed and developed, these innovations are crude and expensive. However, once perfected through limited use by special populations, the broader benefits are usually recognized. The products or technologies are then transformed into mass manufactured products for the general market. The AT market and other special markets can be viewed as a "proving ground" in which unique needs justify the higher cost of innovation. The best contemporary example is the OXO Good Grips utensils with oversized handles made from nonslip, easy-to-grip materials (Figure 6.4). The handle design was based on the built-up handles that occupational therapists have used with their clients for decades. This line of products transformed the industry so that all manufacturers today offer lines with such handles.

Often the transformation from AT to UD is instigated by consumer adoption rather than a business plan. A good example is captioned television. The original captioning systems were housed in a separate device that plugged into a television and cost $200–$300. In the mid 1980s, federal law required that new televisions include a system to caption text. Although mandated for accessibility reasons, people who did not have hearing impairments enthusiastically adopted captioned text. It is now in use wherever noise levels are too high to hear the sound on a television or where it is desirable to reduce the background noise level. Airports, sports bars, fitness centers, and spouses going to sleep at night when their partners want to watch TV, all turn on closed captioning (Figure 6.5).

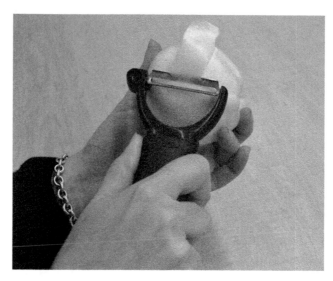

FIGURE 6.4
OXO Good Grips utensil.

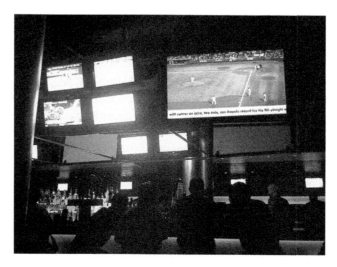

FIGURE 6.5
Closed captioning used in a pub.

Typically AT ideas emerge as individual practitioners develop new ideas for specific individuals with disabilities and realize it in prototype form as a one-off custom device, for example, a new cane handle, navigational aid, or a computer input device. If the solution works well, then it becomes the basis for an AT product. These products are usually manufactured and distributed through companies that target populations with specific disabilities. They are often expensive since these narrow markets are limited and after-market services, like training and tech support, can be very intensive for people with special needs. The reliability of products, interoperability with other systems, and frequency of updates is often below the standards for mass marketed products because the companies themselves do not have the investment capital or cash flow of large consumer product companies. Finally, the aesthetics of AT products are usually compromised for many reasons, for example, the lack of involvement of professional designers, cost considerations, lack of competition in the market. Users of AT have a major functional need for the devices they use and are more willing to accept the limitations of an AT device because of the great benefits they realize. However, abandonment of AT over time is recognized as a serious problem for all the reasons listed earlier and more.

6.4.3 Participatory Action Research Methodology

Implementing a design process that considers people with disabilities and others with functional limitations requires an understanding of (1) how physical, behavioral, and cognitive impairments or social and economic factors result in functional limitations and (2) what mechanisms groups and individuals use to resolve problems they encounter. Consulting with experts who understand the array of issues that different groups face in their daily activities can be extremely helpful. For example, occupational therapists receive fundamental education in the human and natural sciences along with practical clinical training to deal with people with the widest ranges of disabilities. Thus, therapists can be very valuable as consultants or collaborators in the design phase of product development. However, even well-versed and experienced professionals cannot replace the knowledge and daily living experience of people with disabilities.

PAR has been formally articulated and promoted in rehabilitation research and development for most of a decade. PAR facilitates knowledge translation during development activities by including professionals and end users in the process directly [17]. PAR also enables scientists and the user community to exchange information early in development cycles to assure that needs of the target population(s) are addressed [18,19]. This is very consistent with the fundamentals of usability testing methodologies [20–22].

PAR, however, raises an interesting paradox related to UD. PAR is typically implemented with specific diagnostic or functional population groups to target designs specific to their needs. Consequently, the outcomes of PAR often result in identifying focused specifications and design characteristics. As mentioned earlier, the target population for UD is everyone, including people with all different types of disability and impairments. Consequently, the execution of PAR in the context of UD must be expanded and attempt to be inclusive. At a minimum, people with a variety of complete functional impairments such as being totally blind, deaf, nonspeaking, or unable to walk. Additionally, the participating group should include people with partial impairments such as visual loss, hearing loss, poor coordination, partial limb amputation, or intellectual or behavioral impairments (such as reading or attention deficits). Finally, it should represent different people with a variety of socioeconomic characteristics.

Including all impairments becomes a philosophical and practical challenge. Finding and including participants from such broadly defined usability groups seems to confound the common design assumption that usability testing only requires a relatively small number of testers. Nevertheless, the need to increase the size of usability testing cohorts during the design process has support for this approach [23]. It must also be acknowledged that this demand can be burdensome. Ideally, products should be tested across a full range of users, but this can increase cost and extend testing timelines. Thus, alternate strategies to expand the understanding of impairments during interaction with products are needed. In particular, a product or environmental assessment can serve as a proxy for a broad range of people with disabilities [24,34].

6.5 Measuring the Success of a Universal Design

6.5.1 Need for Measurement

The need for measuring universal design is important for many reasons.

1. To supplement limited user participation in design, proxy user perspectives and broad-based bench tests can robustly examine designs for all types of users and assure that all impairments are represented [27].
2. Specific performance criteria for sound, light, or temperature can be developed to assess compliance with guidelines.
3. Measurement of performance can be disseminated, like nutrition information, to inform consumers about products they are comparing.
4. Benchmarking is needed to establish a continuous quality improvement process. This requires methods to measure how well the design works for all user populations in regular use over time.
5. Funding agencies like Medicare and Medicaid require documentation of product performance to meet individual consumer needs to authorize reimbursements [25,26].
6. Measurement methods are needed to identify and document best practices.

6.5.2 Challenges

Measuring universal design has numerous unique challenges, such as (1) measuring outcomes across populations; (2) addressing the needs of specific populations; and (3) meaningfulness to designers, policy makers, and consumers [24,27].

Even when using accessibility codes as a measurement tool, the results leave room for interpretation. For example, if an accessible portion of a reception counter is installed at the mandated height, an ornamental flower pot could sit on counter space blocking the view and access to the space; does this meet the minimum standard of accessibility? Or if a website meets basic accessibility design requirements, including written text equivalent "alt text" for illustrations, but the alt text descriptions are not adequate (e.g., a line drawing of the State of Wisconsin to depict its shape is described with an alt text of "picture of a state"), is it acceptable?

The products and populations for which performance measures are needed are virtually countless [28]. If we consider the number of types of products, possible product features, and specific impairment combinations a person might have, the quantity of measurement tools or the extent of a single measurement system needed to assess individuals quickly becomes overwhelming. Strategies to simplify the measurement approach must be implemented to create realistic assessments.

Measures must also address the fact that a device could be 100% accessible to one individual and 0% to someone else. And establishing priorities adds another challenge. For example, audio output is essential for a blind person but the location of the audio output jack may be less essential. Therefore, each design feature does not necessarily carry the same weight in terms of significance for access and use.

Faced with these challenges, many universal design experts question whether it is even possible to measure universal design. Today, there is no defined set of criteria to even develop a measurement model. Thus, with only the availability of accessibility regulations and a widely scattered literature, the field still depends on expert judgment and wise designers. Fortunately, there has been some progress in measuring accessibility and usability related to populations of people with disabilities that suggest directions for the future.

6.5.3 Current Attempts

There are three basic approaches to outcomes research in accessibility and universal design. The first uses outside observers to assess observable behaviors associated with usability and social participation. The second uses self-report data to provide a subjective perspective of the end user. The third is the use of instrumented data collection devices. While this third direction is preferred, the field is a long way from implementing such approaches widely except, perhaps, with interactive technologies. Progress in the first two methods includes work by Steinfeld and Danford [29] who developed a set of three scales for use in the built environment. In the mid-2000s, work by Mendonca et al. [27,30–32] created a framework for measuring the accessibility of medical devices. A document listing past and current instruments by category resides at the website Access-Mainstreet [33]. More recently, Lenker et al. [34] developed a usability rating scale for universal design that is specifically designed for use by end users and designers as an inexpensive way to assess universal design outcomes during prototype development and testing. Park et al. [35,36] prototyped a restaurant accessibility instrument using a trichotomous scoring system. While there are some existing instruments, considerably more work is needed, particularly in analytical methods for using recorded user interaction with "smart" systems to evaluate usability from a universal design perspective. Steinfeld et al. [37] are using video and motion capture to study the usability of simulated buses and ramps. These methods provide both quantitative measures such as time of task completion, range of motion and acceleration of movement, as well as graphic evidence of usability problems.

6.5.4 Status of the Evidence Base

Smith [38] provided an overview and description of the nascent nature of evidence-based practice in the universal design field from its grounding in medicine. More recently, Steinfeld and Maisel [3] completed a review of the evidence base for universal design for a new textbook on the subject. In this book, the authors divided the knowledge on the subject into three parts: design for human performance, design for health and wellness, and design for social participation. From their review, they derived many guidelines that can be used in universal design practice, but they also noted that there are many gaps in our knowledge. Many of those gaps are related to the lack of knowledge translation from research into guidelines that can be used in practice and others are due to the lack of knowledge or lack of closure in certain research areas. Their development of a better definition of universal design and clarification of goals are the first step in compiling a better evidence base.

Steinfeld and Maisel [3] noted that it is more difficult to develop general design guidelines for health and wellness and social participation outcomes than for human performance issues. The literature on these two outcomes is closely tied to specific contexts and populations, for example, neighborhood, age and income of end users, etc., so design guidelines are more difficult to develop without knowing the nature of a project and the people served. Often the literature suggests adopting approaches to design process rather than specific strategies, for example, using PAR methods. Nevertheless, there are many evidence-based sources of design guidelines for designing specific building types. For example, the Academy of Design and Health has pioneered in disseminating design guidelines for health facilities. As early as 1975, Clare Cooper Marcus [39] reviewed the housing research literature and compiled a lengthy set of guidelines for design of public housing. Gerontologists studying housing and other facilities for aging have produced an extensive evidence base with guidelines (see, for example, [40]).

A major gap in the literature is that there is limited research available on the relationship between social participation and consumer product design, precisely the kind of information that would be useful in developing QoLTs. The knowledge base on consumer health and safety issues like the impact of electromagnetic radiation or noise is extensive, reflected by consumer product safety regulatory activities, but there is less known about how product design contributes to other health-related outcomes of universal design. For example, while it is known that using mobile phones while driving is a dangerous behavior, we do not understand the trade-offs. Mobile phone use during driving may have other important quality of life outcomes like successful use of 911 or lifetime friendship formation and social maintenance activities. Likewise, there is growing literature on the impact of design on emotional response, but we do not know whether positive emotional responses carry through to improved health behavior or social interaction. Research on the outcomes of product use needs to expand past usability to provide a stronger evidence base for universal design. As part of R&D in QoLTs, assessment of impacts on health, wellness, and social participation should be an important agenda item.

6.6 Improving the Adoption of Universal Design

6.6.1 Barriers to Adoption

There are three major barriers to adoption of universal design:

- Clarifying the concept
- Establishing the legitimacy of UD practice
- Lack of incentives

Research into the process of innovation diffusion has identified clarification of an innovation as one of the most important issues in improving adoption [41]. As described earlier, there is a difference between accessible design and AT on one hand, and universal design on the other. In the early stages of UD practice, not enough distinction was made between these terms. In fact, UD has been too often associated solely with design for people with disabilities and frail elders. A recent focus group conducted by the Boomer Project and funded by the AARP [42] demonstrated how difficult it is for consumers to distinguish between the two. Part of the problem is the lack of good precedents. Another is the lack of a consistent message from the community of practice in this field.

Universal design practice has to be viewed as an important and integral aspect of design practice to achieve legitimacy in the design and engineering community. At present, anyone can claim to be an expert on universal design; thus, there is really no added value to having expertise in the field. Legitimacy can be achieved by two means: (1) clarifying the knowledge base underlying universal design and (2) introducing the topic as part of design and engineering education both within the academy and in practice. Three precedents demonstrate the value of this approach. The first is the World Wide Web Accessibility Consortium. The W3C developed guidelines for web accessibility that became the benchmark for insuring website access. Knowledge of the standards and how to achieve them in web design became a clear topic of professional expertise and is now an important knowledge area for web designers. The second is the accreditation program developed for sustainable design by the Green Building Council. By being accredited through training and testing, LEED certified professionals have recognized credentials for implementing sustainable design. The third is the Center for Health Design, which also has developed an accreditation program for design professionals who would like to establish credentials in the field of health facilities design and is actively assembling a knowledge base of evidence for design decisions in health care settings.

Perhaps the most important barrier is the lack of incentives. Unlike accessible design, which is mandated by regulations, there are no mandates for incorporating UD. In fact, it is questionable whether that would be a good idea. UD is about continuous improvement and regulations are about achieving legal minimums. Regulation usually results in minimum compliance rather than higher goal seeking behavior. In the field of sustainable design, there are measurable results like reduced energy costs, reduced storm water runoff, and public relations benefits. Likewise in evidence-based health care design, new research is demonstrating significant savings in operating costs by adoption of design guidelines. The best example is the impact on single-bed hospital rooms on lowering the costs of managing infection [43]. Universal design needs similar incentives. Research has demonstrated that it results in increased usability [29] but the field needs evidence that it reduces costs, increases revenue and other business oriented measures. An example is the adoption of elder friendly design features in the Kaiser supermarket chain. The chain reported that after it introduced these features, revenues increased 25% beyond that estimated by forecasts [44]. Even without such data, however, the adoption of universal design has public relations value, just like sustainable design. It means a commitment to the "customer" and to diversity. Thus, it provides value to business simply through social branding, if there is a way to communicate that to the public.

6.6.2 Labeling and Ratings

Labeling, certification, and accreditation activities can help to address the three barriers to adoption described earlier. There are some early explorations into labeling for UD. One is the development of a UD symbol to be used on products and services (Figure 6.6). The symbol was developed at the IDeA Center at the University at Buffalo, SUNY, through the Universal Design Identity Project, sponsored by the National Endowment for the Arts (NEA). Its intent is to "promote increased understanding, acceptance, and the use of universal design by a broader audience of consumers, design professionals, industry and government leaders, and academics" [45]. The IDeA Center will give permission for the use of the symbol if conditions of use are met (see http://udeworld.com/udlogo.html).

Another study focused on the value of labeling for accessibility compared to other factors in product purchases [46,47]. Mendonca and Smith [24] asked individuals with disabilities to choose home medical devices based on cost, opinion, and accessibility ratings. Accessibility statistically dominated cost and opinion as the most important variable. Clearly, information about accessibility is an important variable for guiding consumer decision making for purchases by people with disabilities. It is likely that usability would be viewed similarly by the general public as well.

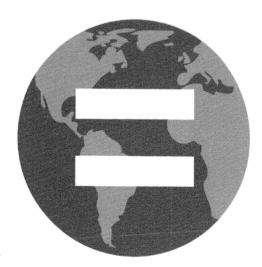

FIGURE 6.6
Universal Design Symbol™.

6.6.3 Standards, Certification, and Accreditation

Standards for universal design are being developed through a relatively new organization, the Global Universal Design Commission (GUDC) (www.globaluniversaldesign.org). The GUDC standards are designed to encourage adoption of universal design through a certification program, similar to the successful Leadership in Energy and Environmental Design (LEED) and Green Globe standards for sustainable design. Once consensus standards are established, they will be the focus of a certification program that recognizes the adoption and implementation of UD. Unlike accessibility standards, the GUDC UD standards are designed to be easy to implement and are not encumbered by highly technical material. Points will be awarded for inclusion of UD features; different levels of certification can be established based on the total points achieved in a project, thereby publicly recognizing achievement of universal design. To obtain certification by the GUDC, project teams will be required to include the participation of qualified professionals. The GUDC plans to establish an accreditation program that, through training and testing, will provide organizations with the expertise they need to implement the standards.

The first GUDC standards will be for public buildings, but plans are under way to develop UD standards for product design in the near future. The standards will be supported with compilations of research evidence and related technical design guidelines. This compilation of knowledge can serve as a focus for research and help to improve communications between practitioners and researchers. The knowledge base will be designed to facilitate the use of the standards in an iterative manner as design proceeds from conception through development of final products and environments. Like the Green Globes and the World Wide Web Accessibility initiatives, design teams will use a computer interface to obtain guidance as they develop their projects, including links to the knowledge base and precedents, and a running "score" of their incorporation of UD features. A program of post occupancy evaluations of buildings constructed with the UD standards is also planned to measure the impact of the standards and obtain baseline data to compare UD features with comparable conventional designs.

Another approach to certification recognizes the achievements of an organization rather than specific products. The "Flag for All Cities" initiative of the Design for All Foundation is the first implementation of this type of strategy for universal design. The program is targeted for municipalities. Governments pledge to devote a certain percentage of their budget to universal design activities within their city over a specified time period. The Foundation will audit their activities and certify their compliance with the program guidelines. If successful, the city will have the right to fly a flag demonstrating their achievement. Communications of innovations in the adopting cities will help to spread innovation and identify creative and effective approaches.

6.7 Success Stories

6.7.1 Good Grips

The kitchen utensils sold under the OXO Good Grips brand are often used as an early example of success in the market place (see Figure 6.4). Earlier in this chapter, we noted that the key Good Grips design concept, large slip-resistant handles, was based upon a practice in AT. The Good Grips handles are larger than conventional utensil handles and the gripping surface is a durable, slip-resistant, and resilient material that is both easier to grasp and high tech looking. The more complex products like the kettle and the salad spinner include additional innovative ideas. The kettle has a hinged handle that, when tilted, opens the cover so that it could be used with only one hand. The salad spinner has a large paddle-type handle that can be pushed down to activate the spinner, which also allows one-handed use and reduces the range of motion needed to shake water off greens.

The Good Grips products are more expensive than the conventional products, but they offer greater value and the price differential is commensurate with that value. A few more dollars obtains a product that is easier to use and has a high-tech modern style as well. Producing a full range of products leads to synergy in marketing and a visible brand identity. Most importantly, the Good Grips products were never targeted for the "elder and disabled" market. They were introduced into the general market directly, eliminating the potential for a stigmatized identity both for the brand and the consumer who purchases them. Their success is demonstrated by the fact that all the company's competitors soon adopted oversized nonslip handles in their own lines.

Lessons learned:

1. AT solutions offer some good points of departure for universal design.
2. Innovative design including an attractive high-tech look enhances emotional appeal.
3. Mass marketing avoids the stigma of design for special markets.
4. Consumers will be willing to pay more when they perceive the added value to be worth the extra cost.

6.7.2 iTunes and Related Devices

The iPod, iPhone, and iPad are truly revolutionary products. While these devices have many design strengths, what really sets them apart from the competition is the ease with which they can be personalized. The simple forms support customization on the outside with the use of third-party cases and sleeves, but the real innovation is personalization on the inside by the downloading of media and applications. Norman [48] uses the Japanese

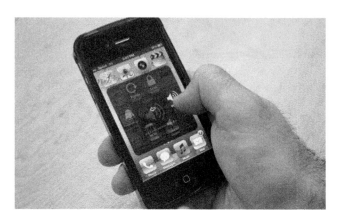

FIGURE 6.7
IPhone showing voice over app.

tradition of the "bento box" as an example of good design for emotional response. A bento box provides a simple package that is attractive on the outside and looks very simple. On the inside, the matrix of compartments holds a very complex mixture of foods. The foods included are endlessly variable and can be customized for each person. The bento box simplifies the presentation and use of a complex menu of options. The screens of the iPhone and iPad even look like bento boxes.

The iTunes website, likewise, provides a simplified delivery system for dealing with the complexity of organizing a vast array of media and apps. It is safe to say that the iTunes website and seamless integration with its devices was the key to Apple's recent success in music players, telephones, and tablets. Taking this concept further, they have now integrated the iTunes store with their Macintosh computer operating system so that even new versions of the Macintosh operating systems, office productivity software, and sophisticated technical software can be downloaded and installed in the same manner as a new song or video. This combination of easy-to-use, standard methods of service delivery combined with the endless variety of personalization opportunities provides a very powerful system design.

It is also noteworthy that Apple produced VoiceOver (See Figure 6.7), an application that creates a sound landscape on a tactile interface to enable use by a broader range of users, namely people who cannot see the screen. A newer application, Assistive Touch, allows individuals who have difficulty making the standard screen interaction gestures to use an alternative set of gestures. It will be interesting to see if uses for these applications are found that were not expected, like the use of closed captioning on television.

Lessons learned:

1. Keep the user experience simple and fun.
2. Provide opportunities for personalization within a structure that clarifies operations.
3. Personalization involves choice, emotional connection, and reconfiguration.
4. Software and hardware must work together seamlessly.

6.7.3 IKEA Stores

IKEA is known internationally for affordable, attractive, and useful products, but their business practices are as important to the company's success as their design initiatives. Here we will focus on their store design and its relationship to business practices.

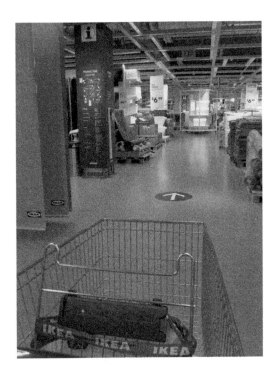

FIGURE 6.8
IKEA store wayfinding system.

The array of goods in IDEA stores could present an overwhelming cognitive challenge to most consumers. But the content and organization of the stores provides a stress-free and comfortable experience for all visitors. The most noticeable feature is the clear linear path through the store from entry to checkout defined by the size of the aisles, signs, lighting, and graphics to simplify navigation (Figure 6.8). This path also exposes customers to all the key departments of the store. There are shortcuts for the shoppers who know what they want and are familiar with the store layout. Rather than organizing the stores by product type, for example, electrical, hardware, and furniture, the organization is primarily by room types, for example, living room, home office, and kitchen, which uses a simple conceptual model for shopping and exposes the shopper to products they might otherwise not notice. The stores incorporate a combination of traditional shopping and "warehouse" shopping. Smaller items are collected while traveling through the store, but larger items are recorded on a form from information on tags attached to the showroom goods. At the end of the linear path, the customer stops at the "warehouse" part of the store to pick up the items on their list. These are often designed for self-assembly, which reduces costs and also facilitates self-delivery to the home. IKEA stores also pioneered child-friendly environments including babysitting, a pleasant dining environment, and, recently, "play spaces" for husbands.

The IKEA stores simplify the shopping experience for the user but also provide a pleasant experience to make the shopper and related family members comfortable and happy, demonstrating that they really care about their customers. Their stores reflect the overall business approach stated in their "Guiding Principles": "The IKEA business shall have an overall positive impact on people and the environment."

Lessons learned:

1. The challenges created by increasing choice and diversity can be reduced by a spatial organization that mirrors everyday experience.
2. A pleasant and exciting environment increases customer interest and satisfaction.
3. A lifespan approach is more user friendly for everyone and recognizes that shoppers are members of families with diverse interests.
4. Business practices that are consumer centric should be integrated into store and product design.

6.8 Conclusions

Universal design is a process that represents an ongoing commitment to designing things that work for people with all abilities, including the full range of disabilities. It incorporates methods that consider the full spectrum of user abilities early on and, through an iterative process, confirms effectiveness during the stages of design and testing. It follows through with business practices and services that improve the experience of finding, purchasing, and using products. Adoption of universal design not only can reduce costs but also increase profitability through improved usability and increased market share. Today, determining the level of accessibility and usability of designs in the prototype and testing stage of development is heavily dependent on experts. However, new practical, responsive, and valid measures are being developed both for application during the development cycle to facilitate the incorporation of universal design features by design teams and also to provide consumer information to improve recognition and awareness of these features. It is essential to recognize that we all benefit from products that are universally designed.

The old paradigm of accessibility promoted development of two markets, the general consumer market and niche markets for people with specific disabilities. Universal design breaks down artificial barriers between these two markets and recognizes that everyone can benefit from improved usability and safety and opportunities to have a closer fit between our abilities, preferences, and the unique challenges of life. It acknowledges that disability and other challenges are part of everyone's life. Technologies that address quality of life issues will impact each of us as we engage our environment, interact with other people, and adjust to the aging process. Universal design also recognizes that the emotional and social aspects of design are as important as the functional and provides strategies to reduce stigma due to differences of any type and increase acceptance of enabling technologies.

The need for incorporating universal design into the daily work of researchers, developers, manufactures, instructors, and academic programs is pressing. Every device-, environment-, or technology-oriented service that fails to incorporate universal design creates risks to manufacturers and service providers—missing market opportunities, increased costs to catch up in future development cycles, and losing market share to competitors who understand and invest in universal design strategies. The more we ignore universal design, the greater the burden for providing assistance to individuals, specialized products, and services. These are public costs as well as individual costs. Design education programs that include instruction about the range of human performance, especially at the extremes, will graduate next generation design experts who can create successful QoLTs that civil societies need and demand.

References

1. B. R. Connell, M. Jones, R. Mace, J. Meuller, A. Mullick, E. Ostroff, J. Sanford, E. Steinfeld, M. Story, and G. Vanderheiden. The principles of universal design. 1997 [Online]. Available: http://www.ncsu.edu/www/ncsu/design/sod5/cud/about_ud/udprinciplestext.htm
2. E. Steinfeld and B. Tauke. Universal designing. In: *Teaching Universal Design—17 Ways of Thinking and Teaching*, J. Christopherson and T. Ronnevig, Eds. Oslo, Norway: Norwegian State Housing Bank, 2002.
3. E. Steinfeld and J. L. Maisel. *Universal Design: Creating a More Inclusive World*. Hoboken, NJ: Wiley, 2012.
4. E. Steinfeld and K. Seelman. World disability report. Geneva, Switzerland: World Health Organization, 2011.
5. E. Steinfeld. Universal design. In: *International Encyclopedia of Rehabilitation*, J. H. Stone and M. Blouin, Eds. 2009 [Online]. Available: http://cirrie.buffalo.edu/encyclopedia/article.php?id=107&language=en
6. World Health Organization. *ICF: International Classification of Functioning Disability and Health*. Geneva, Switzerland: World Health Organization, 2001.
7. K. Pizur-Barnekow, M. Lemke, R. O. Smith, M. Winter, and R. Mendonca. MED-AUDIT impairment categories: Working towards mapping AMI usability. 2005 [Online]. Available: http://www.uwm.edu/CHS/r2d2/rerc-ami/archive/impairments.pdf
8. G. C. Vanderheiden and K. R. Vanderheiden. A brief introduction to disabilities. From accessible design of consumer products: Guidelines for the design of consumer products to increase their accessibility to people with disabilities or who are aging. 1991 [Online]. Available: http://trace.wisc.edu/docs/population/populat.htm
9. R. Mendonca and R. O. Smith. Development of a methodology to measure accessibility. *Proceedings of the RESNA 34th International Conference on Technology and Disability: Research, Design, Practice and Policy*, Arlington, VA, 2011.
10. G. C. Vanderheiden. Thirty-something million: Should they be exceptions? *Human Factors*, 32, 383–396, 1990.
11. K. H. E. Kroemer. *Extra-Ordinary Ergonomics*. Boca Raton, FL: Taylor & Francis, 2006.
12. P. Desmet. Measuring emotion: Development and application of an instrument to measure emotional responses to products funology. *Human-Computer Interaction Series* 3, 111–123, 2005.
13. M. Nagamachi. *Kansei/Affective Engineering*. Boca Raton, FL: CRC Press, 2011.
14. D. Norman. *Emotional Design: Why We Love (or Hate) Everyday Things*. New York: Basic Books, 2004.
15. Garmin. Voices [Online]. Available: http://www8.garmin.com/vehicles/voices/
16. The Classic Typewriter Page [Online]. Available: http://site.xavier.edu/polt/typewriters/tw-history.html
17. G. W. White, M. Suchowierska, and M. Campbell. Developing and systematically implementing participatory action research. *Archives of Physical Medicine and Rehabilitation*, 85(2), S3–S12, 2004.
18. M. Viswanathan, A. Ammerman, E. Eng, G. Gartlehner, K. N. Lohr, D. Griffith, S. Rhodes et al. Community-based participatory research: Assessing the evidence. Evidence Report/Technology Assessment No. 99 (Prepared by RTI–University of North Carolina Evidence-based Practice Center under Contract No. 290-02-0016). AHRQ Publication 04-E022-2. Rockville, MD: Agency for Healthcare Research and Quality, July 2004.
19. N. Khanlou and E. Peter. Participatory action research: Considerations for ethical review. *Social Science and Medicine*, 60, 2333–2340, 2004.
20. J. S. Dumas and M. C. Salzman. Usability assessment methods. *Reviews of Human Factors and Ergonomics*, 2, 109–140, 2006.
21. M. J. Smith, G. Salvendy, D. Harris, and R. J. Koubek, Eds. *Usability Evaluation and Interface Design: Cognitive Engineering, Intelligent Agents and Virtual Reality*. Mahwah, NJ: Lawrence Erlbaum Associates, 2001.

22. R. Jeffries, J. Miller, C. Wharton, and K. Uyeda. User interface evaluation in the real world: A comparison of four techniques. *Proceedings of the ACM Computer Human Interaction*, New Orleans, LA, 1991.

23. L. Faulkner. Beyond the five-user assumption: Benefits of increased sample sizes in usability testing. *Behavior Research Methods, Instruments, and Computers*, 35(3), 379–383, 2003.

24. R. J. Mendonca and R. O. Smith. Effects of providing accessibility product information to people with disabilities. *Proceedings of the FICCDAT International Conference*, Toronto, Ontario, Canada, 2011.

25. Department of Health and Human Services: Inspector General. Medicare payments for power wheelchairs. April, 2004 [Online]. Available: http://oig.hhs.gov/oei/reports/oei-03-02-00600.pdf

26. RERC-AMI. Rehabilitation Engineering Research Center on Accessible Medical Instrumentation (RERC-AMI) Homepage [Online]. Available: http://www.rerc-ami.org/ami/

27. R. O. Smith, K. Barnekow, M. R. Lemke, R. Mendonca, M. Winter, and T. Schwanke. Development of the MED-AUDIT (Medical Equipment Device—Accessibility and Universal Design Tool). In: *Medical Instrumentation Accessibility and Usability Considerations*, J. M. Winters and M. F. Story, Eds. Boca Raton, FL: CRC Press, 2007, pp. 283–296.

28. R. O. Smith. Measuring the outcomes of assistive technology: Challenge and innovation. *Assistive Technology*, 8(1), 71–81, 1996.

29. E. Steinfeld and G. S. Danford. Theory as a basis for research on enabling environments. In: *Measuring Enabling Environments*, E. Steinfeld and G. S. Danford, Eds. New York: Kluwer Academic/Plenum, 1999.

30. R. Mendonca and R. O. Smith. Assessing the usability and reliability of MED-AUDIT. *The 29th Annual Great Lakes Biomedical Conference, Biomedical Informatics: Applications, Achievements, and Frontiers: The Milwaukee Chapter of IEEE EMBS*, Milwaukee, WI, 2005.

31. R. Mendonca and R. O. Smith. MED-AUDIT (Medical Equipment Device-Accessibility and Universal Design Information Tool): Usability analysis. *Proceedings of the 29th International Conference on Thriving in Challenging Times: The Future of Rehabilitation Engineering and Assistive Technology*, Atlanta, GA, 2006.

32. R. Mendonca, R. O. Smith, M. Lemke, and J. Winters. Expert validation of the MED-AUDIT (Medical Equipment Device-Accessibility & Universal Design Information Tool). *Proceedings of the RESNA 31st International Conference on Technology and Disability: Research, Design, Practice and Policy*, Arlington, VA, 2008.

33. Rehabilitation Research Design & Disability (R₂D₂) Center. Tools and resources. ACCESS Main Street, 2011 [Online]. Available: http://access-mainstreet.r2d2.uwm.edu/Tools_Resources/Checklists_Evaluations/

34. J. A. Lenker, M. Nasarwanji, V. Paquet, and D. Feathers. A tool for rapid assessment of product usability and universal design: Development and preliminary psychometric testing. *Work*, 39, 141–150, 2011.

35. M. Park, R. O. Smith, and K. Liegl. The Restaurant Accessibility and Task Evaluation Tool (RATE-IT). *Proceedings of the FICCDAT International Conference*, Toronto, Ontario, Canada, 2011.

36. M. Park, K. P. Liegl, and R. O. Smith. Preliminary validation of the Restaurant Accessibility and Task Evaluation Information Tool (RATE-IT). *AOTA 91st Annual Conference*, Philadelphia, PA, 2011.

37. E. Steinfeld, V. Paquet, J. Lenker, C. D'souza, J. Maisel. Universal design research on boarding and using buses. *TRANSED 2010 Conference Proceedings*, Hong Kong, June 2010.

38. R. O. Smith. Evidence-based practice (EBP) in universal design. In: *The State of the Science in Universal Design: Emerging Research and Developments*, J. L. Maisel, Ed. Sharjah, U.A.E.: Bentham Science Publishers Ltd., 2010, pp. 31–46.

39. C. C. Marcus. *Easter Hill Village: Some Social Implications of Design*. New York: Free Press, 1975.

40. V. Regnier. *Design for Assisted Living. Guidelines for Housing the Physically and Mentally Frail*. Hoboken, NJ: Wiley, 2002.

41. E. Rogers. *Diffusion of Innovation*. New York: Free Press, 2003.

42. Boomer Project. Presentation on results of focus groups with 50+ consumers, 2010.

43. National Health Service. *Ward Layouts with Single Rooms and Space for Flexibility*. Harrogate, U.K.: National Health Service, 2005.
44. K. Badley. Supervalues, *Metropolis Magazine*, 2007. Available: http://www.metropolismag.com/story/20070620/super-values
45. IDeA Center (n.d.). UD E-World. IDeA: Center for Inclusive Design and Environmental Access [Online]. Available: http://udeworld.com/udlogo.html
46. R. O. Smith (n.d.). Program R3/Accessibility Measurement. *RERC on AMI* [Online]. Available: www.rerc-ami.org/rerc-ami/r3/r3-accessibility.htm
47. R. O. Smith and R. Mendonca. New methodology to evaluate the consequences and usefulness of providing accessibility information. *Proceedings of the RESNA 32nd International Conference on Technology and Disability: Research, Design, Practice and Policy*, New Orleans, LA, 2009.
48. D. A. Norman. *Living with Complexity*. Cambridge, MA: MIT Press, 2011.

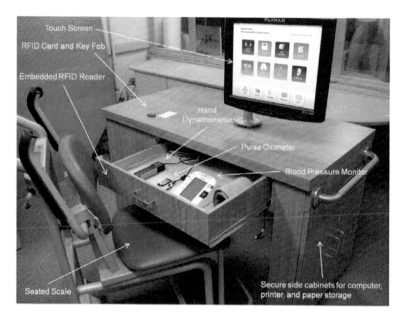

FIGURE 5.2
Multiuser health kiosk.

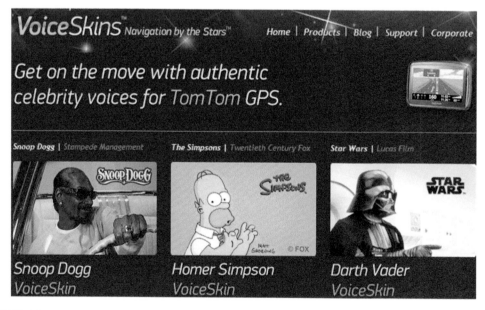

FIGURE 6.3
Garmin navigation device with personalized voice.

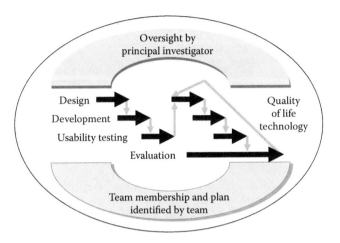

FIGURE 7.1
QoLT dynamic leadership model.

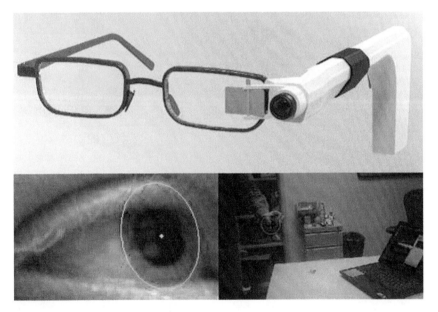

FIGURE 9.1
Example of vision device attached to eyeglasses (top) and gaze-tracking example taken with the system (bottom).

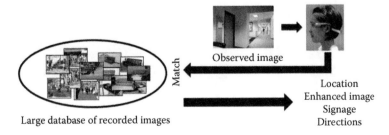

FIGURE 9.3
Localization approach: matching observed images with a large database of recorded images.

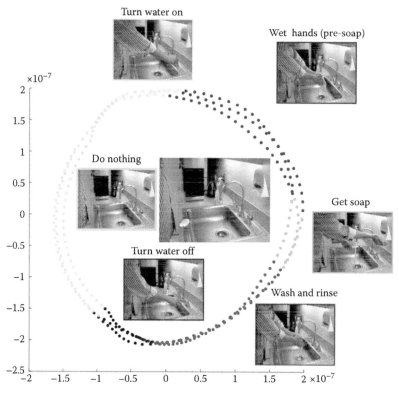

FIGURE 9.7
Segmentation of hand-washing video into distinct phases visualized in a two-dimensional projection of the feature space. The text label for each phase is added manually.

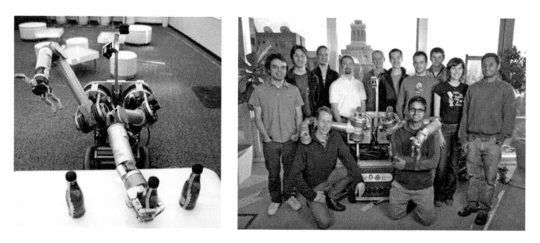

FIGURE 10.1
(Left) HERB: The home exploring robotic butler. (Right) The Personal Robotics Lab at Carnegie Mellon University.

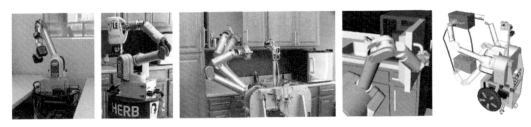

FIGURE 10.4
HERB executing paths planned by our constrained manipulation planning framework.

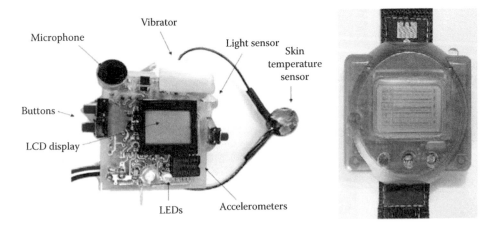

FIGURE 11.2
eWatch multisensor platform.

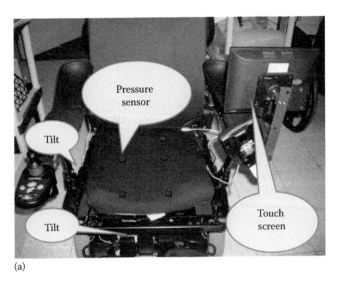

FIGURE 11.4
Power wheelchair virtual coach sensors and touch screen: (a) front view.

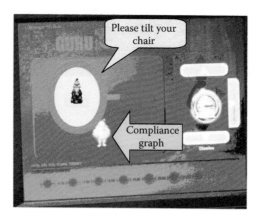

FIGURE 11.8
Virtual coach screen with a reminder to tilt. The compliance graph shows color coded hourly compliance.

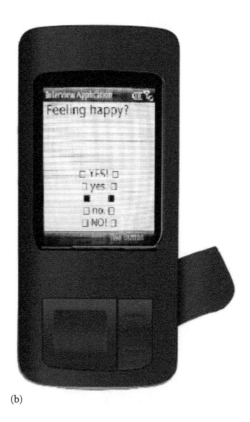

(b)

FIGURE 11.23
(b) a smartphone with a silicon sleeve button interface (right). Both platforms are displaying an example question of the interview application.

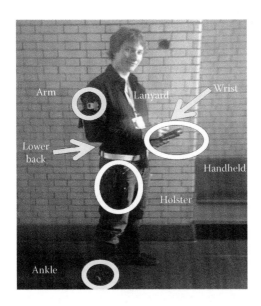

FIGURE 11.28
Multiple sensor placement.

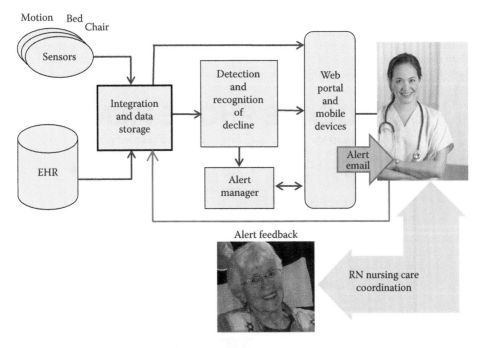

FIGURE 12.3
Integrated sensor network used for early illness alerts sent via email. Nurses provide feedback on each alert as a rating on the clinical relevance.

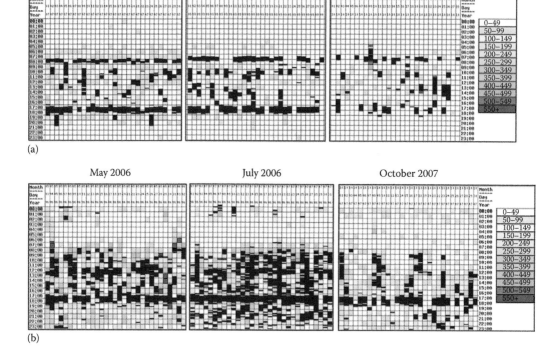

FIGURE 12.6

Motion density maps from two TigerPlace residents. Each column represents one day. The vertical axis ranges from midnight at the top to 11 pm at the bottom. Black indicates out of the apartment. The color scale shows the motion density from low density (white, gray) to high density (blue). (a) A resident who was diagnosed with depression. The density maps show decreasing activity as the resident's depression increased. (b) A resident with an irregular activity pattern indicating possible cognitive problems also shows a changing pattern in the density map.

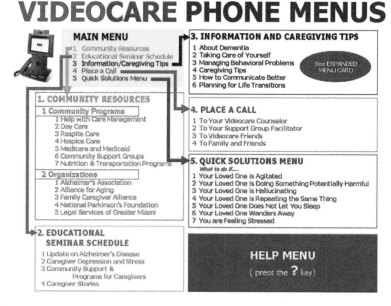

FIGURE 13.5

VideoCare caregiver program: phone menus.

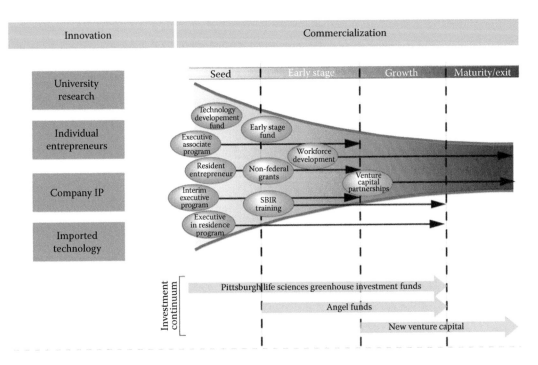

FIGURE 15.2
Innovation and commercialization in start-up companies.

7

Fostering Teamwork and Community Partnerships

Judith T. Matthews and Karen L. Courtney

CONTENTS

7.1 Introduction

Advancing a quality of life (QoL) technology from initial concept to robust and usable end-product requires effective leadership, multidisciplinary collaboration, and community partnership. Best achieved with clarity of purpose, the process of engaging team members, end users, and other stakeholders in such a creative endeavor can and should serve the diverse interests of all concerned. What may appear to require little more than common sense and intuition actually calls for the ability to nurture constructive relationships among the many people and organizations involved in a novel, multifaceted project.

This chapter focuses on how to form effective teams, foster fruitful collaboration, and cultivate community partnerships while moving emerging technologies from the realm of the possible toward invention and innovation. Drawing upon aspects of team building and project management, we offer strategies that support the cohesion necessary to facilitate and inform design, development, and evaluation of QoL technologies. Moreover, we provide examples of their implementation.

7.2 Building the Team with Dynamic Leadership

The complexity and multiplicity of needs among older adults and persons with disabilities, as well as the sophistication required to produce safe, reliable, and customizable QoL technologies for their use, necessitate involvement of many disciplines. As with any ambitious undertaking, assembling the right mix of people willing to devote time and talent to the enterprise can be both challenging and rewarding. For the person who takes the lead in spearheading the project, the challenge lies in fostering a shared vision of the invention among all collaborators. The reward comes from realizing that vision through synergies activated by their collaboration. On the other hand, for persons joining as members of the project team, the challenge is to complement others' efforts by offering unique expertise and being valued for it. For these individuals, reward derives from satisfaction in making a meaningful contribution to the project and achieving personal career objectives.

7.2.1 Gauging Interest and Motivation

The benefits of multidisciplinary teamwork to achieve innovation and improve health and function are evident in the monumental advances made in recent years in the disciplines of genomics, oncology, and prosthetics, among others. These advances have been made by researchers from diverse disciplines who have generously pooled their talents. Their successes have undoubtedly been fraught with many of the challenges to collaboration posed by the emerging field of QoL technology.

In this field, not only is it important for the project leader to begin by identifying persons with the core knowledge, skill, and judgment needed for the project, it is also crucial for that individual to understand what motivates prospective team members and what they hope to gain by participating. Frank discussion of these issues at the outset permits assessment of the extent to which individual goals and motivations may be mutually beneficial. Determining whether factors such as societal impact, intellectual and technical challenge, career ambition, or inescapable obligation drive potential collaborators' interest can help in gauging their level of commitment and their willingness to persevere through completion of the project.

7.2.2 Understanding Diverse Disciplinary Perspectives

Carefully selecting team members and exploring their particular goals and incentives may seem self-evident and not uniquely applicable to the burgeoning field of QoL technology. Yet these actions are particularly salient because project teams in this arena are often drawn from a wide array of disciplines and organizations that may not typically interact with one another or understand each other's cultures. It is not unusual for teams to comprise three general categories of members: technologists, social scientists, and clinicians (see Table 7.1). These individuals are typically recruited from the ranks of engineering, computer science, robotics, human factors, human–computer interaction, social psychology, information and decision sciences, nursing, rehabilitation science, and medicine. They are often based in different academic institutions or work in the clinical, business, or industrial sectors. Bringing together people with such disparate aptitudes and interests inevitably results in them influencing one another. The cross-fertilization of ideas that occurs enriches their understanding of users' needs, the end-product's desired features and functionalities, and the context in which it will be used.

TABLE 7.1

Disciplines with Expertise Relevant to Design and Development of QoL Technologies

Discipline	Relevant Expertise
Engineering	Building hardware (i.e., structure, machine, apparatus) that will achieve the functionality desired under anticipated operating conditions
Computer science	Constructing software algorithms that enable operation of desired functionalities
Robotics	Devising intelligent systems and devices capable of interpretation and actuation based on sensor data
Human factors	Understanding the adequacy of fit between a person's capabilities and the demands of a task, given the environment in which the task is performed and the technologies, processes, and training available to accomplish it
Human–computer interaction	Evaluating human responsiveness to various interfaces (e.g., haptic, auditory, visual, olfactory) featured in technologies encountered
Social psychology	Interpreting how people interact and influence one another in the context of life circumstances and relationships
Information and decision sciences	Organizing information systems to enable effective decision making by users ranging from professionals in a given field to naïve consumers
Nursing	Connecting developers with older adults and persons with disabilities, to enhance mutual understanding of the practical, daily implications of health and functional impairments and to assess the impact of QoL technology on their physical, cognitive, and emotional well-being
Rehabilitation science	Identifying and evaluating how therapeutic modalities and assistive technologies, imbued with intelligence, could preserve, restore, or improve recovery of optimal motor, sensory, cognitive, and perceptual functioning
Medicine	Advising developers regarding acceptable ways to summarize and integrate remotely acquired and self-monitored data into their workflow and channels of communication with patients and family caregivers

Such diversity ensures that multiple perspectives and methodologies will inform the project. However, inherent differences among groups may impede communication and make collaboration more complex, if not more difficult. Roles and responsibilities, professional jargon, sources of funding, and venues for dissemination vary widely across disciplines. Likewise, contractual agreements, allocation of resources, productivity expectations, and guidelines for promotion and remuneration often differ markedly by discipline, organization, and sector. These differences, though not entirely insurmountable, may contribute to misunderstanding and frustration among team members, potentially hampering smooth project management and delaying attainment of important project milestones.

Further complicating interpersonal dynamics is the likelihood that the team will consist predominately of senior-level researchers or executives who are used to being in charge due to their domain expertise, vision, and confidence. The propensity to be at the helm may serve them well in their home institutions or organizations. But these high-ranking individuals may find it difficult to relinquish or share power over the long term in a team of like-minded peers.

7.2.3 Embracing a New Paradigm

We contend that developing QoL technologies requires a new leadership paradigm, one that abandons the traditional top-down approach to assemble and manage a team, in favor of one that enables leadership to shift among members as the project progresses. Such an approach

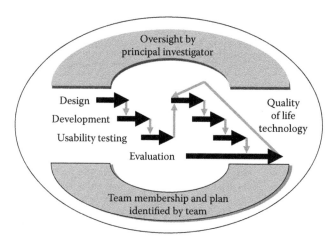

FIGURE 7.1
(See color insert.) QoLT dynamic leadership model.

would capitalize on individual team members' competencies, and do so in a timely fashion. Though several lines of work are likely to proceed in parallel on an ongoing basis, different team members should assume the lead at different points, resulting in the intensity of their involvement varying over the course of the project (see Figure 7.1). Our view is that this new paradigm would encourage the creativity, shared commitment, and flexibility needed to lead teams of peers from different disciplines and organizations, without spawning chaos.

In this model, the project leader serves as both instigator and administrator, with responsibility for assembling the core team, garnering and allocating resources, monitoring progress, and keeping the original vision within collaborators' sights. This individual initiates the project, creates the environment in which multidisciplinary collaboration can flourish, and shepherds the project to its completion. The entire team then develops and implements an operational plan based on consensus reached regarding the team's composition, workflow, strategies for problem solving, and assessment of progress.

Since no individual has all of the necessary expertise to complete the project, evaluation of the team's composition and its work plan requires deliberate consideration and periodic reconsideration. Together the team leader and team members determine the capabilities and resources needed for project success, identifying when additional expertise is needed and who should be recruited to provide it. Together they determine a detailed plan, or roadmap, for the project, specifying what is to be done and in what order, who agrees to take the lead on various aspects of the project, and when important milestones are to be achieved. Together they identify points of intersection when progress on work being done in parallel is to be shared among team members, so that the overall project can proceed. Thus, together they evaluate progress toward milestones, problem solve, and modify the plan when necessary. In so doing, the team ensures that components of the project essential for success are developed in logical sequence, with ample opportunity for quality control, testing, and refinement.

This new leadership paradigm acknowledges that team members should have equal voice, although they may differ in many respects that are not readily apparent or understood by all when the project commences. An important part of the project leader's role is to encourage individual members to explain their disciplinary and organizational perspectives that may be unfamiliar to others. Understanding the context in which each team member considers the project helps the group to coalesce, to recognize each other's vested interests, and to capitalize on their strengths.

Team members should share with one another three key pieces of information:

- Why the project is important to their discipline in terms of its potential to advance science or technology
- What their discipline or organization values are with respect to dissemination (e.g., journal articles, conference proceedings, monographs, book chapters, conferences, invited workshops, or media coverage) and funding (e.g., NSF, NIH, foundations, and industry)
- What they need from the project to make their contribution and meet their professional and personal goals

Transparency should prevail, permitting individuals to gauge when to anticipate the yield from each aspect of the project and enabling them to understand the motivations behind periodic urgency or inaction by others on the team. With knowledge of other individuals' competing demands and upcoming deadlines, team members can better interpret each other's behaviors and, if possible, accommodate their priorities. For instance, team members can be more supportive of each other when they are aware of one another's pressing deadlines or their requirements and timelines for achieving tenure or promotion. Similarly, armed with this insight, they can be more responsive to others' requests for preliminary data or other specific content to include in grant applications, Institutional Review Board (IRB) protocols, and manuscripts or reports in preparation.

7.3 Managing the Project

Teams developing QoL technology may have limited experience working with one another. They may also lack experience managing the range of activities that these projects entail. Adhering to several general guidelines can help to maintain focus and momentum, thereby promoting team cohesion:

- Establishing the significance of the project—A convincing case should be made that the proposed QoL technology would solve a clinical, functional, or QoL issue affecting individuals in the target population, or that it would solve a community or organizational challenge. Similarly, the proposed technology should represent a potential business opportunity that offers a competitive advantage over existing technologies or services.
- Defining the purpose and scope of the project—The team should articulate and agree upon the specific aims and objectives for each phase of the project, including formulation of the design concept, design of the technical specifications, demonstration of proof-of-concept, development of a prototype model, and establishment of a timeline for various types of evaluation such as simulation, laboratory testing, usability studies, and trials in naturalistic settings.
- Developing a detailed plan—The plan should specify the consensus reached by the team regarding critical milestones for each phase of the project. Further, it should stipulate whether the phases are to be completed concurrently or sequentially and estimate the resources (personnel and materials) and amount of time each phase is

likely to take. This is particularly important when one group's work is dependent upon progress made by another group on the team. Gantt charts or other systems may be used to illustrate major features of the plan and to track progress.

- Ensuring motivation—All team members should have at least one researchable question or technical challenge that reflects their vested interest in the project.

- Communicating in a timely manner—Brief, targeted exchanges between the project leader and individual team members or summary updates to the entire team should occur regularly in order to facilitate project oversight and keep all apprised of progress on concurrent lines of work.

- Respecting team members' time—In addition to making reasonable accommodation for the competing demands and pending deadlines that affect team members at different times, the team should schedule meetings only when necessary, primarily for focused deliberation and planning or problem solving. Agendas should be distributed and followed, and requests for information should allow ample time for response.

7.3.1 Example 1: Team Building for First-Person Vision Technology

QoL technologies that enable remote monitoring of health and functional status appeal to informal caregivers who may work or live far from frail or disabled family members and want to provide supervision or mobilize assistance when needed. Though inferences can be made about where people are and what they are doing using motion, heat, and light sensors, among others, cameras installed throughout the home provide the most direct evidence of day-to-day self-management. However, many older adults and persons with disabilities prefer not to have their images captured by QoL technologies that perform in-home monitoring (Beach et al. 2009).

Researchers are exploring alternate methods by which to infer personal activity patterns and behavior. Building upon prior work in first-person vision (FPV; Choudhury et al. 2006; Hodges et al. 2006; Maurer et al. 2006; Havlena et al. 2009; Spriggs et al. 2009; Sundaram and Mayol-Cuevas 2009; Van Laerhoven et al. 2009), a robotics team from Carnegie Mellon University developed a wearable, FPV device that attaches to eyeglasses and is equipped with tiny cameras which capture the user's eye movements and field of view.

Interested in learning potential users and other stakeholders' thoughts about this device, the lead roboticist attended a meeting at which attitudes toward emerging QoL technologies were explored using the group–individual synthesis method described by Downs et al. (2010) that combined individual interviews with group discussion. He demonstrated the device in its alternate forms (i.e., attached to eyeglasses or worn [without eye tracking] as an earbud, headset, or pendant), discussed its software that makes inferences from the images captured, and solicited attendees' input. Positive, if cautious, feedback suggested that both potential end users and other stakeholders considered this technology to be a plausible solution for gauging how well a person is managing and when assistance may be needed at home.

The roboticist then teamed up with investigators from the University of Pittsburgh, whose expertise included nursing, gerontology, and research methodology, to design a usability study of the first-person vision (FPV) device with community-residing older adults, with or without mild cognitive impairment, and their spouses. Together the roboticist and the nurse identified the specific aims of the study and crafted a detailed plan for usability testing. While the roboticist took the lead in making sure that the prototype hardware and software functioned properly, the nurse developed the human subjects protocol for submission to the IRB at their respective universities.

Once IRB approvals were obtained, the nurse organized implementation of the usability study, recruiting study participants through the Gerontology Registry managed by the gerontologist. During single-session home visits, one interviewer (or two, if a couple took part) engaged study participants in performing a series of randomly ordered tasks (e.g., setting the table, retrieving items from the refrigerator, showing where daily medications were stored, reading a newspaper) while they wore the eyeglass version of the FPV device and an engineer provided technical support as needed.

Shifts in leadership for various aspects of the study continued after data collection was complete. The nurse and research methodologist managed data entry and cleaning of all self-report and interview data, while the engineer prepared the video files for review and interpretation. The nurse, in turn, summarized salient qualitative and quantitative findings and shared them with team members. Suggestions for improving the design and functionality of the FPV device were incorporated into its next iteration, ensuring that the eyeglass version would be lighter and capture sound as well as a larger field of view. Motivating this team was the novelty of their work and the recognition that their combined talents were contributing to a new tool for objective assessment of functional capacity, interpersonal interaction, and need for assistance.

7.4 Cultivating Community Partnerships

Efforts to develop QoL technologies would be remarkably shortsighted, if not flawed, without input and evaluation from representatives of the target user populations and the organizations that serve their interests. Involving older adults and persons with disabilities is essential from the early ideation stage to the final evaluation of end-products designed for their use. Likewise, eliciting perspective and inviting participation of individuals from organizations with a vested interest in improving the health, independence, and QoL of these constituent groups is important. Involving these potential end users and stakeholders increases the likelihood that the QoL technology solutions developed will be usable and provide a welcome alternative to existing technologies or practices.

As important as it is to assemble a team of capable collaborators to achieve success, it is crucial to cultivate partners who are willing and able to provide honest, constructive appraisal of QoL technology during design and development and during evaluation of safety, efficacy, and effectiveness. These partnerships may build upon prior, mutually beneficial collaborations with various members of the project team. Or they may require a new initiative that begins with the team identifying community contacts whose interests are likely to dovetail with the project idea, and then requesting exploratory meetings to determine their level of interest. Either way, initial discussion between the project team and potential community partners must allow for the possibility that the original vision for a QoL technology solution will be modified, if not abandoned, should the needs assessment that pointed to the inadequacy of current solutions be deemed shortsighted or faulty.

7.4.1 Being Realistic with Community Partners

Establishing willingness to work together and reaching consensus on project aims are but first steps in community partnering. Agreement is also needed regarding who will be responsible for implementing various components of the plan (e.g., posting advertisements, recruiting study participants, making space available for consent and data collection procedures, reporting findings) within a timeframe considered reasonable by all parties involved. Likewise, developers of QoL technologies and their community partners need to achieve mutual understanding about how the project will be funded, which decisions will be made unilaterally or jointly, and who from each entity will collaborate on logistics and scheduling. These steps underscore the importance of deliberate and collaborative goal setting, joint evaluation of progress on the project, and timely communication by the project leader or other team members as they undertake activities with community partners.

The primary mission of community partners is service to their clientele. That statement, plain and simple, cannot be ignored, nor should it be. Community partners may enthusiastically welcome involvement in QoL technology research projects, and they may graciously agree to provide access to their staff, clients, and family members. But their usual priorities are unlikely to change and, understandably, must take precedence over the program of research. Members of the project team need to respect these priorities and be proactive about learning the workflow in place for administration and delivery of client services. By doing so, team members are less likely to disrupt processes that are important to both staff and clients. They are also more likely to strengthen the partnering relationship, nurturing its potential to extend from a single study focused on a single QoL technology to a series of studies for an array of emerging QoL technologies.

Team members should frequently express appreciation for their community partners' generosity in facilitating recruitment of study participants, for their input and observed reactions will undoubtedly help improve the design and advance the development of a QoL technology. Likewise, team members should be vigilant about scheduling project-related activities as far in advance as possible, to ensure that the time is convenient for community partners and their clients and, if applicable, the space required to conduct the activities is available.

In addition to providing community partners with an overview of the project when exploring their interest in collaborating, the project leader should explain the typical ebb and flow of project activities given the iterative nature of the user-centered design process (see Chapter 5). Specific time points or intervals when researchers and community partners can realistically anticipate active engagement should also be described, as should circumstances when community partners may experience extension of the timeline. Reasons for slower-than-expected progress should be explained. For instance, delays frequently occur when developers encounter difficulties rendering a novel QoL technology sufficiently robust and reliable for use in human studies.

The often lengthy process of obtaining necessary approvals prior to commencing studies warrants explanation and exploration as well. The project leader or a designated member of the project team may be required to make a formal presentation to a community partner's board of directors or in-house research or ethics committee prior to receiving a letter of support or approval for participation. Inquiring about whether this step is required by a community partner will expedite the process.

The next hurdle may entail obtaining IRB approval from the home institution of the principal investigator for studies involving human subjects, which typically takes additional weeks to secure. An IRB approval is also needed from all other academic institutions where research activities related to the project, such as data management, storage, and analysis, will take place. Similarly, research funded by the military or industry sponsors requires separate IRB approval. Depending on the number of entities affiliated with the project, the various submission formats used, and the questions each may ask, it can take months before all IRB approvals are in hand. At times, modifications may have to be made to a previously approved protocol, consent form, or other supporting materials when interpretation of mandated human subject protections differs across IRBs, despite all being bound to adhere to the same federal guidelines.

7.4.2 Example 2: Engaging Community Partners in a Multiuser Health Kiosk Project

Like most challenging endeavors, implementation of the best-laid plans is often easier said than done. Convergence of two lines of research focused on enabling community-residing older adults with or without disability to be proactive about their health provides an example of our work with community partners. As is evident in the following summary, the resulting project moved forward at times because of, and at other times in spite of, our partnering efforts.

Research has demonstrated that when people actively monitor key parameters of personal health and function such as weight, exercise, and dietary intake, they tend to adhere more closely to recommended health habits and enjoy better health outcomes (Van Achterberg et al. 2010; Burke et al. 2011). Telehealth and web-based interventions that permit self-monitoring of health and functional status, either alone or in combination with remote monitoring by clinicians in distant locations, are not widely available to low-income individuals, many of whom are older with cognitive, emotional, or physical disabilities.

Older adults make up the vast majority of individuals living in congregate housing or naturally occurring retirement communities. They tend to make disproportionate use of health care resources, and they have less computer and Internet access than younger adults or more affluent, better-educated age peers (Schoenborn and Heyman 2009; Smith 2010). Health care providers often manage these older individuals' chronic conditions based on information obtained during office visits. Otherwise they rely heavily on self-report—despite its inherent potential for recall bias—to explain what has transpired between visits.

Development and testing of a multiuser health kiosk was the goal of two separate groups affiliated with our Quality of Life Technology Center, each working with different community partners. The envisioned kiosk would be situated in residential communities or senior centers for older adults. It would enable the intended users to monitor parameters such as blood pressure, weight, and oxygen saturation at frequent intervals of their own choosing (perhaps daily or several times per week) or as prescribed by their health care providers.

The first group involved a cadre of researchers from engineering, computer science, occupational therapy, and nursing, along with administrators and clinicians from two aging services organizations and an industry partner. Originally formed to brainstorm about an array of possible projects, this group's momentum faltered over an 18 month period due to ill-defined leadership and lack of follow-through on plans to develop a prototype kiosk that would undergo usability or pilot testing. Efforts to make meetings more productive (e.g., setting and following agendas, identifying desired features and functionalities for the kiosk, developing a proposal specifying measures and procedures for usability and pilot feasibility testing with community partners) by those in the group who endorsed the vision but lacked the wherewithal to develop the technology were unsuccessful in moving the project forward. Interest waned and community partners became understandably frustrated by lack of progress. To preserve the community partnership for future collaboration, the group agreed to suspend meetings until a working prototype was available for testing in residential and other community-based settings.

The second group working on a multiuser health kiosk included faculty researchers in nursing and an administrator from the aging institute that operates under the auspices of the university medical center. This team implemented a pilot feasibility study with older adults in congregate housing, in collaboration with a community agency that provides case management to residents of several senior housing sites in the Pittsburgh area. Using a commercially available kiosk for goal setting and self-monitoring of selected health parameters (i.e., blood pressure, weight, and time spent walking), this group demonstrated that older adults could and would use such a device, despite its limitations. In contrast to the first group, the second group was led by the principal investigator for the commercial kiosk trial who embraced the leadership role. She called meetings whenever the pace of progress slackened and to clarify near-term and long-term objectives as well as a timeline for meeting those objectives.

Frustration with the commercial kiosk's poorly designed interface, few measurement options, and lack of customizability and reliability led to joint discussions involving both groups. It was decided that the proposed kiosk would become the focus of a project-based, rapid prototyping course in human–computer interaction. Over the next 15 months, prototype hardware and software and the graphical user interface were developed in close collaboration with the community partner.

Initial usability testing of the prototype health kiosk was conducted with older adults in a laboratory setting. Following revision of selected features and functionalities, more rigorous community-based usability testing is currently being conducted with 40 independently living older adults recruited from four sites. The administrator in charge of each community site has endorsed the aims and accommodated the proposed methods for recruitment, consenting of study participants, and data collection. A point person has been designated by each site administrator to handle the research team's requests and to facilitate logistics for timely delivery and retrieval of the health kiosk. In collaboration with community partners at each site, the project team has determined the most convenient and least disruptive times to conduct study activities on the premises, negotiated ample space to ensure study participants' privacy during data collection, and confirmed when the comings and goings of team members are acceptable to site staff. Table 7.2 illustrates the timeline for research activities with one of the community partner sites where community-based usability testing has been completed.

7.5 Conclusion

Creativity and technical know-how are essential for transforming novel ideas into workable technological solutions that address the myriad challenges associated with aging and disability. Yet these aptitudes alone are insufficient for successful development and deployment of emerging technologies in this arena. Developing a system or device capable of making a meaningful difference in the daily lives of older adults or persons with disabilities necessitates counterbalancing the *technical* side with the *people* side of the equation.

Unlike development of technology for manufacturing that focuses on solutions for individuals who presumably have the requisite knowledge and skills to perform specific tasks in predictable environments, QoL technology development tackles problems for people with diverse capabilities whose task performance occurs in highly variable and often unpredictable home and community environments. The complex problems that often beset intended users of QoL technologies—such as difficulty with ambulation and transfers, medication taking, and falls—rarely result in simple solutions. Indeed, one-size-fits-all solutions are rare.

TABLE 7.2

Timeline for Community-Based Usability Testing of the Health Kiosk at a Community Partner Site, by Month

Activity	Month 1	Month 2	Month 3	Month 4	Month 5	Month 6	Month 7
Invitation to community partner to participate in project	■						
Agreement by site administrator, board, ethics committee	■	■					
Letter of support from site for IRB protocol		■					
Preparation/submission of IRB protocol to lead institution		■	■				
IRB approval from lead institution			■				
Submission and approval to additional IRBs			■	■			
Site visit by project team to meet point person, see available space, learn workflow/preferred communication				■			
Recruitment using IRB-approved strategies (e.g., talks with groups; fliers/ads; emails; staff-obtained OK to contact)					■	■	■
Screening clients for eligibility in person or by phone					■	■	■
Session #1: Informed consent and baseline data collection procedures completed with eligible and willing clients					■	■	■
Delivery of health kiosk to site					■		
Session #2: Usability testing of health kiosk 2 weeks after baseline with enrolled clients (i.e., study participants)						■	■
Integration of improvements to hardware, software, and interface design based on input/observations from testing						■	■
Weekly communication with point person regarding participant accrual and study progress					■	■	■
Retrieval of health kiosk upon completion of community-based usability testing							■

Ensuring that the people, tasks, and context for which a QoL technology is being developed remain front and center requires effective leadership that sustains a shared vision and motivates teamwork among persons who may not ordinarily work together or implicitly understand one another's domain perspective or expertise. We contend that the efforts of the unique multidisciplinary teams assembled to develop QoL technologies can be optimized by adopting a new dynamic leadership paradigm, one that potentiates the synergies among team members by harnessing their diverse knowledge and skills and exploiting their leadership capabilities for particular portions of the project. Shifting the lead among team members at various points facilitates concurrent development of different components of systems or devices while moving the project forward.

Just as important as effective leadership and teamwork is cultivation of strong partnerships involving the project team and key personnel at community agencies or organizations that are willing to collaborate to achieve the shared vision. Not only do community partners enrich a project with their input, they facilitate important access to potential end users whose views and reactions are invaluable during all phases of the project. In the process, potential end users and other stakeholders may become champions of the technology developed, while team members may deepen their commitment to solving the challenges faced by their target users. By working together with knowledge and mutual respect for what each individual or entity brings to the enterprise, development of usable, acceptable, and helpful QoL technology can flourish.

References

Beach, S., R. Schulz, J. Downs et al. 2009. Disability, age, and informational privacy attitudes in quality of life technology applications: Results from a national web survey. *ACM Trans Access Comput* 2, Article 5. http://portal.acm.org (accessed October 20, 2011).

Burke, L. E., M. B. Conroy, S. M. Sereika et al. 2011. The effect of electronic self-monitoring on weight loss and dietary intake: A randomized behavioral weight loss trial. *Obesity* 19:338–344.

Choudhury, T., M. Philipose, D. Wyatt et al. 2006. Towards activity databases: Using sensors and statistical models to summarize people's lives. *IEEE Data Eng Bull* 29:49–58.

Downs, J., R. Schulz, S. R. Beach et al. 2010. Group-individual synthesis: A novel approach to garnering stakeholder input for engineered systems. Unpublished manuscript.

Havlena, M., A. Ess, W. Moreau et al. 2009. AWEAR 2.0 System: Omni-directional audio-visual data acquisition and processing. *Conf Comput Vis Pattern Recognit Workshops* (June):49–56, http://ieeexplore.ieee.org/stamp/stamp.jsp?tp=&arnumber=5204361

Hodges, S., L. Williams, E. Berry et al. 2006. SenseCam: A retrospective memory aid. *MUM Int Conf Mob Ubiquitous Multimed* 4206:177–193.

Maurer, U., A. Rowe, A. Smailagic et al. 2006. eWatch: A wearable sensor and notification platform. *International Workshop on Wearable and Implantable Body Sensor Networks*, Cambridge, MA, pp. 142–145.

Schoenborn, C. A. and K. M. Heyman. 2009. Health characteristics of adults aged 55 years and over: United States, 2004–2007. *Natl Health Stat Rep* 16:1–31.

Smith, A. 2010. Home broadband 2010. Pew Research Center Internet & American Life Project, pp. 1–28. http://pewinternet.org/2010/Home-Broadband-2010.aspx (accessed November 19, 2010).

Spriggs, E. H., F. De La Torre, and M. Hebert. 2009. Temporal segmentation and activity classification from first-person sensing. *IEEE Workshop on Egocentric Vision, CVPR 2009* (June), Miami, FL, pp. 17–24, http://ieeexplore.ieee.org/stamp/stamp.jsp?tp=&arnumber=5204354

Sundaram, S. and W. Mayol-Cuevas. 2009. High level activity recognition using low resolution wearable vision. *IEEE Workshop on Egocentric Vision, CVPR 2009* (June), Miami, FL, pp. 25–32, http://ieeexplore.ieee.org/stamp/stamp.jsp?tp=&arnumber=5204355

Van Achterberg, T., G. G. J. Huisman-De Waal, N. A. B. M. Ketelaar et al. 2010. How to promote healthy behaviors in patients? An overview of evidence for behavior change techniques. *Health Promot Int* 6:1–15, doi:10.1093/heapro/daq50

Van Laerhoven, K., E. Berlin, and B. Schiele. 2009. Enabling efficient time series analysis for wearable activity data. *Proc Int Conf Mach Learn Appl* (December):392–397. http://ieeexplore.ieee.org/stamp/stamp.jsp?tp=&arnumber=5381499

8

Evaluating Quality of Life Technologies*

Annette DeVito Dabbs, Scott R. Beach, Karen L. Courtney, and Judith T. Matthews

CONTENTS

8.1 Introduction

Involving users in the evaluation of quality of life (QoL) technologies is as important as their participation in the initial user-centered design process. The National Science Foundation defines evaluation as "…a systematic investigation of the worth or merit of an object" (Westat 2002, p. 3). This definition places the focus on conducting evaluations for action-related reasons, such that data gathered and information gleaned can be used to facilitate decisions about a course of action. Evaluation of QoL technologies provides evidence regarding whether project goals and objectives are met. It also enables assessment of the fit among different features and functionalities of the technology in relation to the user and the task in a given environment.

---

* Portions of this chapter appear in *Proceedings of the IEEE* (Schulz et al., in press).

The evaluation process frequently reveals new insights that designers and developers had not anticipated. It also helps to determine whether the use of a system or device ultimately makes a positive difference in the outcomes of interest, including QoL. As an integral component of the iterative design process, evaluation requires a practical, hands-on approach to empirical testing, which is crucial for establishing how well QoL technologies address the needs of their intended users.

In this chapter, we discuss a variety of methods for evaluating the usability, efficacy, and effectiveness of QoL technologies in either laboratory or naturalistic settings. We describe several strategies for assessing the impact of these technologies on health and function as well as QoL. Further, we offer a case example outlining the series of evaluations conducted in laboratory and community settings during development and testing of a novel technology aimed at promoting self-care and reducing adverse outcomes following lung transplantation.

8.2 Types of Evaluation

Evaluation methods vary depending on the stage of development for a QoL technology, and they can be broadly categorized as formative, summative, or both (see Table 8.1). *Formative evaluation* refers to the process of collecting data to judge the acceptability or functionality of incremental changes in the features of a technology during development. This type of evaluation begins early and is conducted at several points throughout the development life cycle for the purpose of improving usability. In contrast, *summative evaluation* refers to the process of collecting data to judge the usefulness of a mature technology or its features in achieving specified goals. Summative evaluations are typically reserved for real-world or translational settings and may be more structured and controlled than formative evaluations. Summative evaluations examine safety and efficacy or effectiveness, thereby providing evidence to inform decisions about dissemination and distribution of a technology.

8.2.1 Formative Evaluation

Initial usability testing is typically performed with users in controlled settings such as laboratories or contrived environments intended to simulate certain conditions. Later usability testing may be conducted in naturalistic environments such as homes or other community settings. The aims of the testing sessions are to ascertain how well the technology works and to identify usability problems. Ideally, individuals participating in these formative evaluations should be representative of the population targeted for the QoL technology. Through their responses, users help developers in several ways by shaping the questions to be addressed, identifying credible criteria for evaluation, providing feedback regarding form and function as well as aesthetic and ethical concerns, validating the interpretation of findings, and enabling further refinement of the technology.

Prototypes, or early versions of a system or device, are often used to evaluate iterative designs of technologies before reaching a final design decision, so that testing may proceed with minimal investment (Tullis and Albert 2008). Prototypes represent aspects of the technology that can be validated quickly by the user without construction of an entire system or functionality. For instance, users are often provided with scenarios that describe a task and the context in which it might be performed, and then asked to comment on its acceptability, helpfulness, or usefulness. They may be also asked to "test" various features

TABLE 8.1

Formative and Summative Evaluation Methods

Method	Purpose and Description	Formative	Summative
Card sort	To gather user(s) input on content, organization, language, labeling or categorizing by sorting cards with content, images, or other depictions relevant to aspects of user interface	X	
Comparison tests	To learn user(s) reactions and views regarding advantages/disadvantages of different interface styles, elements, or features	X	
Heuristic evaluation	To evaluate aspects of the design using accepted principles and practices conducted by domain, usability, or human factors experts	X	
Prototyping	To obtain feedback quickly and inexpensively from users about the content, flow, sequencing, navigation, intuitiveness, and expectations pertaining to user interfaces prior to full-fledged operability and functionality, using low fidelity paper mock-ups or wireframe drawings or a high fidelity prototype that is closer to the final product and functionality (e.g., Wizard of Oz experiment in which a man-behind-the-scenes operates a system that appears to be functional though, unbeknownst to the end user, it is not)	X	
Field testing	To evaluate performance of tasks by representative end users in naturalistic environments using the technology or any of its features for a fixed time period in order to expose usability issues and improve design	X	X
Efficacy trials	To determine whether a mature technology or its features produce an expected result under ideal circumstances specified by a research protocol	X	X
Effectiveness trials	To determine the degree of beneficial effect of a mature technology or features of a technology when deployed in real-world settings	X	X
Comparative effectiveness trials	To evaluate the effects of a mature technology compared to nontechnological options or alternate technologies to determine which works best, for whom, and under what circumstances		X
Adoption studies	To ascertain usability, utilization, and real-world strengths and weaknesses of a mature technology after formal release into the marketplace		X

of a prototype or an intermediary product by performing certain tasks while being observed. Their observed reactions to the prototype, coupled with their stated views about it, allow users to change designers' initial understanding of the work.

8.2.2 Summative Evaluation

Summative evaluation of technology is often measured in terms of efficacy, effectiveness, utilization, and adoption. For a QOL technology, evaluation needs to extend beyond utilization and adoption to include assessment of more distal outcomes. Distal outcomes typically include the relative advantage and whether the use of the technology improves task performance (e.g., driving independently), promotes intended behaviors (e.g., self-monitoring), or prevents untoward events (e.g., falls, wandering, and medication errors).

Other outcomes that warrant consideration include acceptable trade-offs (e.g., less privacy for independent living), the degree of burden (e.g., effort to learn or stigma associated with use), cost (e.g., reimbursable or out-of-pocket expenses), and QoL, as is discussed at length in the following section. This type of evaluation typically begins by testing a technology within a small group of targeted users or settings. It expands over time to include greater diversity among groups and settings, in order to enhance the generalizability of findings.

8.3 Impact of Technology on Quality of Life

Given that QoL technologies are, by definition, intended to enhance QoL among older adults and persons with disabilities, attention must be paid to this complex construct and how it can be evaluated. Over the last two decades, researchers investigating human responsiveness to disease and its treatment have widened their interest beyond objectively measured outcomes (e.g., tumor size, blood pressure, and length of hospital stay) to include subjective assessment of health-related QoL in terms of symptoms and sensations: physical, emotional, cognitive, and social function and general perceptions of health. A multidimensional construct, QoL, reflects how affected individuals appraise the impact of many facets of their situation on daily life and function. The Preface contains an introduction to the QoL construct, including a definition, basic measurement approaches, and application to assessing the impact of QoL technologies on QoL outcomes. In this chapter, we provide further examples and discussion of the measurement of QoL in the conduct of summative evaluations of QoL technology.

8.3.1 Measurement of Quality of Life

As noted in preface, definitions of QoL vary considerably, with measures traditionally categorized as either *generic* or *condition-specific* (see Table 8.2). Generic measures are applicable to all populations and conditions and thus enable cross-population comparisons. Four of the most widely used measures are the MOS 36-item Short-form Health Survey (SF-36; also available as a 12-item version, the SF-12), the Sickness Impact Profile (SIP), the Nottingham Health Profile (NHP), and the World health Organization Quality of Life Assessment (WHOQOL-100; also available as a 26-item version WHOQOL-BREF), which are summarized in Table 8.2. All four instruments assess physical, emotional, and social domains, although the specific aspects of these domains covered differ across instruments. Each of these generic instruments also covers somewhat unique domains not covered by the others. The important point for those evaluating QoL technology is the choice of a generic QoL assessment tool that best measures the specific domains targeted by the technology. For example, if the technology targets pain reduction (e.g., a wheelchair or scooter designed to reduce mobility-related pain), the SF-36 or the NHP should be used. If social function is the primary functional domain targeted (e.g., social networking technology), even though all four generic instruments cover the domain, the SIP (which assesses communication and recreation and pastimes) may be the best option.

Many other generic QoL measurement instruments are available. An excellent resource that summarizes health measurement instruments from various domains in addition to general health status and QoL (including physical disability, social health, psychological well-being, anxiety, depression, pain, and mental status) is provided by McDowell (2006).

TABLE 8.2

Selected Generic and Condition-Specific Quality of Life Measures

Source	Quality of Life Measure	Dimensions
Generic measures		
Ware and Sherbourne (1992)	MOS 36-item Short-form Health Survey (SF-36)	Physical functioning, role limitations due to physical health, bodily pain, social functioning, general mental health, role limitations due to emotional problems, vitality/energy/fatigue, general health perceptions
Bergner et al. (1981)	Sickness Impact Profile	Ambulation, mobility, body care and movement (physical); social interaction, alertness behavior, emotional behavior, communication (psychological); sleep and rest, eating, work, home management, recreation, and pastimes (other categories)
Hunt et al. (1980)	Nottingham Health Profile	Physical abilities, energy level, sleep, pain, social isolation, emotional reactions
The WHOQOL Group (1998)	WHO Quality of Life Assessment (WHOQOL-100; WHOQOL-BREF)	Overall QoL/general health, physical health, psychological health, level of independence, social relations, environment, spirituality/religion/ personal beliefs
Utility-based measures		
Horsman et al. (2003)	Health Utilities Index	Sensation, mobility, emotion, cognition, self-care, pain, fertility (HUI 2); vision, hearing, speech, ambulation, dexterity, emotion, cognition, pain (HUI3)
Perneger and Courvoisier (2010)	EuroQol EQ-5D	Mobility, self-care, usual activities, pain/discomfort, anxiety/depression (health attributes); self-perceived health (visual analog scale—direct utility assessment)
Condition-specific measures (disease)		
Meenan et al. (1980)	The Arthritis Impact Measurement Scale (AIMS)	Physical, social, and emotional well-being related to dexterity, mobility, pain, physical and social activity, depression, and anxiety
DCCT Research Group (1988)	Diabetes Quality of Life Questionnaire (DQOL)	Life satisfaction, diabetes impact, worries about diabetes, social/vocational concerns
Lundqvist et al. (1997)	Spinal Cord Injury Quality of Life Questionnaire (SCIQL-23)	Anxiety, depression, social interaction, body care and movement, mobility
von Steinbuchel et al. 2010	Quality of Life After Brain Injury (QOLIBRI) scale	Cognition, self, daily life and autonomy, social relationships, emotions, physical problems
Ritvo et al. (1997)	MSLQI: Multiple Sclerosis Quality of Life Inventory	Set of generic and disease-specific QOL instruments assessing fatigue, pain, sexual satisfaction, bladder control, bowel control, visual impairment, cognitive dysfunction, mental health, social support
Condition-specific measures (domain)		
Ventry and Weinstein (1982)	Hearing Handicap Inventory for the Elderly (HHIE)	Emotional impact, social and situational effects

(continued)

TABLE 8.2 (continued)

Selected Generic and Condition-Specific Quality of Life Measures

Source	Quality of Life Measure	Dimensions
Melzack (1975)	McGill Pain Questionnaire (MPQ)	Pain description on 20 dimensions (e.g., temporal, spatial, dullness, tension, sensory), change in pain over time, pain intensity
Simets et al. (1995)	Multidimensional Fatigue Inventory (MFI)	General fatigue, physical fatigue, reduced activity, reduced motivation, mental fatigue
Radloff (1977)	Center for Epidemiologic Studies Depression Scale (CES-D)	Depression symptoms: depressed mood, feelings of guilt and worthlessness, feelings of helplessness, psychomotor retardation, loss of appetite, sleep disorders

This book includes copies of the actual instruments, discussions of the conceptual basis and domains covered, and a summary of available psychometric data for each measure.

Utility-based approaches, exemplified by the Health Utilities Index (HUI) (Horsman et al. 2003) and the EQ-5D (Kind et al. 2005; Perneger and Courvoisier 2010), elicit preferences for different health states in terms of both health status and the value of that health status to the individual. While these instruments may cover similar domains as the generic QoL instruments described earlier, utility measures are often used in cost-benefit analyses of the impact of medical interventions, and scores are converted to a universal metric known as the "utility," with possible scores ranging from 0 (representing death) to 1 (representing "perfect health"). The utility represents a preference for a particular health outcome, for example, one that results from an intervention, and it is typically used to calculate "quality adjusted life years" (QALY). QALYs are a combination of length of life the intervention will allow (in years) multiplied by the utility or value placed on the "quality" of the health state produced by the intervention. Thus, an intervention that prolongs life by 5 years and produces a health state with a utility of .9 results in a QALY of 4.5, while one that prolongs life by 7 years with a health state utility of .6 would result in a QALY of 4.2. In such a scenario, the first intervention would presumably be preferred even though it results in fewer years of life but a higher QoL for year lived.

It should be noted that the EQ-5D and the HUI use standard survey question approaches to derive the utilities (0–1) indirectly. For example, the EQ-5D obtains reports on mobility, self-care, usual activities, pain/discomfort, and anxiety/depression (three possible levels each), resulting in a potential 243 health state profiles. Each health state profile can be translated into a utility scale using an algorithm derived from a large-scale, population-based study in which independent samples provided values for a subset of the 243 profiles using direct utility assessments methods. Direct utility assessment relies on more complicated methods like the "standard gamble" (SG) or "time trade-off" (TTO) in which people are asked how much risk they would be willing to endure SG or how many years of life they would be willing to give up TTO to be free of a particular health state (e.g., living with pain and disability). Another approach is to ask how much someone would be willing to pay for a particular intervention that produces a specific health outcome ("willingness to pay"). Finally, some instruments measure utilities directly by using 100-point visual analog scales with 0 ("worst imaginable health state") and 100 ("best imaginable health state") as endpoints for individuals rating either their own health or a hypothetical health state. It is beyond the scope of this chapter to describe these utility-based approaches for measurement of QoL in detail, but the interested reader is referred to Torrance and Feeny (1989) for a detailed introduction.

Condition-specific QoL measures pertain to particular diseases (e.g., cancer, arthritis, and asthma) or domains (e.g., disability, anxiety, depression, pain, and fatigue). A few examples are shown in Table 8.2. These measures are more relevant and sensitive to the specific situation and, therefore, permit detection of important effects that generic instruments might miss. The disadvantage is that condition-specific measures cannot be used for meaningful comparison of QoL across conditions. In the context of QoL technology summative evaluations, technologies targeted to specific diseases should strongly consider supplementing any generic QoL measures with an appropriate disease-specific instrument. In terms of domain-specific measures, although the generic instruments may assess aspects such as depression, pain, and fatigue, if a QoL technology specifically targets a particular domain, the evaluation team should consider a more detailed assessment tool like the Center for Epidemiologic Studies Depression (CES-D) Scale, the McGill Pain Questionnaire (MPQ), or the Multidimensional Fatigue Inventory (MFI).

In summary, most experts recommend using a combination of generic and condition-specific approaches, for the best of both worlds: comparability and specificity. Measures, whether generic or condition specific, should be selected based on psychometric performance and practical considerations. Instruments should be reliable and valid for use with the target population, and they should be adequately sensitive to change over time. They should be scrutinized for their relevance to the target population. Additionally, measures should be appropriate with respect to respondent burden (length and complexity), mode of administration (self-administered vs. interviewer-administered or performance-based), and complexity of scoring.

A third category of measures relevant to QoL technology consists of *technology-specific* outcome measures. These are measurement instruments that focus on the impact that a particular technology has on the user's QoL. Those conducting summative evaluations of QoL technology should consider using a technology-specific measure in addition to the generic and condition-specific tools discussed earlier. This approach maximizes coverage of the range of potential effects of technology on QoL.

Over the past decade, work has been supported by the National Institute on Disability and Rehabilitation Research (NIDRR) in the area of assistive technology outcome assessment methodology. Specially, the Assistive Technology Outcomes Measurement System (ATOMS) Project (www.r2d2.uwm.edu/atoms/) and the Consortium for Assistive Technology Outcomes Research (CATOR) (www.atoutcomes.com) have developed technology-specific outcome instruments, resource repositories, and methodologies. These projects are good resources for QoL technology developers seeking or developing technology-specific outcome assessment instruments to be used in conjunction with more traditional generic or condition-specific QoL measures.

8.3.2 Diverse Perspectives: Direct Users, Health Care Providers, and Family Members

It is important to elicit the perspective of multiple stakeholders affected by QoL devices and systems. Older adults and persons with disabilities who are direct users may be more or less enthralled with a particular QoL technology than their family members, health care providers, or health insurers who experience indirect effects of use. For instance, direct users may disagree with other stakeholders about the benefits and costs of use on different dimensions of QoL. Or they may value outcomes differently, such as the time required for providing assistance or the convenience associated with obtaining health or functional status information for clinical decision making. A delicate balance must be struck among all users' preferences in order to ensure acceptance and adoption.

8.3.3 Cognitive and Physical Impairment

Consideration should also be given to the cognitive and physical capabilities of individuals asked to complete QoL measures. Depending on the stage and degree of impairment, cognitively impaired individuals may be able to respond to standardized QoL instruments using specialized assessment strategies. These strategies are designed to minimize frustration and behavioral symptoms such as agitation, restlessness, and aggression. Strategies include providing simple directions, using simple response formats, relying on performance-based measures, and using multiple measurement methods. Family caregivers may serve as proxy respondents for objective data, but they should not be relied upon for subjective evaluation of QoL since they tend to underestimate perceptions of QoL for older or disabled family members receiving their care. Persons with physical impairments may also require special approaches or accommodation to enable completion of QoL measures. These include offering Braille versions of questionnaires and survey forms or switching to interviewer-administered forms for blind individuals, providing larger font versions of forms to those who are visually impaired, and using paper-and-pencil forms or special telephone amplification or other augmentative communication devices when interviewing individuals who are hearing impaired.

8.4 Example of Formative and Summative Evaluation: Pocket PATH®

People who actively engage with clinicians in managing their chronic health conditions tend to experience better health outcomes than those who do not (Bondeheimer et al. 2002; Coleman and Newton 2005; Kruelen and Braden 2004; Lorig et al. 2001; Martin et al. 2003). That is, they are less apt to endure symptoms and more likely to detect or prevent complications, thereby avoiding unnecessary hospitalization, functional disability, or even premature death. However, like many people with a chronic illness, individuals who undergo lung transplantation often fail to recognize signs and symptoms that may be early indicators of serious and potentially life-threatening complications such as organ rejection or infection. Even when cognizant of these signs and symptoms, they may be unsure about what and when to report condition changes to their health care providers in a timely manner.

Clinical observation of self-management practices (or lack thereof) among lung transplant recipients, coupled with the aforementioned scientific evidence, suggested that some of these adverse health outcomes could be mitigated, if not avoided altogether, with a portable technological solution to enhance self-monitoring. DeVito Dabbs and colleagues (2009a,b), thus, developed the Personal Assistant for Tracking Health, known as Pocket PATH®. This handheld device provides lung transplant recipients with customized data recording, trending, and decision-support software that assist recipients in self-monitoring transplant-related health parameters and promotes their self-care. Guided by an adaptation of the model of usability testing throughout the product lifecycle proposed by Rubin and Chisnell (2008), this team harnessed its expertise in nursing, social science, human–computer interaction, software engineering, communication, graphic design, and research methodology to develop and evaluate this novel QoL technology. The adapted model (see Figure 8.1) is firmly grounded in principles of user-centered design and specifies three phases: (1) establishing the need and specifications for a particular system or device for

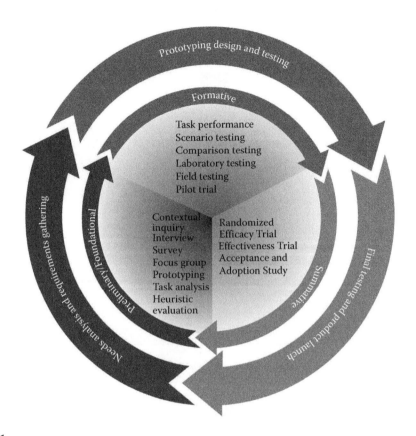

FIGURE 8.1
Model of usability testing throughout the product life cycle. (Adapted from Rubin, J. and Chisnell, D. *Handbook of Usability Testing: How to Plan, Design and Conduct Effective Tests*, 2nd edn., John Wiley & Sons, Hoboken, NJ, 2008, and used to guide evaluation of PocketPATH®.)

the target population (i.e., needs analysis and requirement gathering); (2) building and iteratively refining prototypes based on their appeal and performance with an array of users in varied settings (i.e., prototyping, design, and testing); and (3) rigorous scrutiny of the impact of the end-product in both well-controlled studies and general use (i.e., final testing and product launch).

To date, the Pocket PATH project has included several studies for either formative or summative evaluation of the device and its novel software at various stages of design and development. The timeline presented in Table 8.3 shows that these investigations have spanned many years. It further reflects the team's foresight and perseverance in methodically building the case for a well-designed, usable QoL technology that is both capable of satisfactorily addressing the identified needs of its users and producing desired health outcomes.

8.4.1 Assessment of the Need for Pocket PATH

The development team established the need for a novel technological solution by supplementing its clinical observations and knowledge of the benefits of self-monitoring with information regarding characteristics of lung recipients that could affect their use of computer-based technologies. Characteristics included demographic factors such as age,

TABLE 8.3

Timeline for Development and Evaluation of Pocket PATH for Lung Transplant Recipients

Activity	2000	2001	2002	2003	2004	2005	2006	2007	2008–2012
Literature review of health benefits of self-management after transplant	■								
Focus groups with clinicians to learn self-management expectations (e.g., health indicators, threshold values)		■							
Contextual inquiry to assess self-management at home		■							
Need and features identified for technology to aid self-management			■						
Institutional Review Board approval obtained for human subjects research							■		■
Pocket PATH prototype developed based on iterative usability sessions with recipients in laboratory setting				■	■				
Field trial to evaluate Pocket PATH prototype for usability					■	■			
Refinement of Pocket PATH prototype based on field trial findings						■	■		
Randomized, controlled pilot trial to estimate efficacy of Pocket PATH vs. standard care for self-management							■	■	
Full-scale, randomized, controlled trial to determine efficacy of Pocket PATH vs. standard care for self-management and transplant-related health outcomes									■

gender, and race or ethnicity; proficiency reading English; and experience with computers. Other relevant characteristics were symptoms including blurred vision and numbness and functional impairments such as tremors and fine motor limitations that would preclude the use of mobile devices.

The team also conducted a contextual inquiry in order to learn how lung transplant recipients carried out self-monitoring activities in their homes and to elicit their views about how technology might support these tasks (DeVito Dabbs et al. 2009b). This contextual inquiry involved interviews and field observations in the homes of seven lung transplant recipients who were told by the interviewer, "I'm here to learn how you gather and keep track of the information that you consider important for monitoring your health since your transplantation."

Interview responses revealed these transplant recipients' desire for novel technology with several customized functionalities that would facilitate self-monitoring. These functionalities included the capacity to record simply and accurately measures for a variety of objective and subjective posttransplant indicators and to display data in ways that made it easy to recognize subtle changes and trends. These transplant recipients also wanted the technology to issue warnings when critical values were reached and to provide decision support messages that would prompt them to report changes about which their clinicians expected to be notified. Lastly, they envisioned a technology that would help to organize their contact information and provide reminders when necessary to take medications or perform self-monitoring activities. The need for such features would not have been apparent without having conducted the contextual inquiries with persons in their typical surroundings. Results of the contextual inquiry led developers to incorporate various features and functionalities such as displaying data in graphical formats, trending self-monitoring data over time, and providing automatic, data-driven feedback messages into the initial product design.

8.4.2 Usability Sessions in Controlled vs. Field Settings

During the prototyping, design, and testing phase, a variety of formative evaluation strategies were used to assess the usability of Pocket PATH. For these evaluations, end users were purposively sampled—that is, deliberately selected because of their specific characteristics or experiences—to include lung transplant recipients from various age groups, both genders, and diverse racial and ethnic minorities. The sample also included lung transplant recipients with limited computer experience as well as with blurred vision, tremors, and short-term memory impairments. These end users were selected because these side effects are commonly associated with transplant-related medications.

The early usability testing sessions relied on prototypes and scenarios and were conducted in controlled laboratory settings. Lung transplant recipients were given scenarios to simulate tasks they would perform at home with the device. They were encouraged to use the "think-aloud" technique, which entailed providing a running commentary of their thoughts while performing the specified intended tasks. The developers relied on their own observation and on screen-capturing techniques enabled by video and audio recording software loaded on a laptop and synchronized to record how the users made selections and navigated the system's features on the handheld device. For example, during the usability session, lung recipients were shown prototypes of graphical user interfaces and features and asked to interact with the device to perform simple tasks, such as record a blood pressure value, or rate the intensity of a symptom. This investigation enhanced the team's understanding of users' interpretations, and it resulted in modifications to the interface that included better labeling of health parameters to record and easier ways to navigate between features.

After the laboratory evaluation, Pocket PATH was field tested to determine whether lung transplant recipients found it feasible to use independently in their homes, and to assess the functionality of all of its features, including data recording, data display, and data transmission. Six test users were asked to record their measurements: daily spirometry values, blood pressure, pulse, and symptom ratings, among others. The results were displayed on the iPAQ (personal digital assistant) screen in both log and graphical display formats. Normal thresholds were set for each clinical parameter based on clinical expert recommendations and established clinical guidelines. Feedback messages were generated when values outside the acceptable range were entered. Users were also asked to make any suggestions for improving the device, its interface, and the user manual. Following the field study, the six test users returned to the study center to test the final version of Pocket PATH and to provide feedback as they evaluated its features and functionality.

8.4.3 Pilot Feasibility Testing

A subsequent randomized, controlled pilot trial was conducted to evaluate the efficacy of Pocket PATH in promoting self-monitoring among individuals randomized to use Pocket PATH (n = 15) vs. standard care (n = 15) for the first 2 months following hospital discharge after lung transplantation. The platform was updated for smart phones with cellular network capabilities. Based on this pilot trial, Pocket PATH was found to be more efficacious than standard care, insofar as the Pocket PATH group performed daily monitoring and reported condition changes to clinicians in a timelier manner and at significantly higher rates than standard care controls. Effect sizes (r) for these outcomes ranged between 0.45 and 0.57. Moreover, this small-sample intervention trial provided preliminary evidence that lung transplant recipients could and would use Pocket PATH to monitor and manage their condition, and the use of Pocket PATH could improve self-monitoring and other self-care behaviors (Devito Dabbs et al. 2009a).

8.4.4 Evaluation of Efficacy

Based on the success of the pilot trial, the team is conducting a summative evaluation of Pocket PATH's efficacy prior to the product launch phase. A full-scale, randomized, controlled trial (target N = 214) is currently underway to test the efficacy of Pocket PATH in promoting self-care agency, self-care behaviors, and transplant-related health in the first year after transplantation. This clinical trial is designed to demonstrate whether the use of the device significantly improves perceptions of capability in caring for oneself, encourages adherence to recommended self-care behaviors, and results in better health outcomes relevant to transplantation, when compared to patients receiving standard discharge instructions and relying on their own methods to track and interpret changes in their health conditions.

Randomized clinical trials to evaluate the efficacy of a technology are particularly important to third-party payers such as insurance companies and Medicare. These organizations typically require strong evidence that the technology improves health and/or saves money when compared to existing practice for a particular condition. One of the major strengths of randomized trials is that they are able to control for or eliminate biases common in other evaluation strategies, and therefore provide strong evidence of efficacy when they are successful. The downside of randomized trials is that they are typically expensive to carry out, requiring large numbers of study participants and stringent implementation and data collection strategies.

8.4.5 Preparation for Effectiveness Trials

Recently, this process of involving end users in testing throughout the product lifecycle has been repeated with lung transplant clinicians as end users for a complementary web-based interface for clinicians. Pocket PATH Link is being developed to support remote data sharing and communication between lung transplant recipients using Pocket PATH and their clinician partners. Formative testing is also underway to evaluate the feasibility and usability of Pocket PATH Synergy, which integrates Pocket PATH and Pocket PATH Link to support patient–clinician interaction behaviors required for collaborative care. Future summative testing is planned to evaluate the effectiveness of Pocket PATH Synergy in promoting better patient–provider partnerships, collaboration, and, ultimately, health outcomes including QoL. The final stage will be to evaluate acceptance and adoption of Pocket PATH in real-world, clinical settings.

8.5 Conclusion

Both formative and summative evaluations of QoL technology are needed throughout the development life-cycle. As the Pocket PATH exemplar illustrates, comprehensive evaluation can take considerable time. However, this time is well spent because comprehensive evaluation of new QoL technologies is necessary not only for adoption by end users such as patients, clinicians, or family members, but also for building sufficient evidence for future health care reimbursement or funding.

Evaluation of QoL technologies must be more than just a functional analysis of the technology, that is, whether it can perform as designed. The diversity of potential effects of QoL technologies can be captured through careful development of an overall evaluation plan. Different QoL measures may be used depending on whether the purpose of evaluation is formative or summative, but a multifaceted approach should be employed. Part of the evaluation strategy should include careful matching of QoL measures to both direct and indirect users as well as to the technology, with the use of generic QoL measures enabling cross-technology or cross-condition comparisons, while the use of condition- and technology-specific measures will ensure adequate in-depth evaluation of domains specifically targeted by the technology.

References

Bergner, M., R. A. Bobbitt, W. B. Carter et al. 1981. The sickness impact profile: Development and final revision of a health status measure. *Med Care* 19:787–805.

Bondeheimer, T., K. Lorig, H. Holman et al. 2002. Patient self-management of chronic disease in primary care. *JAMA* 288:2469–2475.

Coleman, M. T. and K. S. Newton. 2005. Supporting self-management in patients with chronic illness. *Am Fam Physician* 72:1503–1510.

DCCT Research Group. 1988. Reliability and validity of a diabetes quality-of-life measure for the Diabetes Control and Complications Trial (DCCT). *Diabetes Care* 11:725–732.

DeVito Dabbs, A. J., M. A. Dew, B. Myers et al. 2009a. Evaluation of a hand-held, computer-based intervention to promote early self-care behaviors after lung transplant. *Clin Transplant* 23:537–545.

DeVito Dabbs, A., B. A. Myers, K. R. McCurry et al. 2009b. User-centered design and interactive health technologies for patients. *Comput Inform Nurs* 27:175–183.

Godwin, M., L. Ruhland, I. Casson et al. 2003. Pragmatic controlled clinical trials in primary care: The struggle between external and internal validity. *BMC Med Res Methodol* 3:28.

Horsman, J., W. Furlong, D. Feeny et al. 2003. The Health Utilities Index (HUI®): Concepts, measurement properties and applications. *Health Qual Life Outcomes* 1. http://www.hqlo.com/content/1/1/54 (accessed November 24, 2010).

Hunt, S. M., S. P. McKenna, J. McEwen et al. 1980. A quantitative approach to perceived health status: A validation study. *J Epidemiol Community Health* 34:281–286.

Kind, P., R. Brooks, and R. Rabin, eds. 2005. *EQ-5D Concepts and Methods: A Developmental History*. Dordrecht, the Netherlands: Springer.

Kreulen, G. J. and C. J. Braden. 2004. Model test of the relationship between self-help-promoting nursing interventions and self-care and health status outcomes. *Res Nurs Health* 27:97–109.

Lorig, K., D. Sobel, P. Ritter et al. 2001. Effect of a self-management program on patients with chronic disease. *Eff Clin Pract* 4:256–262.

Lundqvist, C., A. Siosteen, L. Sullivan et al. 1997. Spinal cord injuries: A shortened measure of function and mood. *Spinal Cord* 35:17–21.

Martin, L. R., K. H. Jahng, C. E. Golin et al. 2003. Physician facilitation of patient involvement in care: Correspondence between patient and observer reports. *Behav Med* 28:159–164.

McDowell, I. 2006. *Measuring Health: A Guide to Rating Scales and Questionnaires*. New York: Oxford.

Meenan, R., P. Gertman, and J. Mason. 1980. Measuring health status. The arthritis impact measurement scales. *Arthritis Rheum* 23:146–152.

Melzack, R. 1975. The McGill pain questionnaire: Major properties and scoring methods. *Pain* 1:277–299.

Perneger, T. V. and D. S. Courvoisier. 2011. Exploration of health dimensions to be included in multi-attribute health-utility assessment. *Int J Qual Health Care* 23(1):52–59.

Radloff, L. S. 1977. The CES-D Scale: A self-report depression scale for research in the general population. *Appl Psychol Measurement* 1:385–401.

Ritvo, P., J. Fischer, D. Miller et al. 1997. *Multiple Sclerosis Quality of Life Inventory: A User's Manual*. New York: National Multiple Sclerosis Society.

Rubin, J. and D. Chisnell. 2008. *Handbook of Usability Testing: How to Plan, Design and Conduct Effective Tests*, 2nd edn. Hoboken, NJ: John Wiley & Sons.

Schulz, R., S. R. Beach, J. T. Matthews et al. In press. Designing and evaluating quality of life technologies: An interdisciplinary approach. *Proceedings of the IEEE*.

Smets, E., B. Garssen, B. Bonke et al. 1885. The multidimensional fatigue inventory (MFI): Psychometric qualities of an instrument to assess fatigue. *J Psychosom Res* 39:315–325.

Torrance, G. W. and D. Feeny. 1989. Utilities and quality-adjusted life years. *Int J Technol Assess Health Care* 5:559–575.

Tullis, T. and B. Albert. 2008. *Measuring the User Experience: Collecting, Analyzing, and Presenting Usability Metrics*. New York: Elsevier.

Ventry, I. and B. Weinstein. 1982. The hearing handicap inventory for the elderly: A new tool. *Ear Hear* 3:128–134.

von Steinbuchel, N., L. Wilson, H. Gibbons et al. 2010. Quality of life after brain injury (QOLIBRI): Scale development and metric properties. *J Neurotrauma* 27:1167–1185.

Ware, J. E. and C. D. Sherbourne. 1992. The MOS 36-item Short-Form Survey (SF-36). *Med Care* 30:473–483.

Westat, J. F. 2002. *The 2002 User-Friendly Handbook for Project Evaluation (REC 99–12175 Evaluation of NSF Educational Programs)*. Arlington, VA: National Science Foundation.

WHOQOL Group. (1998). The World Health Organization Quality of Life Assessment (WHOQOL): Development and general psychometric properties. *Soc Sci Med* 46:1569–1585.

Part III

Core Technologies and
Their Application

9

Vision-Based Sensing Approaches to QoLT

Martial Hebert and Takeo Kanade*

CONTENTS

9.1 Introduction

Understanding the user's environment, her behavior, and her intent from sensor data is a key feature of intelligent systems designed to augment the user's capability, for example, to help older adults and people with disabilities in their daily activities. In this section, we explore key technologies in the general area of visual sensing, that is, systems that can automatically extract information from images and videos from cameras.

Broadly speaking, we are interested in systems that can answer three different types of questions from visual input. First, we would like the system to be able to understand what and who is in the user's environment. This includes semantic-free descriptions of the environment's geometry, such as the configuration of potential obstacles, which can be used to provide important mobility information to a blind person or to an intelligent wheelchair. This also includes more detailed information such as recognizing specific objects in the environment, or even semantic information such as the identity of the persons interacting with the user or about their activities. Being able to extract such information opens the door to the development of systems that address a wide range of cognitive and perception deficits.

A second class of questions that a system should address has to do with understanding where the user is located in the environment. The most immediate need is to support the blind population, in particular in indoor environments for which GPS-based localization systems are inoperative, but, more generally, automatic user localization is a foundation for systems that can provide richer information such as directions, access to signage that is not visible from the user's position, or location of the nearest accessible entrance/exit for mobility-limited users.

Finally, visual interpretation systems may need to understand in what activities the user is engaged. This level of information can range from low-level bits (the user is

---

* In collaboration with Byron Boots, Alvaro Collet, Fernando Dela Torre, Michael Devyver, Ed Hsiao, Takeo Kanade, Hongwen Kang, David Lee, Ekaterina Taralova, and Akihiro Tsukada.

walking vs. sitting down) to higher-level semantic description of complex activities (e.g., preparing a meal). Segmenting and recognizing individual user actions and identifying sequences of actions as complex activities are fundamental building blocks of systems that can analyze the user's activities to detect anomalies, predict future tasks, or automatically assess skill level. Detecting anomalies in behavioral routines could be a valuable tool for early identification of individuals who are likely to become demented. Verifying task completion and assessing skill level are useful in guiding cognitively impaired individuals (e.g., TBI) through task completion. They can be used to relearn how to perform tasks that have been lost due to injury or brain lesions. Task sequencing would enable people with cognitive impairments to complete a few simple daily tasks.

While achieving such levels of sensor interpretation capabilities is a very ambitious goal, recent developments in the computer vision and machine learning fields enable the development of these capabilities, as demonstrated by initial implementations of these ideas over the past decade. In addition, rapid progress in hardware and software used in small, low-cost, low-power embedded systems makes the transfer of these ideas from laboratory systems to practical systems usable by client populations a reality. Their quality-of-life technology (QoLT) applications are many and include augmentation systems for people with low vision or blindness, prosopagnosia, and mild cognitive deficits, and systems for improving caregivers' ability to assess patient's status. As discussed later in this section, adding a second camera to the first person vision (FPV) gives us the ability to reconstruct the three-dimensional structure of the scene, which is an important feature for mapping obstacles for mobility.

In the remainder of this chapter, we briefly review the state of the art in support of sensing systems and of interpretation techniques in the aforementioned three areas, illustrated with examples drawn from current research in vision systems for QoLT, and we discuss key barriers and challenges that need to be overcome for practical deployment of QoLT systems. We focus here on visual sensing from cameras as a rich source of information. However, major progress has been achieved in using information from sensors, such as pressure, temperature, motion, sound, vision, tactile, location, position, and accelerometers, which are typically low power, size, and cost. We investigate the possibilities afforded by these nonvision sensors in Chapters 11 and 12.

9.2 Sensing

The rapid explosion in the demand for portable devices such as phones, PDAs, and tablets, has vastly accelerated the development of low-cost, low-power, miniaturized cameras with sufficiently high image quality that they can be used for advanced image and interpretation tasks. For example, CMOS cameras with resolution, field of view, and image quality that were only available in handheld form factor are now available in miniaturized form suitable for embedded systems. In addition to rapid progress in sensing hardware, much progress has been made in storage technology. Indeed, data storage on a single micro-card sufficient for recording an entire day of video data is available commercially now and TB-size storage devices on a small form factor, for example, 1 in 3, will become available in the next few years.

The implication for QoLT systems is that it is now possible to build a sensing system that a user can wear at all times. Such a sensing system should include a camera observing the user's environment at all times in addition to motion sensors (accelerometers integrated in inertial measurement units [IMUs]) to sense the user's motion.

An additional camera can provide the necessary information for real-time gaze tracking, thus providing the key additional information of where the user is looking at any given time. While many systems for eye tracking have been built in the past, advances in sensor technology make it possible to use unobtrusive cameras to track the eye. Advances in image processing algorithms (Devyver et al. 2011) enable gaze tracking without additional projected infrared light, as is the case in conventional eye trackers (Duchowski 2002, Young and Sheena 1975). This is a particularly important consideration for QoLT applications whose primary target populations would not be accepting of devices using active illumination.

Figure 9.1 shows one implementation of this approach, termed FPV. In this example, the device includes a forward-looking camera, an inward-looking camera for eye tracking, a three-axis IMU, onboard storage for 1 day of recording, and communication interfaces (Devyver et al. 2011). This system uses a shape-based pupil tracker that is more robust and requires less parameter tuning than other approaches based on outputs of filters that are characteristic of the eye region (Hallinan 1991, Noris et al. 2011), or based on detecting the characteristic shape of the pupil's edges, approximated by an ellipse (Li et al. 2006, Vester-Christensen et al. 2005).

Because such a sensing system sees the environment from the same perspective as the user's, and because it follows the user's activities, such a sensing system can provide the necessary data for a vision system to analyze the user's environment and his or her activities. This observation has been used through different types of devices for seeing from the user's perspective in a variety of applications (Mayol-Cuevas 2004, Schiele et al. 1999, Starner et al. 2008, Stiefmeier et al. 2008). Here we focus on the implications of this concept to QoLT applications, illustrated through our own work on FPV techniques.

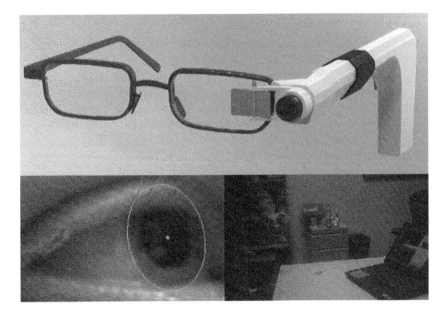

FIGURE 9.1
(**See color insert.**) Example of vision device attached to eyeglasses (top) and gaze-tracking example taken with the system (bottom).

Unlike systems that rely on observing the environment from an outside perspective, such as surveillance systems or instrumented rooms, these wearable sensors enable closer symbiosis between human and computer so that the system can extract richer information directly relevant to understanding the user's true activities and intent. In fact, the importance of capturing and modeling the user's viewpoint, in particular as it relates to behavior and intentions, has been studied extensively (Hayhoe and Ballard 2005, Just and Carpenter 1976). In robotics, models of attention and gaze have been used extensively in the field of active vision (Aloimonos 1990, Aloimonos et al. 1988, Rao and Ballard 2002, Rimey and Brown 1994). The recent advances discussed earlier enable the development of practical systems.

In the rest of this chapter, we show how the use of vision systems is a fertile ground on which to grow new opportunities for QoLT systems. For example, relating the scene viewed by the vision system with prestored data enables automatic localization, recognizing objects supports understanding of the user's interaction with the environment, and people recognition can be coupled with gaze estimation.

Considerable new technical challenges need to be overcome in developing these new applications. In computer vision, algorithms for online interpretation of combined video and IMU data need to be developed. In machine learning, the availability of the vast amount of data from vision systems pose new challenges in developing tractable, efficient approaches to learning, and inference from very large training sets. At the same time, exciting new opportunities emerge as vision data become available to develop algorithms for far more detailed and pertinent representations of the user, her behavior, and her interactions with the environment.

9.3 Recognition: What and Who?

A key goal of vision systems is to provide information that makes the system environment-aware, that is, to recognize the key elements of the scene seen in the camera, including static objects, people, and three-dimensional structure of the scene.

The most basic level of information that can be extracted from visual data is the geometric layout of the user's environment, such as the location of major obstacles and the location of entrances, exits, and pathways. Although this level of interpretation does not convey any semantic information, it is extremely valuable for QoLT systems. For example, systems for the blinds would rely on detecting objects and room layout ahead; systems that use autonomous control of physical devices would benefit from knowing the layout of the environment ahead (short-range sensing solutions exist for reactive control near objects but visual analysis would provide information much further ahead, thus anticipating hazards far ahead).

Estimating layout information from a single camera input is a very difficult task, primarily because the problem is poorly constrained: many different three-dimensional scene layouts can give rise to the same image. This problem has been addressed by computer vision researchers through techniques that combine image features, for example, color or distribution of edges, and geometric constraints, for example, walls are orthogonal to each other or three-dimensional objects rest on the ground plane, into an objective function that is optimized given an input image (Delage et al. 2006, Hedau et al. 2010, Lee et al. 2009, 2010).

While research into the problem of layout estimation from a single image has led to important developments, practical QoLT systems would have access to a continuous stream of video data, not just individual frames. As a result, the environment reconstruction problem can be greatly simplified by taking advantage of tracking of features over time using structure from motion (SFM) techniques. These single-camera techniques are still limited in that they cannot deal easily with combined motion of the camera (i.e., of the user) and of independent agents moving in the environment, for example, in a crowded street or hallway, and they have technical limitations in recovering the absolute scale of scene and motion.

To address these issues, it is well known that by using two cameras instead of one, it is possible to recover the three-dimensional structure of the environment through more direct techniques. Specifically, by using two cameras, we can recover in principle three coupled pieces of information: the three-dimensional structure of the world, the user's motion (termed "ego-motion") in her environment, and the motion of independently moving objects. The three-dimensional structure of the environment can be recovered by stereopsis by identifying image features in common between the two camera views. The motion information can be recovered by matching features across sequences of images.

From a systems viewpoint, as we have noted in the introduction, the cost, size, and power of commercial cameras decrease rapidly at the same time that quality improves dramatically, motivated by the huge consumer market for personal handheld devices. In fact, phone manufacturers are now considering using dual camera systems to be able to capture "three-dimensional photos" from phone cameras. The implication for QoLT systems is that we need to move aggressively in this direction.

From a software standpoint, the problem of simultaneously estimating structure and motion from stereo images has a long history in computer vision: For example, ego-motion and three-dimensional landmark position of static world points can be estimated by using standard filtering techniques (Jung and Lacroix 2003), by tracking blobs in the images (Agrawal et al. 2005, Ess et al. 2009, Talukder and Matthies, 2004), or by using additional data from inertial sensors (Franke et al. 2009). These techniques have been used for detecting and tracking independent motion in crowded scenes (Ess et al. 2009). Stereo vision is also used to provide navigation support to compensate for low vision or blindness (Lu and Manduchi 2005, Sez and Escolano 2008, Treuillet et al. 2007, Zhang et al. 2008).

In one example from our work (Badino and Kanade 2011), we track stereo features and we use temporal filters to estimate their position and velocity, while simultaneously estimating the ego-motion of the camera using a robust method. We integrate the tracking algorithm in a wearable mobile system that provides information of three-dimensional structure, independent motion, and ego-motion to augment the perception of the user in complex environments. As the user navigates in her environment, the system detects and tracks image features and computes their corresponding stereo disparities. The features and disparities of consecutive frames are used to compute the ego-motion of the camera using a robust least squares algorithm. A filter then fuses feature tracking, stereo disparity, and extracted ego-motion to iteratively estimate the three-dimensional position and three-dimensional velocity of each tracked feature in a user-oriented coordinate system. This system runs in real time on a standard laptop, showing that it will be feasible with moderate additional effort to implement such approaches on real-time systems. These initial prototypes help make a compelling argument that practical systems can be produced for QoLT applications in the near future.

The next level of environment understanding relies on identifying specific objects in the scenes observed by the system. Object identities provide important cues as to the user's activities and guidance as to where key objects relevant to the user's daily routine are located.

In state-of-the-art techniques, models built from collections of images from different views can be used for locating specific objects in the user's field of view. The basic approach is based on finding groups of local features in the image that agree with the model in terms of local appearance and in terms of global geometric consistency. Recently, these recognition techniques (Bay et al. 2008, Collet and Srinivasa 2010, Collet et al. 2009, 2011, Torres et al. 2010) have been shown to support real-time, online recognition of household objects. This includes recognizing objects with which the user has interacted in images as a key step toward understanding activities (Fathi et al. 2011, Ren and Gu 2010). Figure 9.2a shows sample outputs from the recognition system from a typical run of the system. Interestingly, the system is able not only to locate the objects in the image but also to estimate the object's three-dimensional location and orientation within the user's viewing frustum. This enables more elaborate reasoning about the geometric configuration of the user's workspace.

These state-of-the-art approaches suffer from two major limitations. First, results such as the one shown in Figure 9.2a are impressive, but they do not extend to all of the objects that one would find in typical daily activities environments, for example, the home. Specifically, the objects shown in this example are three-dimensional objects with distinctive texture and markings, whereas, in fact, many typical household objects either have no texture content (Figure 9.2b) or have ambiguous appearance due to repeated features. Effective recognition of such objects is difficult as confirmed by formal quantitative evaluation of standard recognition approaches showing poor level of performance on many common objects used in daily activities (Ren and Philipose 2009). This problem is critical for object recognition technology to be applied to everyday living scenarios. Current research addresses this challenge by grouping similar features together prior to comparing image and model to boost recognition performance substantially in cases of ambiguous object appearance (Hsiao et al. 2010), and by using a representation based on contour fragments instead of the standard representations that are based on local histograms of gradients (Lowe 2004). Initial results show that it is possible to recognize objects that can be described only by a few simple contour elements. These "simple" objects are particularly challenging because they can easily generate false detections in scene clutter, yet they are pervasive throughout all of the everyday environments. While considerable progress has been made in these areas, robust recognition remains a considerable challenge.

A second major limitation of the existing recognition approaches is that building the object models requires considerable expert supervision, which would dramatically reduce their applicability. One possible approach to streamlining the model building process is based on the popular concept of crowd sourcing in which images are distributed over the Web along with tools for entering annotations (Sorokin et al. 2010).

The alternative is to somehow automatically "discover" objects in visual data, and to build models of these objects. In this case, visual data mean data acquired by the user as she carries out her normal activities. Here again, the idea is to learn useful information, in this case models of common objects, from the user's experience. In related work, the problem of learning appearance models from unlabeled collections of images has received a lot of attention in the computer vision community, primarily motivated by access to large collections of images on the Web (Lee and Grauman 2010, Payet and Todorovic 2010, Sivic et al. 2005). While this research community focuses on generic categories, in the context of QoLT systems, we are interested in building models of specific objects. While operational systems for object discovery are still far in the future, considerable progress has been made in this area. Specifically, techniques have been developed for grouping regions extracted from a large number of images into clusters, filtering the irrelevant clusters, and selecting those clusters that correspond to individual objects (Kang et al. 2011b).

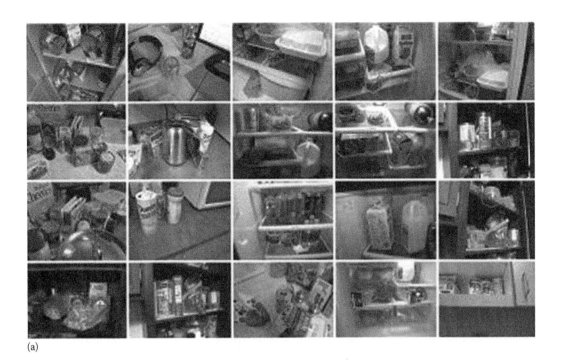

(a)

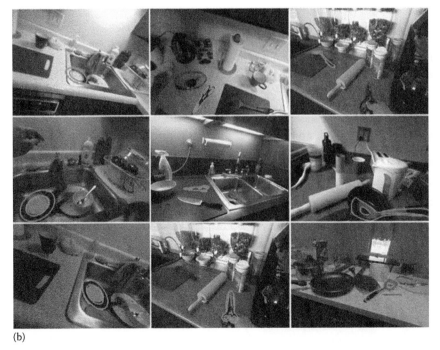

(b)

FIGURE 9.2
Example of recognizing object instances in complex scenes (a) and examples of recognizing common, texture-less objects (b).

Experiments on standard benchmarks from the literature and on our own data from wearable systems show promising performance.

While these results are promising, considerable progress remains to be made. In particular, we need to be able to deal with the huge volume of data that would be produced by an FPV system in continuous use (current approaches handle relatively modest amounts of data). We also need to exploit the gaze information from the eye-tracking part of the system, which would provide guidance as to which part of the image should be emphasized in the discovery process. Despite these challenges, the combined developments in the computer vision community, motivated by mining Web data, and in robotics, motivated by autonomous exploration applications, supported by considerable advances in storage technology make it realistic to expect the advent of practical systems in the future. If we are successful, the benefits of such an approach are immense: We can now imagine systems that can "train" themselves by observing the user's environment and memorizing models of familiar objects without input from the user.

The capabilities described so far generate useful information about the physical interactions between the user and the environment. However, a crucial aspect of people's daily activities involves social interactions. In fact, degradation in the quality of social interactions, for cognitive or physical reasons, is a key factor in increased dependency, depression, and illness. For these reasons, it is important for a system designed to understand the user's environment to be able to provide information relevant to social interactions such as the locations of people in the scene, their identity, and even some indication of their activities and their emotions. All of these cues can then be combined to generate a more complete picture of the user's environment that goes far beyond the mere physical configuration of objects and toward models of human interactions.

To implement these capabilities, real-time techniques for face detection and face recognition are now commercially available (Pittsburgh Pattern Recognition, http://www.pittpatt.com/). Coupled with eye tracking, they enable detection and, possibly, identification of the person(s) viewed in the region of the user's field of view designated by the estimated gaze direction.

9.4 Recognition: Where?

Valuable information can be extracted from vision data without scene reconstruction or recognition by comparing the scene currently seen by the vision system with previously observed data. The basic concept is illustrated in Figure 9.3. Assuming that a large

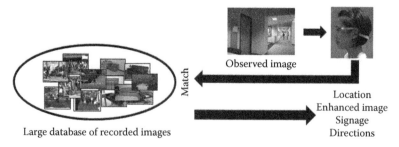

FIGURE 9.3
(See color insert.) Localization approach: matching observed images with a large database of recorded images.

collection of images has been collected in an environment and can be accessed by the system, then, in principle, the image from the database that is most similar to the image seen by the vision system can be retrieved. The information associated with the best matched image can then be retrieved and used. This concept implements the natural idea of searching through past experience—the stored images—to retrieve information associated with the environment currently seen.

The most obvious piece of information that can be retrieved through image matching is the user's location in the environment as was explored in early work on wearable system (Schiele et al. 1999). Figure 9.4 illustrates the output of such a prototype localization system based on image matching. In this example, a building floor is represented by a collection of approximately 80,000 stored images, each of which is associated with the pose (location and orientation) of the camera. At run time, the poses associated with the four best matching images are combined to generate a best estimate of the user's pose based on the current image.

This is an attractive approach to localization because it does not rely on external localization systems, such as GPS, as do most of the existing localization systems and, therefore, can operate in any environment. Beyond the obvious localization application, this concept of image matching can potentially enable the retrieval of richer information from the stored experience. For example, given the viewpoint estimated by image matching, the system can retrieve images with higher resolution in selected regions such as signs, thus revealing parts of the environment not visible from the user's current perspective. Valuable information can be extracted from vision data without scene reconstruction or recognition by comparing the scene currently seen by the vision system with previously observed data. Assuming that a large collection of images has been collected in an environment and can be accessed by the system, then, in principle, the image from the database that is most similar to the image seen by the vision system can be retrieved. The information associated with the best matched image can then be retrieved and used. This concept implements the natural idea of searching through past experience—the stored images—to retrieve information associated with the environment currently seen.

The key building block for this type of system is an algorithm that can find the nearest image to the query image based on a similarity measure. This has been extensively studied in computer vision in the context of image retrieval from image databases (Jegou et al. 2009, Philbin et al. 2007), in which considerable progress was made in designing effective data structures for large-scale indexing. However, most approaches rely on the fact that images are sufficiently dissimilar from each other to be compared based on distributions of local features. In contrast, in QoLT applications, we are interested in comparing images taken in typical daily activities, for example, home or office. In this type of environments, a major obstacle to the development of high performance system is that images tend to be very similar to each other, in that they differ only in small details characterized by few local features, while global image features are very similar. A key research topic is to automatically select distinctive features for image matching. Many images may be similar to the query image, but it may be possible to use localized details, such as a red emergency lever, to disambiguate between the candidate images. Earlier work in information theory (Katayama and Satoh 2001) and experiments on data sets from actual environments suggest that it is indeed possible to perform image matching even in highly ambiguous environments, which is critical in QoLT contexts.

From a systems standpoint, implementing this strategy leads to interesting challenges. A first issue is to build the reference database of images. In our initial work, we collected the images automatically by using a robot roaming the environment and sampling pictures.

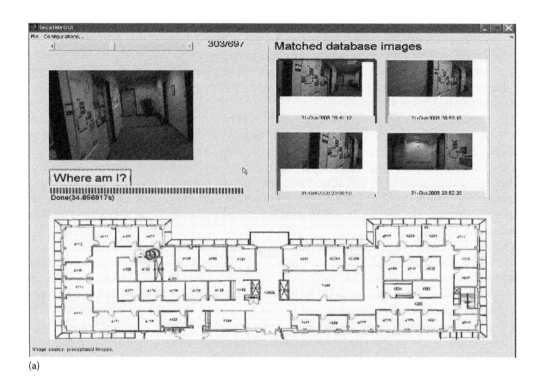

(a)

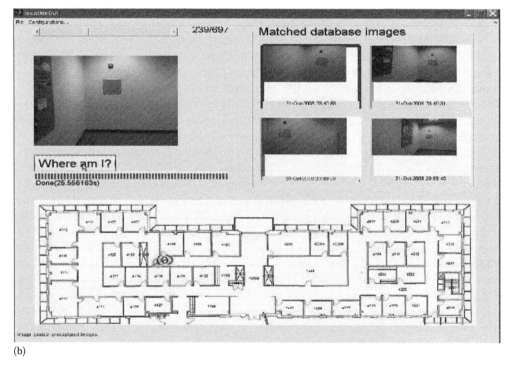

(b)

FIGURE 9.4
Two examples of localization from images: each panel (a) and (b) shows the input image (upper left), four closest matches to the input image (upper right), and estimated localization in the current floor plan.

A more practical approach would be to use images collected by users themselves to populate the database. A second issue is the ability to seamlessly transmit the information relevant to the system. For example, as the user enters a building, all the information necessary for localization would be automatically downloaded to the user's system. This is enabled by advances in distributed systems, networking, and new concepts such as cloudlets.

A third issue is that the environment is not static and may change between the time reference images are collected and the time the current image is observed. This issue is complicated by the fact that direct image differencing is not possible because the images are taken from different viewpoints. Despite the change in viewpoint, it is possible to align the query image with the retrieved reference images sufficiently well to identify regions that are not consistent with the alignment and, therefore, correspond to changes (Kang et al. 2009). This added capability ensures robustness with respect to changes in the environment and enables other functions such as warning the user of hazards that were not documented in the initial mapping of the environment.

9.5 Recognition: What Activity?

The next level of visual data interpretation involves understanding the user's activities. An example is illustrated in Figure 9.5, which shows samples of the ground-truth data used for developing activity understanding capabilities (CMU Kitchen data set 2009). In that example, the vision system observes different meal preparation activities (samples from five recipes are shown). An automatic interpretation system would (1) build models from the activities from training sensor data; (2) recognize the sequence of steps performed by the user in input data (Figure 9.5 [bottom] shows such a sequence from ground-truth manual annotations); and (3) predict future steps from the current understanding of the activity.

Automatic modeling, identification, and prediction of activities would enable a number of augmentation scenarios that are difficult to implement with current technology. For example, anomaly detection in behavioral routines is a valuable tool for early identification

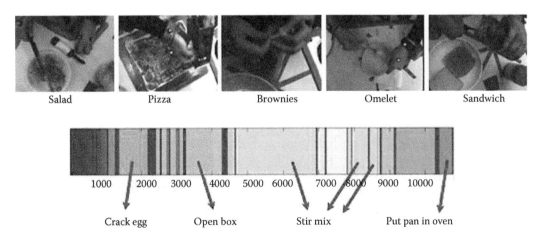

FIGURE 9.5
Example of an activity recognition task: identifying steps in a recipe. Top: Sample video frames from five cooking activities; Bottom: Example of labels used as ground truth for training and performance evaluation.

of individuals who are likely to become demented. Task completion is useful in guiding cognitively impaired individuals (e.g., TBI) through task completion. In particular, it can potentially be used to relearn how to perform tasks that have been lost due to injury or brain lesions. Task sequencing is an important building block for designing an aid that would enable people with cognitive impairments to complete a few simple daily tasks.

There are considerable technical challenges that need to be addressed before activity understanding capabilities from visual data can reach the level of performance that can support an effective augmentation system. Challenges range from building representations of complex video data usable for automatic interpretation, to dealing with large amounts of training data with tremendous variability across samples, to making inference on complex models of activity. At the same time, opportunities for making the problem tractable are afforded by the first-person nature of the data, for example, constrained viewpoint and knowledge of focus of attention, and the large amount of data that can be collected. We briefly review key aspects of current research addressing these challenges in the remainder of this section.

A first challenge is to extract models of activity from sensor data. For example, given sensor data recorded while a person is performing a common activity, for example, cooking, we want to automatically identify temporal sections of the data corresponding to elementary actions, so that we can (1) identify the activity, (2) predict future actions using the techniques described earlier, or (3) identify anomalies in the person's behavior. Converting the raw sensor data to useful features and using these features effectively in these three tasks are challenging research issues.

A first approach can be formulated as a straight classification problem in which low-level features extracted from input data (video frames and, possibly, IMU readings) are collected into feature vectors and fed to a standard classifier. In this type of approaches, it is difficult to identify complex activities spanning significant time intervals. Instead, they are normally used for short-duration, atomic actions. Figure 9.6 shows a typical example for three action classes: walking, waiting, and sitting. These actions were used to describe the activities that a user would conduct to take a bus. In this example, the features are built by computing optical flow over each of the video frames (the optical flow at each point of a grid of sampled points is shown in the example frames of Figure 9.6). Because the optical flow pattern is the apparent motion induced in the image by the user's ego-motion, it is an important cue to distinguish between basic motion patterns.

Detecting individual actions is not sufficient for understanding complex activities for which we need deeper models of the interactions between elementary actions and their sequencing over time. This raises a host of issues regarding how to represent the model, how to learn it from training data, and how to use it to infer activities from input data.

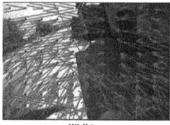
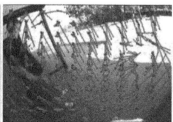
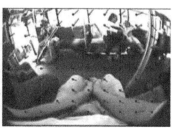

  Walking   Waiting   Sitting

FIGURE 9.6
Optical flow pattern for three different types of motions.

While these problems have been studied extensively in a variety of scenarios for activity understanding, we focus our discussion on these interpretation tasks.

Classical approaches model and recognize temporal sequences as sequences of elementary actions with probabilistic transitions spanning varying time intervals, or they model them as continuous time series. A crucial limitation of these techniques is that they do not scale well to tasks with large state spaces, as would be the case in daily activities and that they cannot represent time horizons longer than a few steps ahead. Alternate models have been proposed to address these limitations (Boots and Gordon 2010, Boots et al. 2010, Siddiqi et al. 2010) showing progress in increasing the complexity of the model, that is, number of actions and states, while keeping the amount of data needed to learn the model limited. Current research challenges in this area include the development of efficient algorithms for learning and applying the models, and for scaling up to complex activity models with many states.

All of these different approaches to activity understanding share the need for representing sensor data in a form that can be used by the learning and classification algorithms. In particular, vision data need to be segmented into samples corresponding to individual actions, and the samples need to be clustered by using some similarity metric. Here, three key challenges need to be addressed.

First, there is enormous variability across subjects performing the same actions in an unconstrained environment. Developing representations that capture features that are common to different subjects but discriminative across different activities is an enormous challenge. Second, in addition to the variability in viewpoint inherent to any vision task, we need to deal with the additional time dimension along which the data may be subjected to considerable temporal variation.

Technically, the first issue complicates its representation through the type of compact vocabulary of visual features that is typically used in state-of-the-art approaches. Specifically, typical approaches quantize feature vectors from a large training set into a compact codebook by relying heavily on clustering algorithms, which, for data with large within-class variability, tend to produce groups of features that belong to individual subjects, rather than groups that encode the desired classes, thus failing to discriminate new examples at test time. One possible approach to this challenge is to modify the standard codebook generation framework for data sets that exhibit such variability by forcing features from multiple subjects to be clustered together (Taralova et al. 2011). Such approaches are inspired by recent advances in the clustering literature (Law et al. 2004, Wagstaff et al. 2001) in which standard clustering strategies are modified to incorporate constraints from domain knowledge (in this case, the subjects from which the data originated). Rather than searching for an optimal clustering, it produces a codebook that generalizes well across subjects and is robust to large within-class variability. Initial experimental results on standard video analysis benchmarks and the kitchen data set validate the benefits of this approach, but the search for effective feature representations remains a key challenge.

A second major challenge in comparing sequences for the purpose of activity identification is the ability to perform temporal alignment of observations, a research area that has recently received increasing attention in machine learning and computer vision (Rao et al. 2003). In general, alignment of data from two or more subjects performing a given activity is a challenging problem. To solve this problem, major challenges include (1) how to compensate for the speed and stylistic variability of actions across and within subjects, (2) how to temporally model the exponential number of possible actions, (3) how to align behaviors that have been recorded with different sensors (e.g., video and motion capture data), and (4) how to develop efficient computational algorithms that scale linearly in the length of the sequences. Approaches to address these challenges attempt to extend standard approaches to temporal alignment, such as dynamic time warping (DTW), to automatically generate feature weights to adapt to different motion style and speed with complexity linear in the length of the sequences, thus guaranteeing computational efficiency (Zhou and DelaTorre 2009, 2011). This also addresses the challenging problem of aligning motions that have been recorded with different modalities (e.g., video and motion data) through feature weighting. Experimental results show that these approaches can efficiently solve the multimodal temporal alignment problem and outperform state-of-the-art methods for temporal alignment of signals with the same modality.

Even assuming good ways of representing and aligning sequences, a final challenge is to segment video sequences and to generate clusters corresponding to individual actions. Solving this challenge would enable the development of systems that can learn activity models from unsupervised data, without the manual annotations based on fixed taxonomies of action sequences, and to more effective activity recognition systems. State-of-the-art approaches combine advanced alignment techniques with unsupervised clustering techniques suitable for high-dimensional feature representations (Nguyen et al. 2011).

Detecting individual actions is not sufficient for understanding complex activities for which we need deeper models of the interactions between elementary actions and their sequencing over time. This raises a host of issues regarding how to represent the model, how to learn it from training data, and how to use it to infer activities from input data.

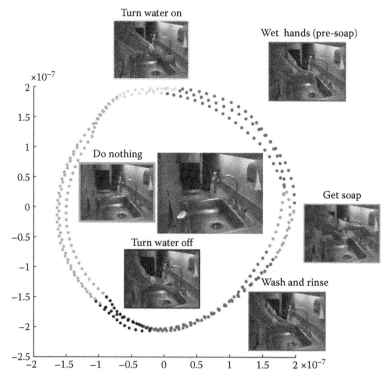

FIGURE 9.7
(See color insert.) Segmentation of hand-washing video into distinct phases visualized in a two-dimensional projection of the feature space. The text label for each phase is added manually.

While these problems have been studied extensively in a variety of scenarios for activity understanding, we focus our discussion to progress in using the FPV data for these interpretation tasks.

Classical approaches model and recognize temporal sequences as sequences of elementary actions with probabilistic transitions spanning varying time intervals as in, for example, classical approaches based on hidden Markov models (HMMs), or they model them as continuous time series as in Kalman filters. A crucial limitation of these techniques is that they do not scale well to tasks with large state spaces, as would be the case in daily activities and that they cannot represent time horizons longer than a few steps ahead.

Different models are needed to address these issues. They include algorithms that can be used in problems with large state spaces but low-complexity transition models (Satinde et al. 2004; Siddiqi et al. 2010). Even more general models are based on dynamical models that allow for mixed discrete and continuous representations and can represent complex distributions with multiple hypotheses (Boots and Gordon 2010, Boots et al. 2010). Current research challenges in this area include the development of efficient algorithms for learning and applying the models, and for scaling up to complex activity models with many states.

Figure 9.7 shows an example of using this type of approaches for analyzing FPV sequences. This example uses video data of hand washing, a common activity of daily living. This activity consists of a number of temporally extended phases (wetting hands, applying soap, rinsing, etc.), each of which varies in appearance and duration. The data are automatically segmented into distinct phases. Interesting perspectives in this area of research is to not only model and recognize actions but also predict future actions. Recent results in learning predictive models in motion prediction and driving application provide a promising foundation for this research direction (Ratliff et al. 2009; Ziebart et al. 2009a,b 2010).

References

Agrawal, M., K. Konolige, and L. Iocchi. 2005. Real-time detection of independent motion using stereo. In *Proceedings of IEEE Workshop on Motion and Video Computing*, Orlando, FL.

Aloimonos, J. 1990. Purposive and qualitative active vision. In *Proceedings of the 10th International Conference on Pattern Recognition*, Atlantic City, NJ.

Aloimonos, J., W. Weiss, and A. Bandyopadhyay. 1988. Active vision. *International Journal of Computer Vision* 1, no. 4:333–356.

Badino, H. and T. Kanade. 2011. A head-wearable short-baseline stereo system for the simultaneous estimation of structure and motion. In *Proceedings of the Machine Vision Applications*, Nara, Japan.

Bay, H., A. Ess, T. Tuytelaars, and L. Van Gool. 2008. SURF: Speeded up robust features. *Computer Vision and Image Understanding* 110, no. 3:346–359.

Boots, B. and G. J. Gordon. 2010. Predictive state temporal difference learning. In *Proceedings of the Advances in Neural Information Processing Systems*, Vancouver, British Columbia, Canada.

Boots, B., S. M. Siddiqi, and G. J. Gordon. 2010. Closing the learning-planning loop with predictive state representations. In *Proceedings of Robotics: Science and Systems VI*, Pittsburgh, PA.

CMU Kitchen data set. 2009. http://kitchen.cs.cmu.edu

Collet, A., D. Berenson, S. S. Srinivasa, and D. Ferguson. 2009. Object recognition and full pose registration from a single image for robotic manipulation. In *Proceedings of the IEEE International Conference on Robotics and Automation*, Kobe, Japan.

Collet, A. and S. Srinivasa. 2010. Efficient multi-view object recognition and full pose estimation. In *Proceedings of the IEEE International Conference on Robotics and Automation*, Anchorage, AK.

Collet, A., S. Srinivasa, and M. Hebert. 2011. Structure discovery in multi-modal data: A region-based approach. In *Proceedings of the IEEE International Conference on Robotics and Automation*, Shanghai, China.

Delage, E., H. Lee, and A. Ng. 2006. A dynamic Bayesian network model for autonomous 3D reconstruction from a single indoor image. In *Proceedings of the Conference on Computer Vision and Pattern Recognition*, New York.

Devyver, M., A. Tsukada, and T. Kanade. 2011. A wearable device for first person vision. In *Proceedings of the International Symposium on Quality of Life Technologies*, Pittsburgh, PA.

Duchowski, A. 2002. A breadth-first survey of eye-tracking applications. *Behavior Research Methods* 34:455–470.

Ess, A., B. Leibe, K. Schindler, and L. Van Gool. 2009. Moving obstacle detection in highly dynamic scenes. In *Proceedings of the International Conference on Robotics and Automation*, Kobe, Japan.

Fathi, A., X. Ren, and J. Rehg. 2011. Learning to recognize objects in egocentric activities. In *Proceedings of the Conference on Computer Vision and Pattern Recognition*, Colorado Springs, CO.

Franke, U., C. Rabe, H. Badino, and S. Gehrig. 2009. 6D-Vision: Fusion of stereo and motion for robust environment perception. In *Proceedings of the DAGM Symposium*, Jena, Germany.

Godfrey, A., R. Conway, D. Meagher, and G. O. Laighin. 2008. Direct measurement of human movement by accelerometry. *Medical Engineering and Physics* 30, no. 10:1364–1386.

Hallinan, P. W. 1991. Recognizing human eye. *Proceedings of SPIE* 1570, no. 1:214–226.

Hayhoe, M. and D. Ballard. 2005. Eye movements in natural behavior. *Trends in Cognitive Sciences* 9, no. 4:188–194.

Hedau, V., D. Hoiem, and D. Forsyth. 2010. Thinking inside the box: Using appearance models and context based on room geometry. In *Proceedings of the European Conference on Computer Vision*, Crete, Greece.

Hsiao, E., A. Collet, and M. Hebert. 2010. Making specific features less discriminative to improve point-based 3D object recognition. In *Proceedings of the Conference on Computer Vision and Pattern Recognition*, San Francisco, CA.

Jegou, H., C. Schmid, H. Harzallah, and J. Verbeek. 2009. Accurate image search using the contextual dissimilarity measure. *IEEE Transactions on Pattern Analysis and Machine Intelligence (PAMI)* 57:888–892.

Jung, I.-K. and S. Lacroix. 2003. High resolution terrain mapping using low altitude aerial stereo imagery. In *Proceedings of the International Conference on Computer Vision*, Nice, France.

Just, M. A. and P. A. Carpenter. 1976. Eye fixations and cognitive processes. *Cognitive Psychology* 8:441–480.

Kang, H., A. Efros, M. Hebert, and T. Kanade. 2009a. Image composition for object pop-out. In *Proceedings of the IEEE Workshop on 3D Representation for Recognition (3dRR-09)*, Kyoto, Japan.

Kang, H., A. A. Efros, M. Hebert, and T. Kanade. 2009b. Image matching in large-scale indoor environment. In *Proceedings of the Workshop on Egocentric Vision (Conference on Computer Vision and Pattern Recognition)*, Miami, FL.

Kang, H., M. Hebert, and T. Kanade. 2011a. Image matching with distinctive visual vocabulary. In *Proceedings of the IEEE Workshop on Applications of Computer Vision (WACV)*, Kona, HI.

Kang, H., M. Hebert, and T. Kanade. 2011b. Discovering object instances from scenes of daily living. In *Proceedings of the International Conference Computer Vision*, Barcelona, Spain.

Katayama, N. and S. Satoh. 2001. Distinctiveness-sensitive nearest neighbor search for efficient similarity retrieval of multimedia information. In *Proceedings of the International Conference on Data Engineering*, Heidelberg, Germany.

Law, M. H., A. Topchy, and A. K. Jain. 2004. Clustering with soft and group constraints. In *Proceedings of the Structural, Syntactic, and Statistical Pattern Recognition*, Lisbon, Portugal.

Lee, Y. J. and K. Grauman. 2010. Collect-cut: Segmentation with top-down cues discovered in multi-object images. In *Proceedings of the Conference on Computer Vision and Pattern Recognition*, San Francisco, CA.

Lee, D., A. Gupta, M. Hebert, and T. Kanade. 2010. Estimating spatial layout of rooms using volumetric reasoning about objects and surfaces. In *Proceedings of the Advances in Neural Information Processing Systems*, Vancouver, British Columbia, Canada.

Lee, D., M. Hebert, and T. Kanade. 2009.Geometric reasoning for single image structure recovery. In *Proceedings of the Conference on Computer Vision and Pattern Recognition*, Miami, FL.

Li, D., J. Babcock, and D. J. Parkhurst. 2006. Openeyes: A low-cost head-mounted eye-tracking solution. In *Proceedings of the Symposium on Eye Tracking Research and Applications*, San Diego, CA.

Lowe, D. G. 2004. Distinctive image features from scale-invariant keypoints. *International Journal of Computer Vision* 60:91–110.

Lu, X. and R. Manduchi. 2005. Detection and localization of curbs and stairways using stereo vision. In *Proceedings of the International Conference on Robotics and Automation*, Barcelona, Spain.

Mayol-Cuevas, W. 2004. Wearable visual robots. PhD thesis, University of Oxford, Oxford, U.K..

Nguyen, M. H., Z. Lan, and F. De la Torre. 2011. Joint segmentation and classification of human actions in video. In *Proceedings of the Conference on Computer Vision and Pattern Recognition*, Colorado Springs, CO.

Noris, B., J.-B. Keller, and A. Billard. 2011. A wearable gaze tracking system for children in unconstrained environments. *Computer Vision and Image Understanding* 115, no. 4:476–486.

Payet, N. and S. Todorovic. 2010. From a set of shapes to object discovery. In *Proceedings of the European Conference on Computer Vision*, Crete, Greece.

Philbin, J., O. Chum, M. Isard, J. Sivic, and A. Zisserman. 2007. Object retrieval with large vocabularies and fast spatial matching. In *Proceedings of the Conference on Computer Vision and Pattern Recognition*, Minneapolis, MN.

Rao, R. and D. Ballard. 2002. An active vision architecture based on iconic representations. *Artificial Intelligence* 78, no. 1–2:461–505.

Rao, C., A. Gritai, M. Shah, and T. F. Syeda-Mahmood. 2003. View-invariant alignment and matching of video sequences. In *Proceedings of the International Conference on Computer Vision*, Nice, France.

Ratliff, N., B. Ziebart, K. Peterson, J. A. Bagnell, M. Hebert, A. Dey, and S. Srinivasa. 2009. Inverse optimal heuristic control for imitation learning. In *Proceedings of the Twelfth International Conference on Artificial Intelligence and Statistics*, Clearwater Beach, FL.

Ren, X. and C. Gu. 2010. Figure-ground segmentation improves handled object recognition in egocentric video. In *Proceedings of the Conference on Computer Vision and Pattern Recognition*, San Francisco, CA.

Ren, X. and M. Philipose. 2009. Egocentric recognition of handled objects: Benchmark and analysis. In *Proceedings of the Egovision Workshop*, Miami, FL.

Rimey, R. D. and C. M. Brown. 1994. Control of selective perception using Bayes nets and decision theory. *International Journal of Computer Vision* 12:173–208.

Satinde, S., M. R. James, and M. R. Rudary. 2004. Predictive state representations: A new theory for modeling dynamical systems. In *Proceedings of the Uncertainty in Artificial Intelligence*, Banff, Alberta, Canada.

Schiele, B., H. Aoki, and A. Pentland. 1999. Realtime personal positioning system for wearable computers. In *Proceedings of the 3rd IEEE International Symposium on Wearable Computers*, San Francisco, CA.

Sez, J. and F. Escolano. 2008. Stereo-based aerial obstacle detection for the visually impaired. In *Proceedings of the ECCV Workshop on Computer Vision Applications for the Visually Impaired*, Nice, France.

Siddiqi, S. M., B. Boots, and G. J. Gordon. 2010. Reduced-rank hidden Markov models. In *Proceedings of the 13th Conference on Artificial Intelligence and Statistics*, Sardinia, Italy.

Sivic, J., B. C. Russell, A. A. Efros, A. Zisserman, and W. T. Freeman. 2005. Discovering object categories in image collections. In *Proceedings of the International Conference on Computer Vision*, Beijing, China.

Sorokin, D., D. Berenson, S. Srinivasa, and M. Hebert. 2010. People helping robots helping people: Crowdsourcing for grasping novel objects. In *Proceedings of the International Conference on Intelligent Robots and Systems*, San Francisco, CA.

Spriggs, E. H., F. De la Torre Frade, and M. Hebert. 2009. Temporal segmentation and activity classification from first-person sensing. In *Proceedings of the Workshop on Egocentric Vision*, Miami, FL.

Starner, T., B. Schiele, and A. Pentland. 2008. Visual context awareness via wearable computing. In *Proceedings of the International Symposium on Wearable Computers*, Pittsburgh, PA.

Stiefmeier, T., D. Roggen, G. Ogris, P. Lukowicz, and G. Tröster. 2008. Wearable activity tracking in car manufacturing. *Pervasive Computing* 7, no. 2:42–50.

Talukder, A. and L. Matthies. 2004. Real-time detection of moving objects from moving vehicles using dense stereo and optical flow. In *Proceedings of the International Conference on Intelligent Robots and Systems*, Sendai, Japan.

Taralova, E., F. Dela Torre, and M. Hebert. 2011. Source constrained clustering. In *Proceedings of the International Conference Computer Vision*, Barcelona, Spain.

Torres, M., A. Collet, and S. Srinivasa. 2010. MOPED: A scalable and low latency object recognition and pose estimation system. *Proceedings of the IEEE International Conference on Robotics and Automation*, Anchorage, AK.

Treuillet, S., E. Royer, T. Chateau, M. Dhome, and J.-M. Lavest. 2007. Body mounted vision system for visually impaired outdoor and indoor way finding assistance. In *Proceedings of the Conference and Workshop on Assistive Technologies for People with Vision & Hearing Impairments*, Granada, Spain.

Vester-Christensen, M., D. Leimberg, B. K. Ersbøll, and L. K. Hansen. 2005. Deformable models for eye tracking. In *Proceedings of the Den 14. Danske Konference i Mønstergenkendelse og Billedanalyse*, Copenhagen, Denmark.

Wagstaff, K., C. Cardie, S. Rogers, and S. Schroedl. 2001. Constrained K-means clustering with background knowledge. In *Proceedings of the 18th International Conference on Machine Learning*, Williamstown, MA.

Young, L. and D. Sheena. 1975. Survey of eye movement recording methods. *Behavior Research Methods* 7:397–429.

Zhang, J., S. Ong, and A. Nee. 2008. Navigation systems for individuals with visual impairment: A survey. In *Proceedings of the International Convention for Rehabilitation Engineering and Assistive Technology*, Bangkok, Thailand.

Zhou, F. and F. De la Torre. 2009. Canonical time warping for alignment of human behavior. In *Proceedings of the Neural Information Processing Systems*, Vancouver, British Columbia, Canada.

Zhou, F. and F. De la Torre. 2011. Generalized time warping (GTW). In *Proceedings of the International Conference on Machine Learning*, Washington, DC.

Ziebart, B., J. A. Bagnell, and A. Dey. 2009a. Purposeful adaptive behavior modeling for robotics. In *Proceedings of the Workshop on Learning from Multiple Sources with Applications to Robotics*, Whistler, British Columbia, Canada.

Ziebart, B., J. Bagnell, and A. Dey. 2010. Modeling interaction via the principle of maximum causal entropy. In *Proceedings of the International Conference on Machine Learning*, Haifa, Israel.

Ziebart, B., N. Ratliff, G. Gallagher, C. Mertz, K. Peterson, J. A. Bagnell, M. Hebert, A. K. Dey, and S. Srinivasa. 2009b. Planning-based prediction for pedestrians. In *Proceedings of the International Conference on Intelligent Robots and Systems*, St. Louis, MO.

10

HERB: Personal Assistive Mobile Manipulator in the Home

Siddhartha S. Srinivasa

CONTENTS

10.1 Introduction

Humans effortlessly perform remarkable manipulation tasks that our robots find impossible. We push, pull, slide, throw, pick up, catch, and play with our environment. Our robots, on the other hand, treat the world like the Towers of Hanoi: a geometry problem that is solved by search. While this paradigm has produced remarkable, automated factories and world-beating chess programs, it constrains the dexterity of our robots. At QoLT, we want our robots to perform useful tasks in the home with and around people: to help an elderly person out of bed and help her put on a shirt, to push her wheelchair to the dining table, and to prepare a meal (Figure 10.1).

The lack of abundance of robots in our homes might seem puzzling at first: surely, something capable of assembling a car, a task that few of us can claim to be capable of performing, should find the task of clearing a dining table after a meal, a task that almost all of us can claim to be capable of performing, trivial.

In trying to explain this paradox, researchers often claim that factories are structured whereas our homes, with their clutter and messiness, are unstructured. But that is perhaps oversimplifying; a bin of nuts and bolts in a car assembly plant or the inside of a chassis is perhaps as cluttered (if not more) than the average kitchen in our homes. Perhaps a deeper difference is that factories are structured for robots, whereas our homes are structured for humans. One might argue that we might be as confused in a car factory as a factory robot is in our kitchen. But, given time, we adapt to the structure that is presented

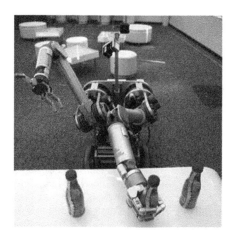
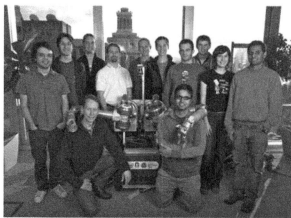

FIGURE 10.1
(See color insert.) (Left) HERB: The home exploring robotic butler. (Right) The Personal Robotics Lab at Carnegie Mellon University.

to us. Likewise, we would like robots in our homes to understand, adapt to, and eventually utilize the structure that is present in our homes.

Another key difference is generality. A car factory is massive, with hundreds of robots spread over hundreds of square feet, each performing a few specific tasks. In contrast, a car mechanic's workshop is small, with a few skilled mechanics spread over a few square feet, each performing a multitude of tasks. The confines of a human environment, built for a general-purpose manipulator like the human, compel robots in such environments to also strive to be general purpose: there just is not enough space for hundreds of specific-purpose robots.

At the Personal Robotics Lab at Carnegie Mellon University, we are developing algorithms to enable robots to perform useful tasks for and with people in human environments. To this end, we have designed and built a series of increasingly capable mobile manipulators starting from the BUSBOY [1]: a mobile base coordinating with a fixed arm, HERB [2]: an integrated mobile base and arm, to the current version HERB 2.0: a bimanual mobile manipulator.

The two paradigms, of structure and generality, resonate through all of our decisions, from the design of the hardware and software architecture to the algorithms for cognition and planning. In the sections that follow, we will reveal the structure present in everyday environments that we have been able to harness for manipulation and interaction, comment on the particular challenges on working in human spaces, and describe some of our lessons learned from extensive testing in kitchens and offices with our integrated platform.

10.2 Hardware Architecture

HERB 2.0's base is comprised of a Segway RMP with a rear caster installed for passive balancing. The Segway was chosen because of its high payload capacity, smooth velocity control, reliable operation, low noise, convenient USB interface, and open-source host interface software. HERB 2.0 manipulates its environment with a pair of Barrett 7-DOF WAM arms and Barrett hands. The WAM arms have proven themselves to be great choices for working

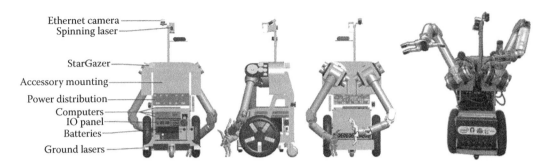

Ethernet camera
Spinning laser

StarGazer
Accessory mounting
Power distribution
Computers
IO panel
Batteries
Ground lasers

FIGURE 10.2
Rear, side, and frontal renderings of the latest HERB design, and the completed robot.

alongside humans, due to their comparatively low mass, backdriveability, and hardware-implemented safety system. Additionally, we have further enhanced their safety by sensing and reacting to position disturbances that indicate physical collisions and by keeping the operating speeds to a reasonable level so that humans are not surprised by sudden motions. The configuration of the two arms with respect to the base was chosen after careful consideration of a number of alternatives. With the two arm bases mounted side by side facing forward, HERB 2.0 maximizes the workspace in which both hands can reach the same point while still remaining narrow enough to fit through a 28 in. wide doorway. The mounting height allows HERB 2.0 to grasp objects from both the floor and from high shelves in overhead cabinets (Figure 10.2).

An array of three miniature laser rangefinders mounted just above ground level gives HERB 2.0 360° perception of obstacles that pose a hazard to navigation. A fourth higher-power laser is mounted on a custom-built spinning base to produce full 3D point clouds of the surrounding environment.

The spinning mechanism allows for variable spin rates in order to control the overall cloud resolution and features dedicated hardware to capture the precise rotation angle for each laser scan so that the 3D points can be accurately assembled. The resulting point clouds are used to avoid collisions with unexpected obstacles in the work area such as nearby people and moveable furniture.

HERB 2.0 features three camera-based sensors for object recognition and localization. HERB 2.0 has a monochrome gigabit ethernet camera for recognizing household objects in the workspace. This particular camera model was chosen for its high sensitivity so that even when restricted to the lighting conditions present in typical indoor environments we can take short exposures in order to minimize motion blur. HERB 2.0 also has an upward facing infrared camera for localizing the base with respect to ceiling-mounted retro-reflective markers. The self-contained unit includes infrared LEDS for lighting the markers and features an overall resolution of 2 cm position and 10° rotation. Finally, HERB 2.0 uses a Microsoft Kinect RGB-D gaming camera located in the environment to track humans in the environment.

Additionally, HERB 2.0 makes extensive use of the sensors built into the Segway base and the WAM arms and hands. The Segway odometry is synthesized with the StarGazer output in order to provide a pose estimate that outperforms either sensor working alone. The WAM is equipped with both joint position sensors and an end-effector force/torque sensor that detect disturbances applied by the environment, while the fingers on the Barrett hands feature position, strain, and tactile sensors that produce critical feedback while manipulating objects.

HERB 2.0's onboard power system allows it to operate untethered for hours at a time, even when fully active. Recharging occurs at twice the discharge rate, so HERB 2.0 can operate indefinitely at a 67% duty cycle. The battery packs offer a serial interface for monitoring charge level and current flow; and 7-segment LED displays mounted on the rear panel give the user a quick indication of battery voltage and current draw. A bank of software-controlled relays provide several contacts for each voltage level so that individual loads can be turned on or off through software control. The power system was designed for hot-plug recharging, which is currently provided by a manually connected tether and plug but which will be replaced by a docking system for autonomous recharging.

10.3 Software Architecture

A key challenge for robot systems in the home is to produce safe goal-driven behavior in a changing, uncertain, and dynamic environment. A complex system like HERB 2.0, that has a host of sensors, algorithms, and actuators, must address issues ranging from software robustness (sensors failing, processes dying, and communication failure) to problems that emerge from inaccurate or unknown models of the physical world (collisions, phantom objects, and sensor uncertainty). To address this challenge, HERB 2.0 uses a software architecture loosely based on the sense-plan-act model to provide safe and rich interaction with humans and the world. Abstract components in Figure 10.3 show the interaction between the different components of our architecture. We gather information about the world which is composed of fixed and dynamic objects, agents like humans and other robots, and semantics like HERB 2.0's location in the home. We gather data from a wide range of sensors including high-definition cameras, the Microsoft Kinect, laser scanners, a localization system (StarGazer), Segway encoders, as well as HERB 2.0's joint encoders and force sensors. Analysis of the sensor data over time allows us to perceive and model both objects and actions in the world.

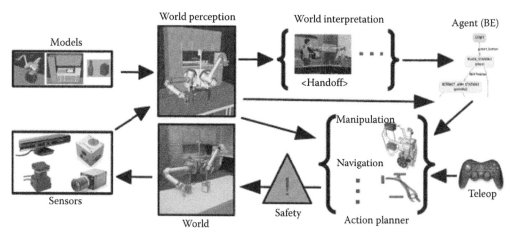

FIGURE 10.3
The HERB software architecture.

HERB 2.0 has three classes of plan components that can make decisions: safety, agent, and teleop. Safety components ensure that HERB 2.0 does not harm humans, the environment, or itself. Some examples of safety components include the limitation of forces that the arm is allowed to exert and the limitation of joint velocities. Safety limits cannot be overridden by other components. Agent components try to accomplish goals based on HERB 2.0's perception of the world. These goals include manipulating objects in the world, expressing via gestures, and physically interacting with humans. Much of the agent programming deals with edge cases where the robot tries to correct for perception errors or system failures. The teleop components are human interfaces where the human can explicitly tell the robot what to do; both at a low level like moving single joints or at a high level like grasping an object. Teleop components override agents but cannot override safety components. Finally, the act components perform actions to accomplish the tasks commanded by the plan components. This includes planning trajectories and base motion, serving the motors, making sounds, and interacting with other computer systems. In addition, each act component advertises to the user interfaces the subset of actions it is capable of performing at that given time. For example, if HERB 2.0 is holding an object and moves close to a recycling bin, the action planner advertises the recycle action.

There are some interesting implications to using this system architecture. First, because all actions must go through the safety components before and during execution, it is impossible for higher level components to execute unsafe actions. Second, because of the modularity, the designers can decide at which level the decisions are made. For example, suppose the agent commands the action planner to pick up a full coffee mug. Should the agent also tell the action planner not to tip the mug, should the planner know to not tip the mug from its own information, or should the modeled mug object have a property of not being tippable as identified by the perception system? In this example, HERB 2.0's action planner decides to keep the mug upright based on its own knowledge that the mug may have liquid in it; however, this decision could easily be made by the agent or the perception system without loss of functionality. Third, due to the parallel and modular properties of this system architecture, the designer has control over what kind and how much information each component shares with the other components. One can see the parallels between these system properties and those of software architecture. It would be interesting to see if the same design principles used in software architecture can be used in the design of robot systems and their interactions.

HERB 2.0's software consists of several nodes that operate in parallel and communicate to one another using the Robot Operating System, ROS [3]. ROS provides a framework for internode communication along with an online database of open source nodes. HERB 2.0's nodes are launched over SSH and VNC from an off-board computer. ROS offers modularity and extensibility, and our nodes are written in C++, Python, Lua, and Lisp. ROS has become more stable over the years and some of our nodes, in particular the sensor drivers and visualization tools, are from community-created open-source ROS repositories. The core of HERB 2.0's intelligence—perception, planning, control, behavior engine, and navigation—was developed in our lab. The following sections discuss each of these nodes in greater detail.

Robot systems and software systems, in particular, are in a state of constant flux. We have added and moved around sensors, added an arm, reconfigured lasers, and are constantly updating the software. Core software engineering concepts, of modularity and extensibility, become all the more important when dealing with a system that physically interacts with the world. We have also found the ability to quickly prototype nodes and swap them in at runtime to be of great use.

10.4 Manipulation Planning

Motion planning for a mobile manipulator like HERB 2.0 is difficult because of the large configuration space of the arms and the constraints imposed on the robot's motion. Some of these constraints arise from the torque limits of the robot or the necessity of avoiding collision with the environment. However, some of the most common constraints in manipulation planning involve the pose of a robot's end-effector. These constraints arise in tasks such as reaching to grasp an object, carrying a cup of coffee, or opening a door. As a result, researchers have developed several algorithms capable of planning with end-effector pose constraints [5–10]. Although often able to solve the problem at hand, these algorithms can be either inefficient [5], probabilistically incomplete [6–8], or rely on pose constraint representations that are difficult to generalize [9,10].

We have developed a manipulation planning framework [4] that allows robots to plan in the presence of constraints on end-effector pose, as well as others. Our framework has three main components: constraint representation, constraint-satisfaction strategies, and a sampling-based approach to planning. These three components come together to create an efficient and probabilistically complete manipulation planning algorithm called the Constrained BiDirectional RRT (CBiRRT2). The underpinning of our framework for pose-related constraints is our Task Space Regions (TSRs) representation.

TSRs describe volumes of permissible end-effector pose for a given task. For instance, for a reaching-to-grasp task TSRs can be used to define the set of end-effector poses that result in stable grasps. For picking up a cup of water, TSRs can define the set of poses in which the water does not spill. TSRs are intuitive to specify, can be efficiently sampled, and the distance to a TSR can be evaluated very quickly, making them ideal for sampling-based planning. Most importantly, TSRs are a general representation of pose constraints that can fully describe many practical tasks. For more complex tasks, such as manipulating articulated linkages like doors, TSRs can be chained together to create more complex end-effector pose constraints [11]. TSRs can also be used to construct plans that are guaranteed to succeed despite uncertainty in the pose of an object [12].

Our constrained manipulation planning framework also allows planning with multiple simultaneous constraints. For instance, collision and torque constraints can be included along with multiple constraints on end-effector pose [13]. Closed chain kinematics constraints can also be included as a relation between end-effector pose constraints without requiring specialized projection operators [14] or sampling algorithms [15].

We have applied our framework to a wide range of problems both in simulation and in the real world (Figure 10.4). These problems include grasping in cluttered environments, lifting heavy objects, two-armed manipulation, and opening doors, to name a few.

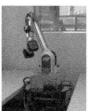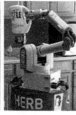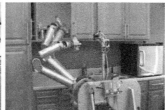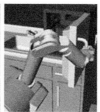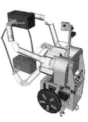

FIGURE 10.4
(See color insert.) HERB executing paths planned by our constrained manipulation planning framework.

These examples demonstrate our framework's practicality, but it is also important to understand the theoretical properties of manipulation planning. Specifically, we would like to understand whether various sampling methods are able to fully explore the set of feasible configurations. To this end, we provided a proof for the probabilistic completeness of our planning method when planning with constraints on end-effector pose [16]. The proof shows that, given enough time, no part of the constraint manifold corresponding to a pose constraint will be left unexplored, regardless of the dimensionality of the pose constraint. This proof applies to CBiRRT2 as well as other approaches [5,17] whose probabilistic completeness was previously undetermined.

One criticism of TSRs is that the constraint representation may not be sufficiently rich. For instance, some modifications to TSR chains are necessary to accommodate constraints where degrees of freedom are coupled (as with screw constraints). Indeed, TSRs and TSR chains cannot capture every conceivable constraint, nor are they intended to. Instead, these representations attempt to straddle the trade-off between practicality and expressiveness. TSRs have proven sufficient for solving a wide range of real-world manipulation problems while still remaining relatively simple and efficient to use in a sampling-based planner. While a more expressive representation is surely possible, we have yet to find one that is as straightforward to specify and as convenient for sampling-based planning.

We also found that, while it was fairly straightforward to generate TSRs for many tasks, the process became quite tedious. Thus, it would be interesting to develop a system that could automatically generate the constraints corresponding to a given task. We have investigated automatically forming TSRs for grasping tasks by sampling over the space of stable grasps, clustering the grasps, and fitting TSRs to these clusters [18]. To generalize to object placement tasks, we would need to develop a different method. For instance, could a robot look at a scene and determine all the areas where a given object can be placed? Such a task would require understanding where the object could be placed (through grounding the idea of placing geometrically) and also taking into account user preferences for where objects should be placed.

10.5 Planning under Clutter and Uncertainty

Robotic manipulation systems suffer from two main problems in unstructured human environments: uncertainty and clutter. Consider the task of cleaning a dining table. In such a task the robot needs to detect the objects on the table, figure out where they are, move its arm to reach the goal object, and grasp it to move it away. If there is significant sensor uncertainty, the hand could miss the goal object, or worse collide with it in an uncontrolled way. Clutter multiplies this problem. Even with perfect sensing, it might be impossible for the hand to wrap around the object for a good grasp. With both clutter and uncertainty, the options for a direct grasp are even more restricted and often impossible.

We address the problems for manipulation in such a context.

Two approaches we have taken are (1) using the mechanics of pushing to provably funnel an object into a stable grasp despite high uncertainty and clutter. We call this *push-grasping*. (2) Rearranging clutter around the primary task with the use of motion primitives such as pushing, sliding, sweeping, and picking up.

A push-grasp aims to grasp an object by executing a pushing action and then closing the fingers [19]. We present an example of push-grasp in Figure 10.5 (top). Here, the robot

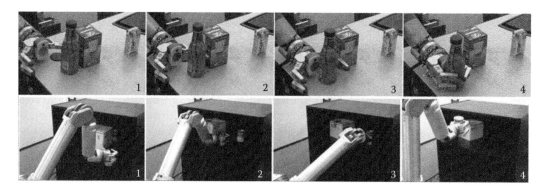

FIGURE 10.5

(Top) An example push-grasp of an object in contact with the surrounding clutter. (Bottom) An example rearrangement plan. The robot pushes the large ungraspable box out of the way before retrieving the goal object.

sweeps a region over the table during which the bottle rolls into its hand before closing the fingers. The large swept area ensures that the bottle is grasped even if its position is estimated with some error. The push also moves the bottle away from the nearby box, making it possible to wrap the hand around it, which would not have been possible in its original location. The robot must predict the consequences of the physical interaction to find the right parameters of a push-grasp in a given scene. For this purpose, we introduce the concept of a capture region, the set of object poses such that a push-grasp successfully grasps it. The concept of capture region is similar to the preimages in the preimage backchaining approach [21]. We compute capture regions for push-grasps using a quasi-static analysis of the mechanics of pushing [22] and a simulation based on this analysis. We show how such a precomputed capture region can be used to efficiently and accurately find the minimum pushing distance needed to grasp an object at a certain pose. Then, given a scene, we use this formalization to search over different parametrizations of a push-grasp to find collision-free plans.

Our key contribution is the integration of a planning system based on task mechanics to the geometric planners traditionally used in grasping. We enhance the geometric planners by enabling the robot to interact with the world according to physical laws, when needed. Our planner is able to adapt to different levels of uncertainty and clutter, producing direct grasps when the uncertainty and clutter are below a certain level.

Tasks is human environments may require rearrangement. Imagine reaching into the fridge to pull out the milk jug. It is buried at the back of the fridge. You immediately start rearranging content—you push the large heavy casserole out of the way, you carefully pick up the fragile crate of eggs and move it to a different rack, but along the way you push the box of leftovers to the corner with your elbow.

We developed an open-loop planner that rearranges the clutter around a goal object [20]. This requires manipulating multiple objects in the scene. The planner decides which objects to move and the order to move them, decides where to move them, chooses the manipulation actions to use on these objects, and accounts for the uncertainty in the environment all through this process. One example scene is presented in Figure 10.5 (bottom). In this scene, the robot's primary task is to grasp the can buried inside the shelf. The planner pushes the large ungraspable box to the side. This creates the space it then uses to grasp the primary goal object.

Our planner uses different nonprehensile manipulation primitives such as pushing, sliding, and sweeping. The consequences of actions are derived from the mechanics of pushing and are provably conservative. Since our planner uses nonprehensile actions, it generates plans where an ordinary pick-and-place planner cannot. This enables HERB 2.0 to perform manipulation tasks even if there are large, heavy, ungraspable objects in the environment, or when there is a large uncertainty about object poses.

Nonprehensile actions can decrease or increase object pose uncertainty in an environment. To account for that, our planner represents the object pose uncertainty explicitly and conservatively. The planner plans backward starting from the primary goal object and identifying the volume of space required to manipulate it. This space is given by the volume swept by the robot links and by the manipulated object, with the object pose uncertainty taken into account. Then, if any other object is blocking this space, the planner plans an action to move the blocking object out of the way. This recursive process continues until all the planned actions are feasible.

The planners we have for push-grasping and for rearranging clutter are open-loop planners. On the one hand this is good because the robot does not depend on a specific sensor input that may be noisy or unavailable at times. But on the other hand the open-loop planners need to be very conservative to guarantee success. For push-grasping this can sometimes result in unnecessarily long pushes. For the rearrangement planner this can result in a quick consumption of planning space the robot can use. The lesson is as follows: build a system that can work open-loop, but that can also integrate sensor feedback when it is available. With this line of thinking we are currently working on integrating visual and tactile sensory feedback into our system.

Clutter is not only a problem for robot actions, but it is also a problem for robot perception. If an object is hidden behind another object on a cluttered fridge shelf, there is little chance that the camera on the robot's head will be able to see it. This problem motivates us to use the rearrangement planning framework, also to move objects with the goal of making the spaces behind them visible to the robot sensors.

10.6 Trajectory Optimization and Learning

A vital requirement for a personal robot like HERB 2.0 is the ability to work with and around people, moving in their workspaces. While the Rapidly-Exploring Random Tree algorithm from Section VI is very good at producing feasible, albeit random motion, we need to start thinking toward predictability and optimality of the paths the robot executes.

With these criteria in mind, motion planning becomes a trajectory optimization problem. However, since manipulation tasks induce a very high-dimensional space, optimizers often struggle with high-cost local minima corresponding to dangerous and sometimes even infeasible paths. In this section, we present two ways of alleviating this issue: one is to improve the optimizer itself, which widens the basin of attraction of low-cost solutions; the other is to learn to initialize the optimizer in the basin of attraction of these low-cost solutions, thus ensuring convergence to a good trajectory.

Most manipulation tasks, such as reaching for an object, placing it on a table, or handing it off to a person, are described by an entire region of goals rather than one particular goal configuration that the robot must be in at the end of the trajectory.

This section extends a recent trajectory optimizer, CHOMP [23], to take advantage of this goal region by changing the end point of the trajectory during optimization [24]. Doing so enables more initial guesses converge to low-cost trajectories.

Our algorithm, entitled Goal Set CHOMP, optimizes a functional that trades off between a smoothness and an obstacle cost, with a prior measuring a notion of smoothness such as sum squared velocities or accelerations along the trajectory, an obstacle cost pushing all parts of the robot away from collision, and a function that capturing constraints on the trajectory.

While CHOMP has an implicit fixed goal constraint, our extension relaxes this assumption and replaces the constraint by an entire goal region rather than a single configuration.

In Ref. [24], we have shown that this extension improves upon CHOMP for a wide range of day-to-day tasks that HERB 2.0 encounters.

With Goal Set CHOMP, we widened the basins of attraction of low-cost solutions, making initialization in such a basin more likely. In this section, we will focus on improving the initialization based on prior experiences by learning to predict the goal at which the trajectory should end.

Because of local minima, the goal choice still has a great influence on result of Goal Set CHOMP: the difference between the best and worst performances is drastic. However, by collecting training data from such scenes, we can learn to predict an initial goal that will place the final cost within only 8% of the minimum [25]. We compared the loss over this minimum cost for five different learners against the baseline of selecting a goal at random. Here, SVM is a Support Vector Machine classifier that attempts to predict whether a goal will be the best. IOC is a Maximum Margin Planning [26] algorithm that attempts to find a cost under which the best cost will be minimum. The Linear Regression (LR), Gaussian Process (GP), and Neural Network (NN) learn to map initial goals to final trajectory costs.

For each of these algorithms, we found it important to make efficient use of the available data: the classifier and the inverse optimal control method, which traditionally focus solely on the best option, should take into account the true cost of the other candidates; at the same time, the regressors, which traditionally focus on all the data, should not waste resources on the poor options. The data savvy version of IOC obtains the best results by combining the focus on predicting the best goal with the awareness of costs from other goals.

In moving away from the random sampling approaches, we are giving up the fast exploration that makes RRTs successful for optimal, predictable motion. Even though CHOMP is armed with an exploration technique derived from the dynamics of physical systems, namely Hamiltonian Monte Carlo, exploring while optimizing is more costly than pure exploration. An idea for merging optimization and randomized sampling is using CHOMP as the extension operator for the tree. However, such an algorithm will spend too many resources optimizing paths that do not contribute to the final solution.

At the core of this work lies the idea that while trajectory optimization in high-dimensional spaces is hard, we can make it easier in the case of manipulation by taking advantage of the structure inherent in the problem: tasks are described by sets of goals that can be exploited, and the repeatability of tasks allows for self-improvement over time. We found that even naive learning methods improve the optimization process, and that the benefit is even greater when using the data in a way tailored to the problem. For future work, we are excited about using other attributes of trajectories, beyond goal choices, to guide this learning process. Due to its predictable nature, trajectory optimization can benefit in a lot of cases from machine learning in overcoming the need for exploration.

10.7 Interacting with People

Personal robots that are intended for assisting humans in daily tasks will need to interact with them in a number of ways. The design of human interaction behaviors on these robots is particularly challenging since the average user will have little knowledge about how they work. It is essential to tune these behaviors for the users' expectations and preferences.

To this end, we have performed a number of systematic user studies with HERB 2.0 [27,28], and we have put its human interaction behaviors to test at a number of public events (Figure 10.6, Left).

In designing HERB 2.0, we are particularly interested in collaborative manipulation with humans, focusing on robot—human hand-overs. Many of the potential tasks for personal robots, such as fetching objects for the elderly or individuals with motor-impairment, involve hand-over interactions. Different aspects of robot—human hand-overs—have been studied within robotics, including motion control and planning [29–32], grasp planning [33], social interaction [34–36], and grip forces during hand-over [37,38]. A few of these report results from user studies involving hand-overs between a physical robot and a human [30,34–36].

The problem of planning a hand-over is highly underconstrained.

There are infinite ways to transfer an object to a human. As a result, it is easy to find a viable solution; however, it is hard to define what a good solution is from the human's perspective. Our approach involves parametrizing hand-over behaviors and identifying heuristics for searching desirable hand-overs in these parameter spaces.

Hand-overs involve several phases starting from approaching the human with an object to retracting the arm after releasing the object. The object and robot configuration at the moment of transfer and the trajectory that leads to this configuration are critical. The hand-over configuration influences how the object will be taken by the human and the trajectory leading to this configuration lets the human predict the timing of the hand-over and synchronize their movements.

10.7.1 Hand-Over Configurations

A hand-over configuration is fully specified by a grasp on the object and a 7-DOF arm configuration. We conducted three user studies to identify heuristics for choosing good hand-over configurations. The first study (10 participants) asked users to configure several

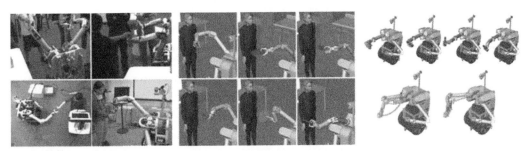

FIGURE 10.6
Robot–human hand-overs with HERB 2.0. (Left) Handing objects to a human during Research at Intel Day and systematic user studies. (Middle) Hand-over configurations learned from human examples (top), and planned using the kinematic model of the human (bottom). (Right) Poses that best convey the intent of handing over (top) and two sample trajectories with high and low contrast between carrying and hand-over configurations.

good and bad handing configurations for five objects through a graphical user interface. Afterward, users were asked to choose between two hand-over configurations that differed by one parameter. We found that the set of good configurations provided by participants are concentrated around a small region in the space of all configurations and has little variance across participants. These good configurations expose a large portion of the object surface and tend to present the object in its default orientation. While confirming these results, the forced-choice questions revealed that participants prefer extended arm configurations that look natural (are mappable to a human arm configuration) [28].

In the second study (10 participants) we compared the configurations learned from good examples collected in the first study, with configurations planned using a kinematic model of the human (Figure 10.6, Middle). The robot delivered each object twice, with the learned and planned configurations, and the participant was asked to compare them. Participants preferred the learned configurations and thought they were more natural and appropriate; however, they had greater reachability over the objects presented with the planned configurations [28].

Besides allowing humans to easily take the object, a handover configuration needs to convey its intention. Our third study (50 participants) involved a survey that asks the participant to categorize the intention of a robot configuration holding an object. We find that the intention of handing an object is best conveyed by configurations with an extended arm, grasping the object from the side opposite to the human and tilting the object toward the human (Figure 10.6, Right) [27].

10.7.2 Hand-Over Trajectories

We parametrize hand-over trajectories by the configuration in which the object is carried while approaching the human. When the robot is ready to deliver the object, it transitions to the hand-over configuration through a smooth trajectory. We conducted a fourth user study (24 participants) to analyze the effects of the carrying configuration. We found that carrying configurations that have high contrast with the handing configuration results in the most fluent hand-overs [27]. These are configurations in which the robot holds the object close to itself, obstructing the human from taking the object (Figure 11.6, Right). They improve the fluency by avoiding the human's early attempts to take the object and by distinctly signaling the timing of the hand-over.

We have made a lot of progress on manipulating objects in real-world environments through novel and improved techniques. However, adding humans into the equation imposes unique constraints, such as usability of interaction interfaces or legibility of the robot's movements that can only be addressed through user studies. We have seen, in the context of robot—human interactions— that such user studies can reveal interesting heuristics that can be used in manipulation and motion planning to produce desirable and human-friendly behaviors.

10.8 Outlook and Challenges

We have presented a snapshot of 2 years of effort on HERB 2.0. The platform is evolving and will forever be evolving. Key to our progress has been a commitment to working in a home environment and understanding the nuances of how humans structure their environments. Understanding this structure has enabled more robust, efficient, and predictable behavior. Some of our observations have surprised us and they point toward much deeper research questions, on understanding human intent, on collaborative manipulation, and on addressing extreme clutter with physics-based manipulation planners. We are now well positioned to move toward new unsolved problem domains.

1. Reconciling geometric planning with physics-based manipulation: Humans have instinct. Robots have search. We are able to pick up knives and forks, stack plates, move objects with our arms, balance dishes, kick open kitchen doors, and load dishwashers. HERB 2.0 has barely scratched the surface of what he can do with his arms and base. Our work on push-grasping clutter is a start toward merging physics-based manipulation with geometric search, but we are excited to go beyond that. There are two immediate questions to answer: (1) how can we incorporate sensor feedback into our strategies, and (2) how can we automatically learn strategies from observation or demonstration? Answering the first question will enable robust execution of existing strategies. The second question is much harder to answer but is critical. There are countless strategies to learn but robots can use their prior knowledge and also learn from their own and other robots' experience.

2. Collaborative manipulation: We envision HERB 2.0 performing complex manipulation tasks with humans: HERB 2.0 should be able to prepare a meal and clear a table with a person or to build an IKEA shelf with them. Human–robot interaction must go beyond dialog management to physical collaboration. Currently, HERB 2.0 is on its way to performing each of these tasks autonomously. But, strangely enough, doing these tasks with a human will be much harder: HERB 2.0 might need to sense human kinematics, human intent, understand turn-taking, and react to the environment and humans in real time. So, do we really need collaboration? There are definitely scenarios in which collaboration is critical: in the battlefield for assembling a mortar or carrying an injured soldier or in the home assisting a patient with disabilities with their activities of daily living. But even in these cases, the role of a robot and the balance of autonomy and collaboration will change dynamically. We are excited to explore this balance and the challenge of humans and robots performing tightly coupled manipulation tasks collaboratively.

3. Sensing and actuation for robotics: Do we really need a $500,000 robot like HERB 2.0 to enable lifelong mobile manipulation? We have been exploring the capabilities of simple hands. Surely, simple hands can do a lot less than more expensive complex hands, but the details of their limits are important. Our results to date have been surprising: we have demonstrated that by shifting the complexity from the mechanisms to the computational algorithms, complex tasks like bin-picking and singulation can be achieved with simple hands.

With robots like HERB 2.0, we now have the ability to excavate these questions and are perfectly positioned to identify, prove, develop, and demonstrate the principles of mobile manipulation that will enable our robots to interact with us in our environment and impact our lives in meaningful ways.

References

1. S. Srinivasa, D. Ferguson, J. Vande Weghe, D. Berenson, R. Diankov, C. Helfrich, and H. Strasdat, The robotic busboy: Steps towards developing a mobile robotic home assistant, in *IEEE International Conference on Intelligent Autonomous Systems*, Baden Baden, Germany, July 2008.

2. S. Srinivasa, D. Ferguson, C. Helfrich, D. Berenson, A. Collet, R. Diankov, G. Gallagher, G. Hollinger, J. Kuffner, and J. Vande Weghe, HERB: A home exploring robotic butler, *Autonomous Robots*, 28(1), 5–20, 2009.

3. M. Quigley, K. Conley, B. P. Gerkey, J. Faust, T. Foote, J. Leibs, R. Wheeler, and A. Y. Ng, ROS: An open-source Robot Operating System, in *ICRA Workshop on Open Source Software*, Kobe, Japan, 2009.

4. D. Berenson, S. Srinivasa, and J. Kuffner, Task space regions: A framework for pose-constrained manipulation planning, *The International Journal of Robotics Research*, 30(12), 1435–1460, 2011.

5. M. Stilman, Task constrained motion planning in robot joint space, in *Proceedings of the IEEE/RSJ International Conference on Intelligent Robots and Systems (IROS)*, San Diego, CA, 2007.

6. Y. Koga, K. Kondo, J. Kuffner, and J. Claude Latombe, Planning motions with intentions, in *SIGGRAPH*, Orlando, FL, 1994.

7. K. Yamane, J. Kuffner, and J. Hodgins, Synthesizing animations of human manipulation tasks, in *SIGGRAPH*, Los Angeles, CA, 2004.

8. Z. Yao and K. Gupta, Path planning with general end-effector constraints: Using task space to guide configuration space search, in *Proceedings of the IEEE/RSJ International Conference on Intelligent Robots and Systems (IROS)*, Edmonton, Canada, 2005.

9. E. Drumwright and V. Ng-Thow-Hing, Toward interactive reaching in static environments for humanoid robots, in *Proceedings of the IEEE/RSJ International Conference on Intelligent Robots and Systems (IROS)*, Beijing, China, 2006.

10. D. Bertram, J. Kuffner, R. Dillmann, and T. Asfour, An integrated approach to inverse kinematics and path planning for redundant manipulators, in *Proceedings of the IEEE International Conference on Robotics and Automation (ICRA)*, Orlando, FL, 2006.

11. D. Berenson, J. Chestnutt, S. S. Srinivasa, J. J. Kuffner, and S. Kagami, Pose-constrained whole-body planning using task space region chains, in *Proceedings of the IEEE-RAS International Conference on Humanoid Robots*, Paris, France, 2009.

12. D. Berenson, S. Srinivasa, and J. Kuffner, Addressing pose uncertainty in manipulation planning using task space regions, in *Proceedings of the IEEE/RSJ International Conference on Intelligent Robots and Systems (IROS)*, St. Louis, MO, 2009.

13. D. Berenson, S. S. Srinivasa, D. Ferguson, and J. Kuffner, Manipulation planning on constraint manifolds, in *Proceedings of the IEEE International Conference on Robotics and Automation (ICRA)*, Kobe, Japan, 2009.

14. J. H. Yakey, S. M. LaValle, and L. E. Kavraki, Randomized path planning for linkages with closed kinematic chains, *IEEE Transactions on Robotics and Automation*, 17(6), 951–958, 2001.

15. J. Cortes and T. Simeon, Sampling-based motion planning under kinematic loop-closure constraints, in *Proceedings of the Workshop on the Algorithmic Foundations of Robotics (WAFR)*, Utrecht/Zeist, the Netherlands, 2004.

16. D. Berenson and S. Srinivasa, Probabilistically complete planning with end-effector pose constraints, in *Proceedings of the IEEE International Conference on Robotics and Automation (ICRA)*, Anchorage, AK, May 2010.

17. S. Dalibard, A. Nakhaei, F. Lamiraux, and J.-P. Laumond, Whole-body task planning for a humanoid robot: A way to integrate collision avoidance, in *Proceedings of the 9th IEEE-RAS International Conference on Humanoid Robots (Humanoids 2009)*, Paris, France, 2009.

18. D. Berenson, Constrained manipulation planning, PhD dissertation, Robotics Institute, Carnegie Mellon University, Pittsburgh, PA, May 2011.

19. M. Dogar and S. Srinivasa, Push-grasping with dexterous hands, in *Proceedings of the IEEE/RSJ International Conference on Intelligent Robots and Systems*, Taipei, Taiwan, October 2010.

20. M. Dogar and S. Srinivasa, A framework for push-grasping in clutter, in *Robotics: Science and Systems VII*, Los Angeles, CA, 2011.

21. T. Lozano-Perez, M. T. Mason, and R. H. Taylor, Automatic synthesis of fine-motion strategies for robots, *International Journal of Robotics Research*, 3(1), 3–24, 1984.

22. S. Goyal, A. Ruina, and J. Papadopoulos, Planar sliding with dry friction. Part 1. Limit surface and moment function, *Wear*, 143, 307–330, 1991.

23. N. D. Ratliff, M. Zucker, J. A. Bagnell, and S. S. Srinivasa, Chomp: Gradient optimization techniques for efficient motion planning, in *IEEE International Conference on Robotics and Automation*, IEEE, Pittsburgh, PA, 2009, pp. 489–494.

24. A. D. Dragan, N. D. Ratliff, and S. S. Srinivasa, Manipulation planning with goal sets using constrained trajectory optimization, in *IEEE International Conference on Robotics and Automation*, IEEE, Pittsburgh, PA, 2011.

25. A. D. Dragan, G. J. Gordon, and S. S. Srinivasa, Learning from experience in manipulation planning: Setting the right goals, in *International Symposium on Robotics Research (ISRR)*, 2011.

26. N. D. Ratliff, J. A. Bagnell, and M. A. Zinkevich, Maximum margin planning, in *Proceedings of the 23rd International Conference on Machine Learning (ICML06)*, Pittsburgh, PA, 2006.

27. M. Cakmak, S. Srinivasa, M. Lee, S. Kiesler, and J. Forlizzi, Using spatial and temporal contrast for fluent robot-human hand-overs, in *Proceedings of the Sixth International Conference on Human-Robot Interaction (HRI)*, Lausanne, Switzerland, 2011, pp. 489–497.

28. M. Cakmak, S. Srinivasa, M. Lee, J. Forlizzi, and S. Kiesler, Human preferences for robot-human hand-over configurations, in *Proceedings of the IEEE/RSJ International Conference on Intelligent Robots and System (IROS)*, San Francisco, CA, 2011.

29. A. Agah and K. Tanie, Human interaction with a service robot: Mobilemanipulator handing over an object to a human, in *Proceedings of the IEEE International Conference on Robotics and Automation (ICRA)*, Shanghai, China, 1997, pp. 575–580.

30. M. Huber, M. Rickert, A. Knoll, T. Brandt, and S. Glasauer, Humanrobot interaction in handing-over tasks, in *Proceedings of the IEEE International Symposium on Robot and Human Interactive Communication (RO-MAN)*, Munich, Germany, 2008, pp. 107–112.

31. E. Sisbot, L. Marin, and R. Alami, Spatial reasoning for human robot interaction, in *Proceedings of the IEEE/RSJ International Conference on Intelligent Robots and System (IROS)*, San Diego, CA, 2007.

32. S. Kajikawa, T. Okino, K. Ohba, and H. Inooka, Motion planning for hand-over between human and robot, in *Proceedings of the IEEE/RSJ International Conference on Intelligent Robots and Systems (IROS)*, Pittsburgh, PA, pp. 193–199, 1995.

33. E. Lopez-Damian, D. Sidobre, S. DeLaTour, and R. Alami, Grasp planning for interactive object manipulation, in *Proceedings of the International Symposium on Robotics and Automation*, 2006.

34. A. Edsinger and C. Kemp, Human-robot interaction for cooperative manipulation: Handing objects to one another, in *Proceedings of the IEEE International Symposium on Robot and Human Interactive Communication (RO-MAN)*, Toyama, Japan, 2007.

35. K. Koay, E. Sisbot, D. Syrdal, M. Walters, K. Dautenhahn, and R. Alami, Exploratory study of a robot approaching a person in the context of handing over an object, in *Proceedings of the AAAI Spring Symposium on Multidisciplinary Collaboration for Socially Assistive Robotics*, Palo Alto, CA, 2007, pp. 18–24.

36. Y. Choi, T. Chen, A. Jain, C. Anderson, J. Glass, and C. Kemp, Hand it over or set it down: A user study of object delivery with an assistive mobile manipulator, in *Proceedings of the IEEE International Symposium on Robot and Human Interactive Communication (ROMAN)*, 2009.

37. K. Nagata, Y. Oosaki, M. Kakikura, and H. Tsukune, Delivery by hand between human and robot based on fingertip force-torque information, in *Proceedings of the IEEE/RSJ International Conference on Intelligent Robots and System (IROS)*, 1998, pp. 750–757.

38. I. Kim and H. Inooka, Hand-over of an object between human and robot, in *Proceedings of the IEEE International Symposium on Robot and Human Interactive Communication (RO-MAN)*, 1992.

11

Architecture and Applications of Virtual Coaches

Daniel P. Siewiorek, Asim Smailagic, and Anind Dey

CONTENTS

11.1 Evolution of Technology

The confluence of several new technologies enabled a new generation of always attentive personalized systems called virtual coaches. Virtual coaches continuously monitor its users' activities and surroundings, detect situations where intervention would be desirable, and offer prompt assistance. Virtual coaches is the latest phase of a technology evolution over the past two decades.

The advent of powerful microprocessors capable of running an operating system with real time responsiveness in small, energy efficient packages in the early 1990s enabled a new generation of personal computing systems that provided access to information anytime anywhere. Handheld personal digital assistant (PDA) that could fit in a shirt pocket gave access to addresses, notes, and schedules via a new interface access modality featuring stylus and hand writing recognition (e.g., graffiti).

Another novel technology, head mounted displays, enabled revolutionary new body worn systems termed wearable computers [Siewiorek, Smailagic, Starner 2008] that were always on providing instantaneous access to reference information in application areas such as complex plant operations, manufacturing, maintenance, and group collaboration.

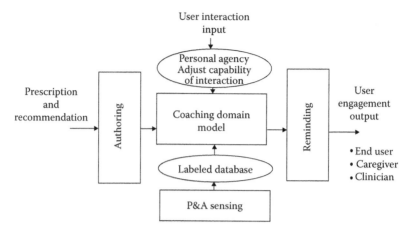

FIGURE 11.1
Virtual coach architecture.

Micro-electro-mechanical systems (MEMS) created low-cost, low-energy sensors that could sense physical parameters such as acceleration, orientation, temperature, and light that when coupled with signal processing and machine learning algorithms allowed personal systems to infer user context in context-aware systems.

Figure 11.1 depicts the elements of a virtual coach. MEMS sensors sample the environment and the users' interaction with it yielding a perception and awareness (P&A) of the surroundings. The data are labeled for interpretation by the coaching domain model. The coach is instructed about what to monitor and how to respond to situations as described by recommendations and prescriptions prepared by medical staff, caregivers, or even the users themselves. The system interacts with the user through a personal agency that adapts to the user's capabilities, which may be diminished by physical and/or cognitive decline. Taking into account the current context and the instructions provided through authoring, the coaching domain model engages the user to remind them of activities they should be doing. Summaries are also prepared for caregivers and clinicians.

The first generation sensors (accelerometers, light, sound, temperature, global positioning system—GPS) combined with statistical machine learning algorithms enabled whole body activity recognition (e.g., running, standing, sitting, walking, climbing stairs) as well as upper body exercises. The amount of physical activity could be measured and calories burned could be estimated. User activity could also be inferred from location. There are several well-established location approaches for outdoor (GPS—resolution of approximately 10 m worldwide, tower cell phone is communicating with—resolution 20 m) and indoor (audio and light fingerprints of rooms) location. There are also biological parameter sensors such as pulse, respiration, and even EKG [Plare et al. 2011; Siewiorek et al. 2010]. Statistical machine learning has been very effective at categorization. First the raw data, often in the form of a two-dimensional wave form of sensor value (such as acceleration) versus time, are segmented into time-based chunks (typically a couple of seconds). Then features of these wave forms (such as area under the curve, peak count, number of zero crossings) are calculated. A set of categories are picked (e.g., whole body activities), and through experience or statistical learning, the features that have the highest probability of differentiating the different categories are selected. During run time the activity is classified into the category that matches the measured features most closely.

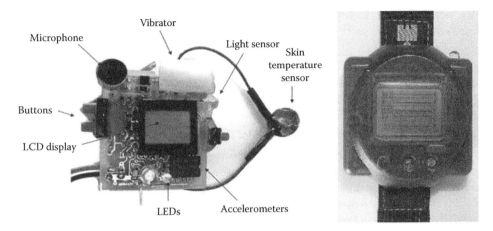

FIGURE 11.2
(See color insert.) eWatch multisensor platform.

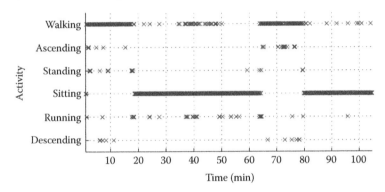

FIGURE 11.3
Real time categorization of whole body activities.

The eWatch is an example of these first generation systems. The eWatch multisensor platform senses acceleration, light, sound, and temperature (Smailagic et al. 2005) as shown in Figure 11.2. When combined with statistical machine learning algorithms, it is possible to identify user activity in real time as shown in Figure 11.3.

Time sequences can be modeled to predict how long you will continue to do an activity. For example, if I have been sitting in a meeting for the last 20 min, chances are very high I will still be in that meeting 5 min from now.

While activity recognition is routine, the next step to identify user intent is still the subject of research. Typically, data are required from multiple sensors monitoring over a period of time.

Keeping users engaged is another active area of research. Interactive games have created the principles that keep users engaged with cyber activities over long periods of time and motivate users to learn more about the game's environment. Online games have motivated distributed users to collaborate to achieve a common goal. How can these principles be applied to virtual coaches.

Virtual coaches integrate elements of wearable computing, context aware computing, artificial intelligence, and user engagement. Section 11.2 provides background on cognitive aids followed by a detailed example in Section 11.3 of a virtual coach that provides advice and reminders for power wheelchair users. Section 11.4 provides several other examples of virtual coaches. A methodology for designing, evaluating, and architecting virtual coaches is given in Section 11.5. Section 11.6 summarizes the virtual coach examples and provides future challenges.

11.2 Virtual Coaches as Cognitive Aids

An important application domain for cognitive augmentation is in assisting individuals whose own cognitive capabilities have been impaired due to natural aging, illness, or traumatic injuries. Recent estimates indicate that over 20 million Americans experience some form of cognitive impairment. This includes older Americans living alone (~4 M), people with Alzheimer's (~4.5 M), people with mild cognitive impairments (~6 M older adults), survivors of stroke (~2.5 M), and people with traumatic brain injury (~5.3 M). Of the many challenges faced by older individuals, declines in memory and cognition are often most feared and have the largest negative impact on themselves and their family members.

Cognitive aids currently available are simplistic, providing only scheduled reminders and rote instructions. They operate open loop without regard for the user's activities or environment. In contrast, virtual coaches monitor how the user performs activities, provides situational awareness, and gives feedback and encouragement matched to her cognitive state and circumstances at the time. Consider the difference between a medication reminder that blindly sounds an alert every day at noon versus a virtual coach that both realizes a user took her pill at 11:58 or in another situation, such as when she is having a conversation, sets itself to vibrate mode.

Other transformative features of a virtual coach include the following:

- As the user learns, it reduces the number and level of detail in the cues it provides.
- It matches its level of support to the user as his abilities change.
- A caregiver can upload new capabilities to the virtual coach, as required, without even an office visit.
- It provides constant and consistent monitoring of adherence to a caregiver's instructions, enabling a deeper and more timely understanding of conditions beyond the episodic patient examinations available today.

Human–system interactions based on understanding of user situations and needs are also effective for applications aimed at larger populations. For example, cognitive support can ensure safe use and compliance with instructions in rehabilitation and management of chronic illness. Many individuals are released from hospital to home with inadequate training for themselves or their family caregivers for the operation of newly prescribed home medical devices or following complex medical regimens. Failure to properly follow directions often results in expensive (to the insurer) rehospitalizations. Similarly, understanding how to effectively motivate people toward healthy behaviors, such as proper diet and physical activity, can benefit broad segments of the general population. Virtual coaches can monitor for compliance, provide cognitive assistance, provide advice that is trusted and followed, and adapt to user capabilities that vary with time and circumstances.

11.3 Example: Seating Virtual Coach: A Smart Reminder for Power Seat Function Usage

Patients with spinal cord injuries have lost feeling in the lower parts of their body. They must shift their positions periodically to prevent the occurrence of pressure sores. Once pressure sores occur they are very difficult to heal.

The power wheelchair virtual coach is an intelligent system that guides power wheelchair users in achieving clinician established goals for body positioning. An array of pressure, tilt, and IR sensors provide data to the virtual coach which monitors user compliance with the clinician's goals and generates reminders for doing past due activities. Clinicians and power wheelchair users were part of the design team from the first day.

Power seat functions (PSFs) allow the user to recline, tilt, elevate the seat and elevated the leg-rest of the chair. Tilt indicates that the entire seating system is shifted backward, but the angle between the back and seat remains constant. Recline changes the backrest angle only, and leg-rest elevation changes the leg-rest angle. The seat elevation raises or lowers the individual in a seated position.

An array of pressure sensors are distributed over the backrest and seat cushion providing the pressure information to the virtual coach, as shown in Figure 11.4. Three tilt sensors determine the tilt angle of the backrest, seat recline, and leg-rest elevation, as illustrated in Figure 11.5. Infrared sensors are used to detect obstacles behind the chair and determine the height of the seat. Pressure sensors are monitored for weight distribution inferring body positions.

Tilt, recline, and leg-rest elevation are monitored for any improper sequences in using seat functions, such as reclining the backrest without tilting the seat, elevating the leg-rests without reclining the backrest, and reclining or tilt angles that are too large, as well as any inappropriate use of seat functions during driving. The user interaction and sensor monitor software run on an embedded computer, attached to the back of the wheelchair seat.

A barrier to wider adoption of QoLT systems that include clinicians and other caregivers (e.g., physical therapy coaches) is the current dearth of techniques and languages appropriate for them to program assistive technology systems, instruct users on the desired behaviors, and assess users' adherence to instructions. Realistically, we cannot expect caregivers to become software programmers, so these interactions should use familiar vocabulary and formats and be flexible to accommodate a variety and range of caregiver specialties and individual styles.

After interviewing clinicians, several attributes of a prescription were identified:

- Activity: Indicates the PSF to be performed. It also includes the pressure activity that is not explicitly performed by the user but is the result of using the chair.
- Parameter: The minimum, ideal, and maximum values per function.
- Duration: Each activity (except pressure) is to be performed for the ideal duration.

However, it is not considered a violation if the duration is between min and max value. Only the max duration for the pressure activity is valid and this indicates the maximum time for which the pressure reading can be above the max value of the parameter.

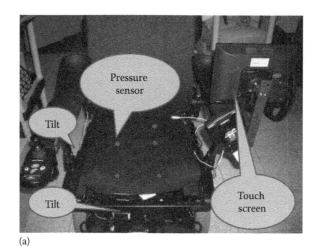

(a)

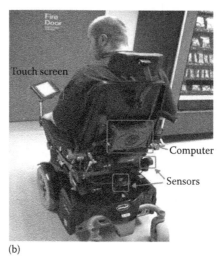

(b)

FIGURE 11.4
(See color insert.) Power wheelchair virtual coach sensors and touch screen: (a) front view and (b) rear view.

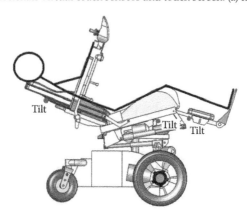

FIGURE 11.5
Tilt function and placement of sensors.

TABLE 11.1

Sample Prescription, Filled by the Clinician

Activity	Parameter			Duration			Gap			Alert after
	Min	Ideal	Max	Min	Ideal	Max	Min	Ideal	Max	
Tilt	25°	30°	35°	25 s	30 s	35 s	20 min	30 min	2 h	10
Recline	10°	15°	20°	4 min	5 min	6 min	4 h	5 h	6 h	15
Feet elevation	25°	30°	35°	50 s	1 min	1 min 10 s	1 h	2 h 30 min	2 h 30 min	20
Pressure	0	60 mm	200 mm	0 s	0 s	30 min	0 s	0 s	0 s	5

General tilt angle: Min 10°, Ideal 20°, Max 30°.

- Gap: This value represents the time after which each activity (except pressure) is to be repeated.
- Alert after: This value indicates the number of rule violations, after which the notification action takes place.

An Attribute: Value pair approach was selected wherein the clinician fills in the value cells of a spreadsheet (Table 11.1) (Siewiorek and Smailagic 2008). It is interesting to note that through students soliciting inputs from clinicians for the power wheelchair virtual coach, the clinicians changed their practice to a more repeatable process.

Data analysis software extracts underlying user patterns. A clinician-friendly interface allows therapists to prescribe rules for proper use of the wheelchair, as well as parameters for user compliance goals. To illustrate how a user would comply with one of the rules, we describe the use of the feet elevation rule:

1. The user tilts to an angle between the min and max of the general tilt angle, aiming for the ideal specified angle.
2. The user then reclines to an angle between the min and max of the general recline angle, aiming for the ideal value.
3. Now, the user elevates the leg-rest to an angle between the min and the max in the feet elevation activity parameter, aiming again for the ideal value.
4. The user maintains this position for the duration specified in the prescription.
5. This completes the compliance of the feet elevation rule and the user can wait for more reminders or resume daily activity.

Clinician settings, user data, and sensor data are stored in a database, and a web service component securely transfers data from the clinician's computer to chair-side system. A web portal is designed to provide quick access to all frequently needed information to a clinician.

After entering a usage prescription, the clinician can periodically monitor the wheelchair user's compliance to those recommendations. An example alert as seen by the clinician is shown in Figure 11.6. The shape of daily, weekly, or monthly Kiviat graphs, makes it easy for the clinician to quickly determine the progress of each user, as shown in Figure 11.7. Reminders are generated to prompt the user to comply, while alerts indicate noncompliance and are sent to the user, as shown in Figure 11.8.

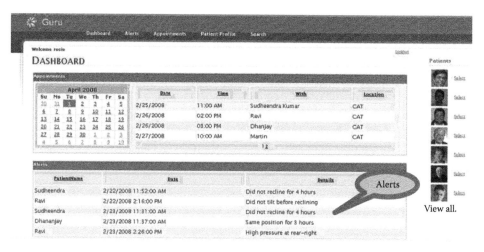

FIGURE 11.6
Dashboard for the clinician showing noncompliance alerts.

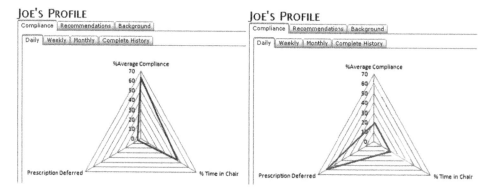

FIGURE 11.7
The clinician can look at daily, weekly or monthly graphs of the wheel chair user's compliance and follow the progress of each user. The shape of the triangle should be orientated towards the right indicating user compliance. On the left, an example of good compliance is shown. On the right, an example of poor compliance is shown.

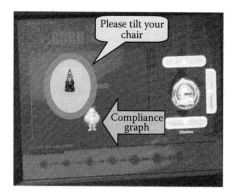

FIGURE 11.8
(See color insert.) Virtual coach screen with a reminder to tilt. The compliance graph shows color coded hourly compliance.

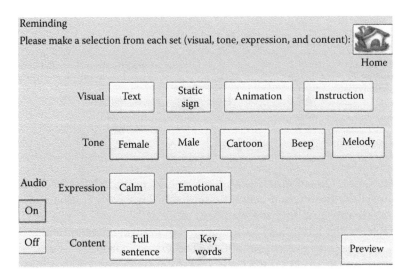

FIGURE 11.9
Menu for selecting features for virtual coach interaction design.

11.3.1 Laboratory Test

An important part of the design process is to obtain user feedback. The feedback can be gathered in the laboratory even before the virtual coach is operational. A Wizard of Oz user preference study was used to determine the appropriate interface modalities and coaching strategies. A survey program (Figure 11.9) was created allowing participants to select different interface modalities/stimuli for four types of coaching scenarios: reminding (e.g., when a user forgets to change the seating position for an hour), warning (e.g., when a user accesses PSFs in an incorrect sequence), guidance (e.g., when a user attempts to access pressure relief positions), and encouragement (e.g., when a user responds to the message with appropriate actions) (Liu et al. 2010).

Nine participants who use power wheelchairs equipped with PSFs and six clinicians experienced in prescribing PSFs showed that speech was the most frequently selected modality for the reminding theme and beeping was the most frequently selected modality for the warning theme. Most subjects gave monotonic speech the lowest ranking. Male face animation received the lowest ranking. Most subjects gave cartoon animations or PSF task animations higher rankings than human face images. The participants preferred to have cartoon animation to inform them of the task they need to do, as they are funny and entertaining. They also preferred to have the animated power wheelchair figure to illustrate the instructions for the specific task, which not only conveys the essential point of a message but also makes them feel it is important to follow the instructions. Many power wheelchair users have limited upper extremity functions and strength, and moving arms and hands to navigate on a touch screen is a much more difficult task than using a joystick. An example of participant's rank ordering of the preferred location of notification by vibration is shown in Table 11.2.

11.3.2 Field Study

Subsequent to laboratory tests, the next step is to evaluate the system in the field. A 3 day pilot study was conducted to gather user feedback during actual system operation. The participants were given a demonstration of the virtual coach and supplied with

TABLE 11.2

Rank Ordering of Vibration Output Modality

Ranking of Vibration Location on the Seat	Armrest	Headrest	Backrest around Shoulder Blade	Backrest around Mid of Upper Trunk
1	60.0	6.7	26.7	6.7
2	13.3	6.7	26.7	53.3
3	26.7	6.7	33.3	26.7
4	0	80.0	13.3	13.3

educational material. Questionnaires and interviews provided feedback. Subsequently, the participants took the virtual coach home for 3 days with feedback again solicited through questionnaires and interviews (Liu et al. 2011).

Systems that leave the laboratory to operate in the natural environment must be robust. Of particular concern was system reliability. The virtual coach was exercised over various surfaces to evaluate vibration tolerance including pitch, cement, pothole, crack, grass, gravel, and mud. Location and mounting of the extra hardware, such as the touch screen, were evaluated as well as the repeatability of measurements of PSFs (e.g., tilt angles). For example, the initial screen mounting increased the width of the wheelchair and caused difficulties in traversing doorways. The ball joint that adjusted the screen angle tended to loosen. Power is a critical issue, since once the wheelchair battery is discharged the participant is unable to move. The range of the unmodified power wheelchair was 26.2 miles on a single charge. The addition of the virtual coach electronics reduced the range to 23.2 miles. This provides a comfortable margin since the average daily distance traveled by an active power wheelchair user is 10.7 miles, less than half the range with the virtual coach.

The functionality provided included pressure relief reminders (temporal and postural parameters) and further instructions once the user starts to engage seat functions. There were 12 power seat usage warnings. The warnings and reminders only appeared when the chair was occupied.

It was important to provide participants with support when the researchers were not present. A user's guide described how to use the virtual coach, precautions and limitations of the virtual coach, and how to diagnose problems and contact researchers. The clinician's guide described the default settings for the 17 variables, the relationship between the settings, and how to increase/decrease sensitivity of the warnings.

11.4 Examples of Virtual Coaches

The goal of the PWC coach is to monitor and report on compliance to a clinician authored prescription. Two basic technologies are used to identify the system's context. The power wheelchair coach is a rule-based system and an example rule for feet elevation is given in Section 11.3. The next two sections will provide brief examples of four more coaches. The manual wheelchair propulsion coach monitors for correct arm movement while propelling the chair. IMPACT seeks to motivate users to exercise. Finally, MemExerciser has a goal of improving user memory. The manual wheelchair coach uses statistical machine learning as described in Section 11.4.1. Ergo buddy identifies improper techniques while handling and delivering packages.

11.4.1 Manual Wheelchair Propulsion Coach

The manual wheelchair coach (MWC) explored providing advice to manual wheelchair users to help them avoid damaging forms of locomotion. The primary form of context for this system is the user's propulsion pattern. The contexts of self versus external propulsion and the surface over which propulsion is occurring are used to improve the accuracy of the system's propulsion pattern classifications.

The MWC uses statistical machine learning algorithms to classify propulsion patterns and surface material. The top three acceleration characteristics for six common activities after a linear discriminant analysis (LDA) transformation (Figure 11.10) illustrates spatial clustering that can be exploited (Maurer et al. 2006) to continuously infer physical activity. Both wearable (Figure 11.11) and wheelchair-mounted accelerometers were used to provide contextual information (French et al. 2007). An eWatch was worn on the wrist and a second eWatch was attached to the wheelchair frame.

Four classic propulsion patterns have been identified by a limited user study (Figure 11.12): semicircular (SEMI), single loop over (SLOP), double loop over (DLOP), and arcing (ARC). Of these, the recommended propulsion pattern is semicircular, because the strokes have lower cadence and higher stroke angle. Data were collected using all four propulsion patterns on a variety of surface types. Machine learning algorithms produced accuracies of over 90%. It was also noted that the higher the resistance of the surface traversed, the higher the propulsion prediction accuracy.

Two common machine learning algorithms, k-nearest neighbor (kNN) and support vector machines (SVM) with a radial basis function (RBF) kernel (Maurer et al. 2006), were used to classify propulsion patterns. We also experimented with simplifying the classification

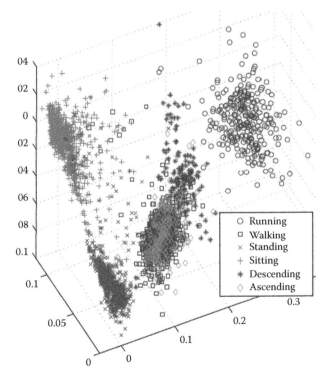

FIGURE 11.10
Feature space after LDA transformation.

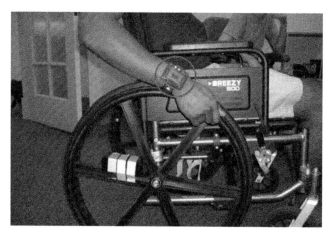

FIGURE 11.11
The eWatch worn on the wrist while the wheelchair was self-propelled.

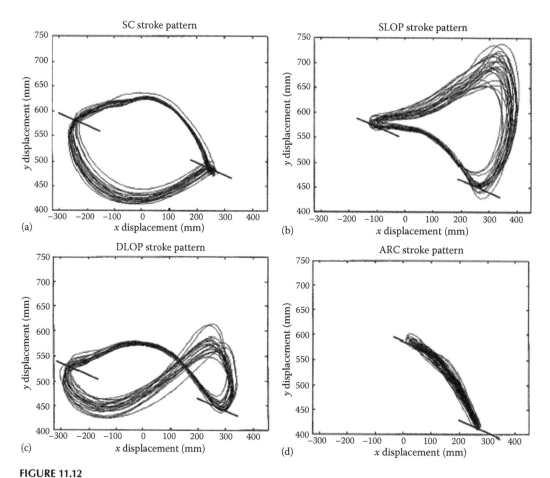

FIGURE 11.12
Four classic propulsion patterns are shown: (a) semicircular (SC); (b) SLOP; (c) DLOP; and (d) arcing. The dark bars to the right of each pattern represent the beginning of the propulsion stroke. The dark bars to the left of each pattern represent the end of the propulsion stroke and the beginning of recovery.

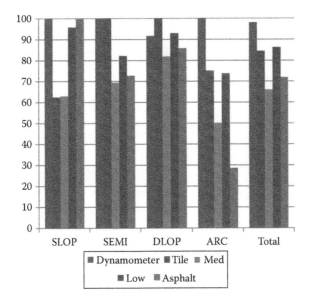

FIGURE 11.13
Classification results using KNN algorithm for various surfaces.

task into an arcing versus nonarcing pattern classification in an attempt to improve classifier accuracy. The justification for this being that arcing patterns are the most damaging to the users. Using this binary classification scheme, we found the average classification accuracy increased to the 85%–95% range.

We were able to differentiate between the resistance levels of the surface over which propulsion was occurring with 70%–80% accuracy (Figure 11.13). It can be seen that the classification accuracy tends to be higher, with less variability across patterns, on surfaces with higher resistance (dynamometer, low carpet), when compared to surfaces with low resistance (tile, asphalt). Classification accuracy for arcing was considerably lower than the other propulsion patterns. Namely, the arcing is a subset of each of the other patterns and, hence, is most susceptible to misclassification.

We found that there is differential classification accuracy across subjects, which seems to be dependent upon the arm length of the subject. Intuitively, this makes sense since the longer the arm, the faster the acceleration of the wrist if the arms are maintaining similar velocities. This also means that in order to develop cross-subject classifiers, we may need to normalize the acceleration profiles with respect to participant arm length.

We were also able to use the acceleration profile of the wheelchair from the frame-mounted accelerometer to differentiate between self-propulsion and being pushed with ~80%–90% accuracy. This type of information will be useful in system management, for example, we do not want to be providing feedback to the user on their propulsion pattern when they are not propelling themselves.

11.4.2 IMPACT: Personal Health Coach

Many physical activity awareness systems are available in today's market. These systems show physical activity information (e.g., step counts, energy expenditure, heart rate) which is sufficient for many self-knowledge needs, but information about the factors that affect physical activity may be needed for deeper self-reflection and increased self-knowledge.

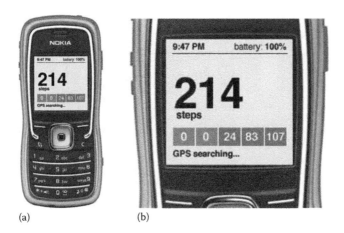

(a)   (b)

FIGURE 11.14
Monitoring device for the second version of IMPACT. Nokia 5500 Sport (a) and detailed view of the display (b).

The IMPACT project explored the use of contextual information, such as events, places, and people, to support reflection on the factors that affect physical activity.

IMPACT uses a mobile phone and GPS to monitor step counts and the user's location (Figure 11.14). The mobile phone also has an easy-to-use interface to input what the user is doing and whom he/she is with. The pedometer application stores the user's step counts per minute and displays the user's aggregate step counts for the day and for each of the past 5 min. The GPS module scans the user's location every minute, which is then stored by the phone application. The phone application collects additional contextual information using activity-triggered experience sampling. When the user is active or inactive, the phone vibrates to prompt the user to select from a list: what they were doing (events) and whom they were with (people). The list is prefilled with five common activities (e.g., grocery shopping, walking) and five usual companions (e.g., friends, family, coworkers), but users can enter new labels. We did not implement automatic labeling of events and people because such classification requires additional sensors that may not be robust enough for a long-term field study or are still not mainstream and widely available.

The IMPACT system also includes a web interface (Figure 11.15) that shows the association between daily activities and step counts on (1) a timeline of the user's steps with time segments labeled with contextual information and (2) a histogram of the total number of steps associated with a particular label (e.g., 400 steps at work, 1300 steps at the grocery store). Instead of manually entering step counts and contextual information on the web site, a desktop application synchronized data between the phone and the new web site. If the user needs to add more contextual information after uploading, they can label periods of time on the visualizations. We also implemented two other versions of the system: *steps-only* and *control*. The *steps-only* system only monitored step counts and the web site only showed daily step counts without any contextual information. The mobile phone still alerted users when they have been active and inactive, but they were just asked to rate how active they were on a 5-point Likert scale (not at all active to very active) to make the interruption comparable to the *IMPACT* version. The *control* system also only monitored step counts, but we removed visualizations on the web site. Essentially, it is similar to an off-the-shelf pedometer.

We conducted an 8 week long study with 49 participants with an age range of 18–60: 4 weeks for a *baseline* phase and 4 weeks for an *intervention* phase. During the *baseline*

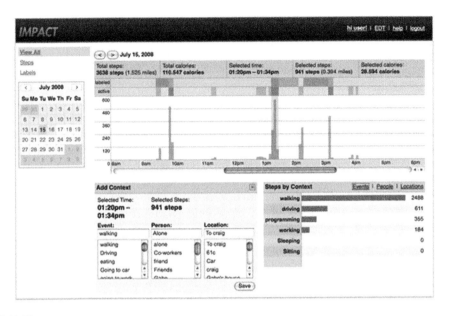

FIGURE 11.15
Visualizations in the IMPACT website showing step counts with contextual information. Detailed step counts graph with contextual annotations (top) and context graph (bottom right).

phase, all participants used the *control* system. During the *intervention* phase, participants were randomly assigned to three types of interventions: *control*, *steps-only*, and *IMPACT*. The evaluation revealed three major findings. First, when given access to contextual information and physical activity information, users can and do make associations between the information helping them become aware of factors that affect their physical activity. Second, reflecting on physical activity and contextual information can increase people's awareness of opportunities for physical activity. Lastly, automated tracking of physical activity and contextual information increases the amount of data collected by the user, which benefits long-term reflection but may be detrimental to immediate awareness.

We believe these results are applicable to the use of contextual information to reveal factors that affect other types of behaviors, for example, diabetes management and energy conservation. These contributions suggest that personal informatics systems should further explore incorporating contextual information.

11.4.3 MemExerciser

People with episodic memory impairment (EMI), such as those with early-stage Alzheimer's disease, struggle with maintaining their sense of self (Conway 1990). While they can still remember experiences from the distant past, recent experiences are difficult to recall. As a result, their window of remembered experiences shrinks as their memory abilities decline, leading to feelings of frustration, anger, or depression (Steeman et al. 2006). Over 36 million people worldwide suffer from Alzheimer's disease (AHAF 2012), but the effects are not limited to these individuals. Rather, the disease also affects the well-being of family caregivers as they have to provide the cognitive support necessary for aging in place. Caregivers usually help the person with EMI remember the details of an experience by providing cues, small details of the experience from which the person with EMI can use to recollect other details and mentally relive the experience. However, caregivers often must repeatedly provide cues for the same experience again and again which can lead to feeling overburdened, burnt out, or even depressed (Almbert et al. 1997).

Lifelogging systems automatically record a log of a user's personal experience in the form of pictures, sounds, actions, activities, or raw sensor data using wearable or embedded sensors such as cameras, audio recorders, location tracking, and bodily sensors. The data collected by lifelogging systems can provide memory cues to help people remember the original experience (Sellen et al. 2007). However, the sheer amount of data collected can also be overwhelming.

MemExerciser, a lifelogging system, is specifically designed for people with EMI and their caregivers. The system records and supports reminiscence for significant personal experiences that the user wants to remember in detail. The goals of the system are to maximize the independence of the person with EMI and at the same time minimize the burden on their caregiver. The system provides an appropriate amount of cueing assistance for the person with EMI to reminisce about the experience without needing to bother the caregiver repeatedly to provide additional cues.

MemExerciser consists of three subsystems (Figure 11.16): passive experience capture, hybrid cue selection (CueChooser), and cue review (CueViewer).

The system captures both the visual and audio content of the experience as well as contextual information such as location, movement, and light levels. People with memory impairment often forget to explicitly trigger a device (e.g., camera) to record. The system uses a passive capture approach that requires the user only to turn it on and allow the system to manage when to trigger recording. The capture system consists of three devices (Figure 11.17): the Microsoft SenseCam (Hodges et al. 2006), an off-the-shelf digital voice recorder, and an off-the-shelf Wintec GPS location tracker. The SenseCam is a wearable digital camera that automatically

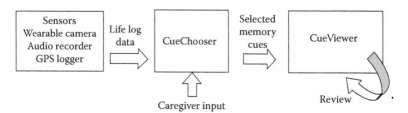

FIGURE 11.16
MemExerciser system design: capture, selection, and review.

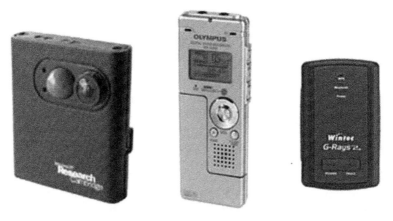

FIGURE 11.17
Capture devices: Microsoft SenseCam, digital voice recorder, GPS logger.

takes pictures when triggered by the onboard light sensor, infrared sensor, accelerometer, or simple timer. With an initial reminder from the caregiver, the person with EMI can switch on these three capture devices before each experience, wear the camera around the neck, place the audio recorder in their top shirt pocket, carry the GPS logger in their pocket, and can simply enjoy their experience without needing to stop and tell the system to record.

With a passive capture approach mentioned previously, the system can capture a large amount of data. To identify the most salient memory cues to present to the person with EMI, the lifelogging system employs a hybrid approach that involves both automated computer analysis of the lifelog as well as the expertise of the caregiver. CueChooser is a software application that assists the caregiver in selecting the most salient memory cues using automated content and context analysis.

Prior work (Lee and Dey 2007) has identified that the most salient memory cues are determined by the type of experience. There are people-based, place-based, action-based, and object-based experiences. The caregiver can specify the type of the experience and CueChooser (Figure 11.18) will apply the appropriate content and context analyses to suggest potentially good cues. For people-based experiences, CueChooser identifies photos with faces using computer vision. For place-based experiences, it uses a combination of GPS data and the SenseCam's accelerometer data to determine when the user enters, is near, or is staying in a particular place. Similarly for object-based experiences, CueChooser can use GPS or accelerometer data to find when the user is standing still and looking at an object of interest. For action-based experiences, image summarization techniques (Doherty et al. 2007) are used to find cues from different scenes. However, good memory cues have other characteristics that computers have difficulty identifying such as distinctiveness and personal significance (Lee and Dey 2007). The CueChooser interface allows the caregiver to browse through the automatically suggested photos to select content to

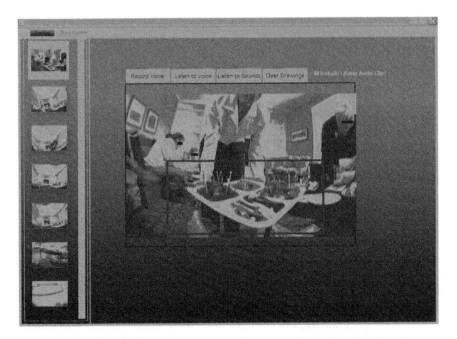

FIGURE 11.18
MemExerciser's CueChooser user interface. The caregiver can view system-suggested cues in constructing a narrative and provide audiovisual annotations to selected cues.

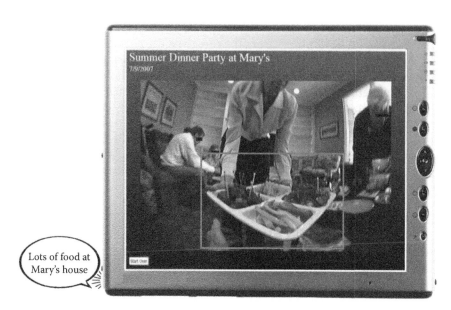

FIGURE 11.19
MemExerciser's CueViewer user interface: tapping on the screen displays pictures and plays back lifelog audio and caregiver's voice annotation.

include in a slideshow narrative. Caregivers can add their own annotation using their voice or drawing on each photo in the slideshow narrative.

The lifelogging system presents the lifelog data in a way that maximizes the opportunities for the person with EMI to think deeply about each cue to trigger his own recollection of the original experience. Caregivers normally reveal cues one at a time to allow the person with EMI to remember the rest of the experience on their own (Lee and Dey 2007). MemExerciser (Figure 11.19) includes a software application designed to run on a Tablet PC. Based on the selection of photos, sounds, and annotations from the caregiver with the CueChooser application, MemExerciser allows the person with EMI to step through all the cues at their own pace. The cue review process is designed to be challenging enough to stimulate their memory processes (acting as a form of mental exercise), but it also can be supportive enough so that people with EMI can feel as if they are mentally reliving the experience. Instead of passively playing back each photo and sound like a movie, MemExerciser shows only one picture at a time and gives the user control over how long they want to examine each picture. Recorded audio and the caregiver's annotation are progressively revealed to facilitate the user's self-recollection. With MemExerciser, the person with EMI can feel as if his caregiver is walking him through the cues but with the benefit of going at their own pace and not repeatedly bothering the caregiver.

A pilot field evaluation was conducted of the lifelogging system with three people with EMI (all associated with the early stages of Alzheimer's disease) and their spousal caregivers. The self-guided review approach of the lifelogging system was compared with a caregiver-guided approach (Hodges et al. 2006) where the caregiver repeatedly guides the person with EMI through only the photos taken with the SenseCam. Participants review the cues every other day during the 2 weeks after their experience. It was found that the self-guided approach resulted in a statistically significantly greater number of details freely recalled 4 weeks after the experience (Figure 11.20) as well as greater confidence in memory when assessed using the metamemory in adulthood questionnaire (Figure 11.21).

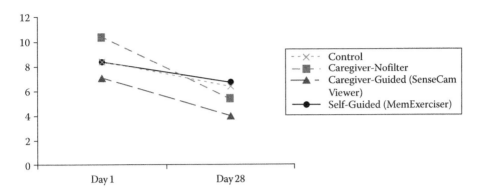

FIGURE 11.20
Mean number of details recalled.

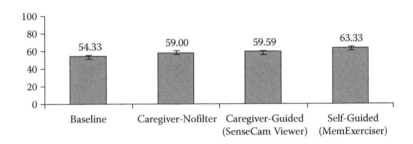

FIGURE 11.21
Participant's self-assessed memory confidence using the metamemory in adulthood questionnaire.

Caregivers expressed that the self-guided approach freed them from repeatedly going through the same cues again and again.

In summary, MemExerciser is a lifelogging system to assist people with EMI to reminisce about recent experiences. The system uses a passive capture approach so that the person with EMI does not have to remember to initiate capture. The system uses both automated computer analysis and the expertise of the caregiver to select out the most salient cues from the lifelog. Finally, the system structures the cue review interaction so that it allows the person with EMI to think more deeply about each cue and remember the details of their experiences without repeatedly burdening the caregiver.

11.5 Design, Evaluation, and Architecture of Virtual Coaches

In the process of designing and deploying virtual coaches we have gained experiences that are transferrable to new virtual coaches. The first is a design methodology where the end user is an integral part of the design team. Many of the coaches described in this paper were designed by an interdisciplinary capstone design class as described in Section 11.5.1.

Traditionally systems are completely designed and built before an evaluation with tens of users. Iterating to improve the design is labor intensive and time consuming. Section 11.5.2

describes how very early in the design process CogTool can be used to accurately predict the user time to complete a task.

Virtual coaches typically have multiple sensors. Section 11.5.3 explores how virtual coaches should be constructed with respect to conserving communications bandwidth and power consumption while maximizing accuracy in the face of errors.

11.5.1 User-Centered Design

Commercial systems go through a formal evolution of increasing functionality and robustness. These releases are typically referred to as Alpha and Beta. The Alpha release, the first functional version, is exercised by knowledgeable users to uncover defects and to suggest functional enhancements. The Beta release is fully functional but may still harbor obscure bugs that may only appear after many hours of user interaction.

Research systems undergo a similar development, although the labor is typically provided by students. Figure 11.22 shows one such pipeline based on user-centered design representing four iterations. With the advent of rapid design methodologies and rapid fabrication technologies, it is possible to construct fully customized systems in a matter of months. Carnegie Mellon has developed a user-centered interdisciplinary concurrent system design methodology (UICSM) in which teams of electrical engineers, mechanical engineers, computer scientists, industrial designers, and human–computer interaction students work with an end user to generate a complete prototype system during a 4 month long course (Siewiorek et al. 1994, Smailagic et al. 1995). The methodology defines intermediary design products that document the evolution of the design. These products are posted on the Internet so that even remote designers and end users can participate in the design activities. The methodology includes monitoring and evaluation of the design process by a dedicated faculty member.

The design methodology proceeds through three phases: conceptual design, detailed design, and implementation. End users critique the design at each phase. In addition, simulated and real application tasks provide further focus for design evaluation. Based on user interviews and observation of their operations, baseline scenarios are created for current practice. A visionary scenario is created to indicate how technology could improve the current practice and identify opportunities for technology injection. This scenario forms the basis from which the requirements for the design are derived as well as for evaluating design alternatives. Both scenarios are reviewed with the end user. A technology search generates candidates for meeting the design requirements. Several architectures, each appropriate to the various disciplines, are generated next: hardware, software, mechanical, shapes/materials, and human interaction modes. User feedback on scenarios and storyboards become an input to the detailed design phase. Designers alternate between the abstract and the concrete; preliminary sketches are evaluated, new ideas emerge, and more precise drawings

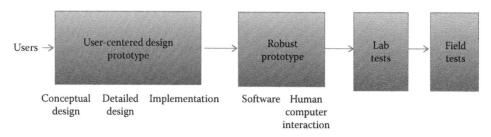

FIGURE 11.22
Project pipeline from prototype to field deployment.

are generated. This iterative process continues with soft mock-ups, appearance sketches, computer, and machine shop prototypes, until finally the product is fabricated.

The iterative evaluation by end users throughout the design process yields the equivalent of a second level (i.e., Beta) prototype that is much closer to deployment than a prototype produced by a traditional design methodology. Further development through the summer semester by selected students from the class yields a prototype suitable for pilot studies. Engagement of between 20 and 25 students from multiple disciplines (computer engineering, electrical engineering, mechanical engineering, computer science, industrial design, and human–computer interaction) yields 4000–5000 engineering hours devoted to an integrated system prototype.

In universities many technical disciplines have capstone design courses wherein senior students are given the opportunity to apply the theory they have learned to a large-scale project. While these courses will approach a project from a focused perspective, taken as a group they provide a measurable improvement. In Figure 11.22 we depict a human–computer interaction capstone that engages end users to evaluate and redesign the user experience and a software engineering capstone that improves the robustness of the software. Example of software improvements could include extending the software architecture to be multithreaded and event oriented, add logging of GUI and application events, customize device configuration; improve error handling by catching and handling hardware problems, automatic disabling malfunctioning assessments; and employing software best practices using styles and templates to separate application and data domains, and design patterns.

Other capstone opportunities may be available depending on the disciplines required for the project. Project development continues through end user testing in the lab followed by end user testing in the field. Multiple replicas of the project enable field deployment at multiple sites, greatly increasing experience and data collection.

11.5.2 Evaluating Virtual Coach Interactions at Design Time

We have explored alternative means of interacting with mobile, sensor-based systems and application of CogTool to evaluate the relative efficiency between interface modalities at design time. The application domain was periodically requesting users to answer a short survey. Reminders and polling of users for input are common features of virtual coaches. There are several possible user interaction modalities, but the selection of an inappropriate interface can lead to several factors longer to complete a task. CogTool can evaluate user interaction designs very early in the design process allowing for quick iteration into an efficient design.

As an example, in one field trial we had 30 participants use different multimedia platforms to answer a questionnaire (French et al. 2010). Each interview consisted of a series of stress-related questions, approximately 200 s in length, asked every 45 min. User input was collected through buttons and gestures. Outputs were either audio or video. Different platforms (Figure 11.23a and b) supporting the various input/output modalities were evaluated. A common state machine was used for all variations of user modalities (Figure 11.24). We also evaluated the interaction designs using CogTool. Once a mockup of the user interaction has been created, a designer can demonstrate the steps of a particular task by directly interacting with the series of screens that represent the user progressing through a task. As the demonstration proceeds, CogTool builds a model of the task (Figure 11.25) that translated into a KLM-like language called ACT-Simple. The language is executed via the ACT-R cognitive architecture to produce a performance prediction and a detailed trace of modeled behavior. (ACT-R is a sophisticated system with a rich theoretical basis and years of use in the

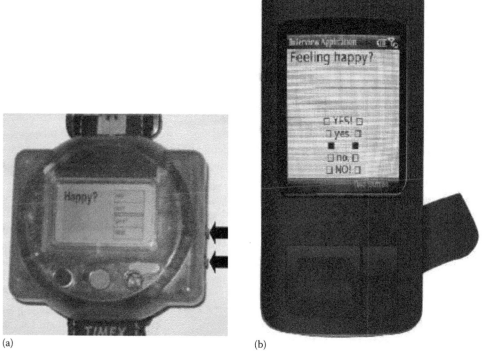

FIGURE 11.23
(See color insert.) Two platforms that were explored during the EMA development process: (a) the eWatch and (b) a smartphone with a silicon sleeve button interface (right). Both platforms are displaying an example question of the interview application.

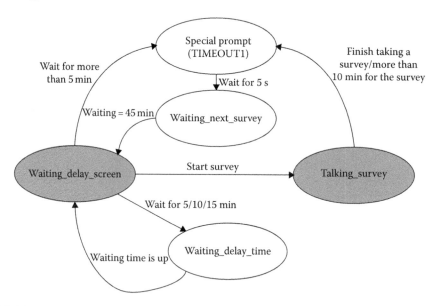

FIGURE 11.24
Stress survey state diagram; the states shaded in gray require user interaction.

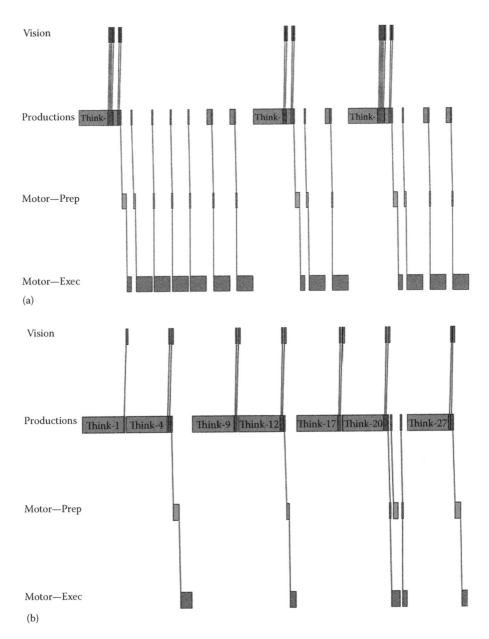

FIGURE 11.25
A visual depiction of the modeled actions of an expert interacting with the first three screens of the interview application using the visual output modality combined with the gesture input modality (a) and the eWatch button input modality (b).

cognitive psychology research community and elsewhere). The CogTool simulation predicted user interaction time typically within 10% of the actual human subject time (Figure 11.26). Surprisingly users were more efficient using buttons to respond rather than gestures, even though using buttons required both hands. These results are predicted by the CogTool model (French et al. 2010).

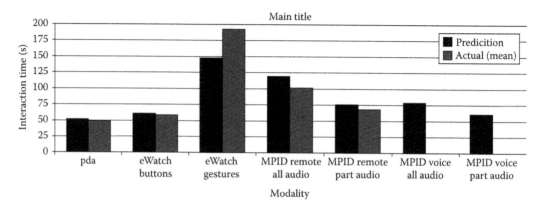

FIGURE 11.26

Interaction time comparison between CogTool model predictions and measured user interaction times. Voice input has yet to be implemented so only the predictions are given.

11.5.3 Virtual Coach Architecture

We will illustrate architectural trade-offs in the context of the design of ergo Buddy, a virtual coach system for package delivery workers to help prevent injury and reinforce trained ergonomic practices. The user activities are inferred from a handheld device (which delivery drivers carry containing the routing information as well as recorder for recipient signatures) and supportive wearable devices. A typical approach in determining the best combination of sensor locations is to have the user wear multiple devices and use only the data from selected devices to evaluate performance for the different configurations.

For example, Figure 11.27 shows accuracy of activity classification for six locations on the user's body: wrist, pants pocket, book bag, lanyard (neck), shirt pocket, and belt. For the majority of activities (running, sitting, standing, walking) any of the locations would give a classification accuracy over 90%. However, if descending stairs was important, a wrist mounted sensor should be added. For ascending stairs, the book bag sensor is most accurate.

For ergo Buddy, there is a single master handheld device and five eWatches (small sensor nodes) worn at the arm, ankle, back, lanyard, and wrist positions (Figure 11.28).

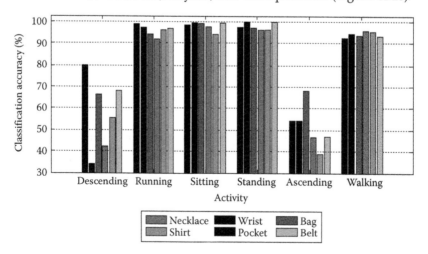

FIGURE 11.27

Activity recognition accuracy at body locations.

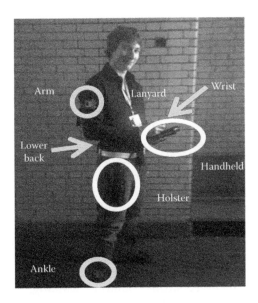

FIGURE 11.28
(See color insert.) Multiple sensor placement.

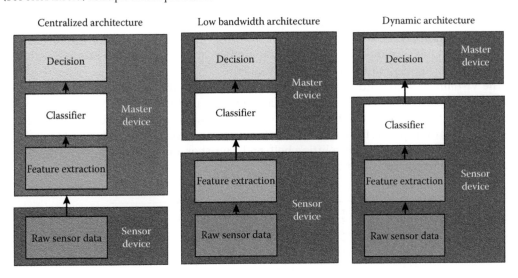

FIGURE 11.29
Classification engine partitions.

For a statistical machine learning classifier, there are four layers of processing: raw sensor data, feature extraction, classifier, and decision. These four layers can be intuitively partitioned into three different architectures shown in Figure 11.29. As expected, there are implications with each partition on how fusion is performed and wireless bandwidth utilization. A brief overview of the three partitions.

Centralized aggregation architecture: This is a commonly used architecture in which raw data from all nodes in a network are transmitted to a master device for feature extraction and classification. In our experiment the amount of data transmitted is a continuous stream at 2 kB/s. This scheme requires a static set of sensors.

Low bandwidth architecture: This architecture requires lower radio bandwidth since feature vectors are transmitted upon completion, yielding approximately 200/tw Bytes/s. This yields the same accuracy performance of a centralized aggregation architecture. Again a static set of sensors is required.

Dynamic architecture: The dynamic architecture further decreases bandwidth usage since only the context and confidence information is transmitted every window. This is approximately 80/tw Bytes/s. Decision fusion differs from the previously described aggregators in that it allows the number of sensors to be dynamic. Accuracy is expected to decrease because only an abstraction of raw data is provided to the final decision maker (fuser), but the system becomes resilient to sensor failure and packet loss faults.

Multiple fusion techniques were used for the study and the best performance was offered by a scheme in which the average probability of all available sensors' confidence is used to fuse the local decisions into a final decision (Fisk et al. 2011). This fusion technique, since it does not require all sensors to be available every time it makes a decision, is resilient to lost packets and node failures. In a perfect environment we achieve up to 90% leave one subject out cross-validation classification accuracy on trained package delivery activities. The activity set included sitting, standing, walking, running, lifting, carrying, sweeping/mopping, using stairs, using a ladder, and using a cart, and there were 11 subjects totally, which yielded approximately 20 h of data. Multiple machine learning algorithms were tested, but best performance, given device constraints, was boosted decision trees on the eWatch (lower memory footprint) and random forests on the MC9500 master device. Additionally we find that performance scales well when data are missing, offering improved performance over a nonfusion method at any packet lose rate and only 2% worse accuracy performance at 0% packet loss rate.

The visualization in Figure 11.30 graphs the F-Measure (harmonic mean of recall and precision) of each for each activity. These data are particularly relevant for a customer who may be specifically interested in detection of activities with ergonomic consequences such as lifting. For example, in the case of lifting the customer would definitely want to include a lower back sensor, perhaps in a lifting belt, and a wrist or ankle sensor to complement the back sensor and capture other activities.

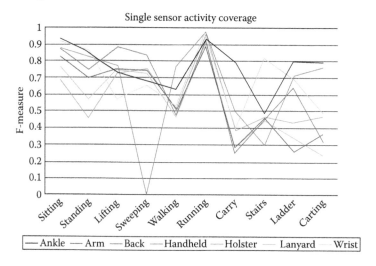

FIGURE 11.30
A visualization of the performance of sensor locations as they vary with activity.

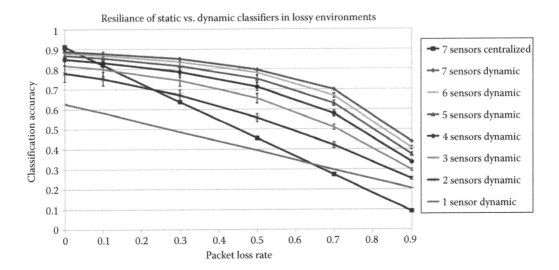

FIGURE 11.31
With the same number of sensors in a 0% loss environment, fusion only provides 2% worse performance than a low bandwidth model.

In order to test the resilience of the classifier, we simulated packet loss from 10% to 90%. For completeness, the best sensor subsets of one to seven sensors were included in the analysis. To visualize the difference in reliability, a low bandwidth scheme was also included. Figure 11.31 illustrates the results from this experiment. The primary takeaway from this chart is that in all nonideal environments, 10% and up of packet loss, better classification performance was achieved with fusion. For example, there is a 35% accuracy increase for fusion in an environment with 50% packet loss. We have discovered that the number of sensors can be reduced in low loss environments for power and bandwidth savings. Seven sensors seems to be overkill based on this dataset, and three sensors is a more appealing configuration in terms of overall encumbrance, power, and accuracy performance.

11.6 Summary

Table 11.3 summarizes examples of virtual coaches and Table 11.4 summarizes over a dozen virtual coaches and the technologies they employ.

Virtual coaches pose several research challenges. In addition to the challenges of interruption, there are also challenges of privacy. The information routinely emitted by wireless

TABLE 11.3

Summary of Example Virtual Coaches

Function	Coach	Technology
Monitoring for compliance	Power wheelchair	Rule
Correct form	Manual wheelchair propulsion	Machine learning
Correct form	Ergo buddy	Machine learning
Motivation	IMPACT	Rule
Cognitive	MemExerciser	Rule

TABLE 11.4

Summary of Technology Employed by Several Virtual Coaches

		Technologies						
Virtual Coach	Status	Sensor Data Processing	Sensor Fusion	Context Aware Sensing	Machine Learning	Ecological Momentary Assessment	Data Visualization	Computer Vision
Seating coach	Current testbed	X	X				X	
Health kiosk	Current testbed	X				X	X	
IMPACT	Technology reuse	X		X	X	X	X	
Personal exercise	Current testbed				X		X	
Ergo buddy	Assoc. project	X	X		X			
Osteoarthritis PT	Assoc. project	X	X		X		X	
Head coach	Assoc. project	X	X		X		X	
Myomo	Pending follow-on proposal	X	X		X	X	X	
Drive cap	Current testbed	X	X	X	X		X	X
Trinetra		X					X	
MemExerciser	Reuse or commercialize	X	X				X	X
Building navigation	Future	X					X	X
Who's that	Future	X					X	X

devices to stay in contact with the network is open to abuse. Some social objectives related to collection and use of personal information may be in conflict. We must determine what information is requested of users, what information is collected through monitoring, how long such information is stored, how it is protected from unauthorized access, who is authorized to examine information associated with an individual, and who is authorized to examine aggregate information on groups of users.

Meeting the needs of users requires revealing personal information in some cases and protecting it in others. One way to meet diverse needs is to allow individuals to state their own preferences to the system. The challenge will be to create a protocol that is complex enough to address the diverse privacy issues, while embedding it in a user interface that is simple enough for the layman to use.

The goal is to employ theory from social science, cognitive science, and economics. Social science models of collaborative behavior can be used as a basis for determining the nature of the social setting. Theories and observations of which clues humans use to interrupt a social situation and gain attention can form the basis for sensor data processing and software decisions in virtual coaches. By mapping observable parameters into cognitive states, the computing system can estimate the form of interaction that minimizes user distraction and the risk of cognitive overload.

References

AHAF (2012). About Alzheimer's Disease, American Health Assistance Foundation, http://www.ahaf.org/alzheimers/about/

Almbert, B., Grafstrom, M., Winblad, B. (1997). Caring for a demented elderly person—Burden and burnout among caregiving relatives, *Journal of Advanced Nursing*, 25 (1), 109–116.

Conway, M. (1990). *Autobiographical Memory*. Open University Press, Milton Keynes, U.K.

Doherty, A.R., Smeaton, A.F., Lee, K., Ellis, D. (2007). *Multimodal Segmentation of Lifelog Data*. RIAO, Pittsburgh, PA.

Fisk, S., Siewiorek, D.P., Smailagic, A. (June 2011). Increasing multi-sensor classifier accuracy through personalization and sensor fusion, *Proceedings of the International Symposium on Quality of Life Technology*, Toronto, Canada.

French, B., Siewiorek, D.P., Smailagic, A., Deisher, M. (2007). Selective sampling strategies to conserve power in context aware devices, ISWC, *Proceedings of the 11th IEEE International Symposium on Wearable Computers*, Boston, MA, pp. 1–4.

French, B., Siewiorek, D.P., Smailagic, A., Kamarck, T. (2010). Lessons learned designing multi-modal ecological momentary assessment tools, *Journal of Technology and Disability*, Special Issue on Quality of Life Technology, IOS Press, 22 (1–2), 41–51.

Hodges, S., Williams, L., Berry, E., Izadi, S., Srinivasan, J., Butler, A., Smyth, G., Kapur, N., Wood, K. (2006). SenseCam: A retrospective memory aid, *Proceedings of the UBICOMP*, Seattle, WA, pp. 81–90.

Lee, M.L., Dey, A.K. (2007). Providing good memory cues for people with episodic memory impairment, *Proceedings of the ASSETS 2007*, Phoenix, AZ, pp. 131–138.

Liu, H., Cooper, R.M., Cooper, R.A., Smailagic, A., Siewiorek, D., Ding, D., Chuang, F. (2010). Seating virtual coach: A smart reminder for power seat function usage, *Journal of Technology and Disability*, 22 (1–2), 53–60.

Liu, H.-Y., Grindle, G., Chuang, F.-C., Kelleher, A., Cooper, R., Siewiorek, D., Smailagic, A., Cooper, R. (2011). User preferences for indicator and feedback modalities: A preliminary survey study for developing a coaching system to facilitate wheelchair power seat function usage, *IEEE Pervasiv Computing*, 10, http://ieeexplore.ieee.org/stamp/stamp.jsp?tp=&arnumber=5744066stag=1

Maurer, U., Smailagic, A., Siewiorek, D.P., Deisher, M. (2006). Activity recognition and monitoring using multiple sensors on different body positions, *Proceedings of the BSN*, Aachen, Germany, pp. 113–116.

Plarre, K., Raij, A., Hossain, S., Ali, A., Nakajima, M., Al'Absiz, M., Ertin, E. et al. (2011). Continuous inference of psychological stress from sensory measurements collected in the natural environment, *Proceedings of the ACM/IEEE International Conference on Information Processing in Sensor Networks (IPSN 2011)*, Chicago, IL, pp. 97–1010.

Sellen, A.J., Fogg, A., Aitken, M., Hodges, S., Rother, C., Wood, K. (2007). Do life-logging technologies support memory for the past?: An experimental study using sensecam. *Proceedings of the CHI*, Irvine, CA, pp. 81–90.

Siewiorek, D.P., Smailagic, A., Lee, J.C. (1994). An interdisciplinary concurrent design methodology as applied to the Navigator wearable computer system, *Journal of Computer and Software Engineering*, 2(3), 259–292.

Siewiorek, D.P., Smailagic, A. (2008). Virtual coach for power wheelchair users. Institute for Complex Engineered Systems Technical Report, Carnegie Mellon University, Pittsburgh, PA.

Siewiorek, D. P., Smailagic, A., Starner, T. (2008). *Application Design for Wearable Computing*, Morgan & Claypool Publishers.

Siewiorek, D.P., Smailagic, A., Courtney, K., Matthews, J., Bennett, K., Cawley, R., Liao, X., Vartak, M., White, N., Yates, J. (June 2010). Multi-user health kiosk, *Proceedings of the International Symposium on Quality of Life Technology*, Las Vegas, NV.

Smailagic, A., Siewiorek, D.P., Anderson, D., Kasabach, C., Martin, T., Stivoric, J. (1995). Benchmarking an interdisciplinary concurrent design methodology for electronic/mechanical design, *Proceedings of the ACM/IEEE Design Automation Conference*, New York, pp. 514–519.

Smailagic, A., Siewiorek, D.P., Maurer, U., Rowe, A., Tank, K. (2005). eWatch: Context sensitive system design case study, *Proceedings of the IEEE Symposium on VLSI*, Tampa, FL, pp. 98–103.

Steeman, E., De Casterle, B.D., Godderis, J., Grypdonck, M. (2006). Living with early-stage dementia: A review of qualitative studies, *Journal of Advanced Nursing*, 54, 722–738.

12

Nonwearable In-Home Sensing for Early Detection of Health Changes

Marjorie Skubic, Marilyn J. Rantz, Steve J. Miller, Rainer Dane Guevara, Richelle J. Koopman, Gregory L. Alexander, and Lorraine J. Phillips

CONTENTS

12.1 Introduction

One aspect of quality of life (QoL) is having the flexibility and freedom (i.e., personal control) over where to live. Thus, an example of QoL technology is in-home sensing that supports aging in the home of choice. This is often called aging in place, in reference to the strong preference of older adults to stay in their own homes rather than move to an assisted living or skilled nursing facility [Rantz et al., 2005a]. This chapter offers an example of QoL technology in the form of sensing and data analysis methods that support aging in place through the detection of early signs of illness and functional decline. Through early detection, while health problems are still small, interventions can be offered more effectively to hold off drastic declines in health conditions and functional well-being.

In the Preface, four attributes of QoL technology were presented. In this chapter, the *functional domain targeted* is proactive health care of older adults through early detection of health changes. In the continuum of *compensatory, preventive and maintaining, or enhancing*, this chapter falls in the middle, focusing on preventing and maintaining health by providing alerts of impending threats to QoL, in this case, due to health changes that may affect the functionality of individuals and force them into hospitalization or nursing homes. In the third attribute of *passive or interactive*, this chapter presents methods and technology that are passive with respect to user involvement of the older adult. Sensors are mounted in the home environment and analysis of the sensor data is transparent to the resident. The resident is not required to wear anything or do anything outside of the normal daily activities. In fact, the objective of the monitoring is to capture normal everyday activity patterns and recognize when these begin to change. Finally, in the attribute of *system intelligence*, this chapter provides an example of a decision support system. Automated reasoning is used to detect changes in the sensor data patterns and send alerts to clinicians. The system then relies on the expertise of the clinicians to determine what is causing the change and whether further actions or interventions are warranted. Throughout the chapter, the focus is on in-home monitoring of older adults; however, much of the work could be applied to other groups with the same motivation to maintain independence.

12.2 Creating an Interdisciplinary Team with a Shared Vision

The work described in this chapter was initiated by the University of Missouri (MU) Sinclair School of Nursing (SSON). The Aging in Place (AIP) project vision was developed in 1996 in the SSON with a diverse team to provide more and higher-quality services at home, allowing people to "age in place" [Rantz et al., 2005, JNCQ]. Residents get services when they need them until regaining independence, and then services are limited or withdrawn, so costs are controlled. Out of this initiative came TigerPlace (named after the MU mascot, shown in Figure 12.1), built by Americare Systems, Inc.: a state-of-the-art independent living facility, built to nursing home standards, licensed as intermediate care so people can use long-term care insurance, and operated as independent housing with services [Rantz et al., 2008]. While TigerPlace is owned and operated by Americare, the SSON owns and manages Sinclair Home Care, the home health-care agency that employs the clinical staff and runs the clinical operations. Thus, TigerPlace is an example of a successful partnership between a private company and a state university.

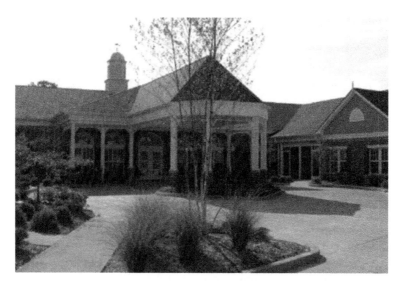

FIGURE 12.1
The TigerPlace Aging in Place facility.

From the beginning, TigerPlace was set up with an infrastructure to support aging-related research. The SSON vision was to be able to conduct research on aging in an environment where people really lived. Standardized instruments for ongoing assessment, stored in an electronic health record (EHR), and informed consent were included for all residents to allow the use of medical data for research projects. The EHR contains a longitudinal database of the standardized assessments, medical diagnoses, medications, nursing interventions, and clinical outcomes. The EHR standardized measures of functional health include the SF-12, MMSE (mini-mentalstate examination), GDS (geriatric depression scale), ADL and IADL from OASIS (home-care-required instrument), and MDS (minimum data set for nursing homes). This type of assessment is unique for independent living environments but necessary to facilitate aging research. The goal in developing TigerPlace was to maximize the living environment, add standardized instruments, and develop and evaluate new interventions to help people age well and age in place.

A timeline of important events in establishing a cohesive interdisciplinary research team is shown in Table 12.1. Two rounds of state legislation were necessary to enable the aging-in-place vision as implemented in TigerPlace. The involvement of the technical collaborators began in early 2002 when SSON professor Dr. Rantz gave a talk in the MU College of Engineering, looking for collaborators to get eldercare technology research started at TigerPlace. The path to funded research projects was not easy. Before a credible research proposal could be written, the group studied related work, assessed the collective strengths and limitations, and brainstormed new ideas. There are several challenges in establishing a truly interdisciplinary research team in which members from multiple disciplines are respected as equal partners, and cutting-edge, archival papers can be published in multiple disciplines. Different disciplines often have different vocabularies, different cultures, and different reward structures. It takes time to build a cohesive, interdisciplinary group in which interest is sustained and members persevere through the initial tough stage into becoming a team.

Early on, the group at MU conducted a series of focus groups at a local senior housing center to gage the interest and acceptance of older adults for technology solutions. The results showed that seniors would accept eldercare technology, provided that it (1) met a real need and provided a perceived benefit and (2) respected the sensory limitations typical of many older adults, such as reduced hearing and vision, and nerve loss in fingertips (haptic sensing), which makes the use of small buttons difficult [Demiris et al., 2004]. In fact, many of the senior participants of the early focus groups offered new ideas that are still innovative nearly 10 years later.

Through this effort, the group also eventually developed a shared model that the clinicians and engineers could both understand. Figure 12.2 conceptualizes this model. The solid line shows a typical stair-step trajectory of decline in functional ability based on research and practice with aging adults [Rantz et al., 2005a]. The typical trajectory includes plateaus where no measurable decline occurs and precipitous step-downs that illustrate dramatic functional decline, often the result of a significant health event or change in health status. To the engineers, the model represents a control system in which the goal is to optimize the area under the curve. To accomplish that, feedback on the current state is needed.

This model has been the basis of the integrated sensor network implemented and tested at TigerPlace. The objective is to recognize or predict the beginning of the decline using sensor data, early enough to offer effective interventions, and, thus, prevent or reduce the decline. The aimed trend (the dotted line) extends the length of the plateaus and reduces the depth of the steps. The key is to identify small health problems early—before

TABLE 12.1

Eldertech Timeline: Anatomy of an Interdisciplinary Research Team

1999	June	Aging in place state legislation passes
2000	Summer	Aging in place state legislation is challenged
2001	June	Round 2 aging in place state legislation passes
2001	Fall	Work with architect on the design of TigerPlace
2002	**Winter**	**Rantz gives a talk in the College of Engineering, looking for collaborators**
2002	**Spring**	**Rantz, Skubic and Tyrer meet with Americare and architect to discuss technology needs of TigerPlace**
2002	Summer	Building plan #1 is scrapped; architect #2 is hired
2002	**Fall**	**Skubic and students meet with Rantz, study related work, brainstorm new ideas**
2003	Winter	Group meets to discuss NIH proposal
2003	Spring	TigerPlace construction begins; discussions of technology infrastructure
2003	June	NIH R01 proposal submitted (Tyrer, PI), rejected with no score
2004	Feb	NSF ITR proposal submitted (Skubic, PI), funded!
2004	**June**	**TigerPlace opens**
2004	Oct	NIH R21 proposal submitted (He, PI), scored but rejected
2004	Oct	NIH RO1 proposal submitted (Tyrer, PI), rejected
2004	**Nov**	**Funded NSF ITR project begins (Skubic, PI)**
2005	Jan	NSF ITR kick-off meeting with UVa
2005	**Jan**	**First collaborative paper published in Nursing Outlook**
2005	March	AOA proposal submitted (Rantz, PI), funded!
2005	May	NSF UA proposal submitted (Skubic, PI), rejected 2005
2005	Sept	AOA project starts (Rantz, PI)
2005	**Oct**	**First sensor network installed in a TigerPlace apartment**
2005	Oct	NIH R21 proposal revision is submitted (He, PI), again rejected but close
2005	Nov	Second sensor network installed in TigerPlace
2006	Jan	Annual meeting for NSF ITR project with UVa. Discover overlap problems with 2 deployed sensor networks
2006	**July**	**Center for Eldercare and Rehabilitation Technology established in the College of Engineering (Skubic, Director)**
2006	July	NIDDRR RERC proposal submitted (Skubic, PI), rejected
2006	June	RAND proposal submitted (Rantz, PI), funded!
2006	Aug	Demiris leaves MU for the Univ. of Washington. Collaboration continues.
2006	Oct	NIH R21 proposal revision is submitted (He, PI), finally funded!
2006	Oct	NSF HCC proposal submitted (Skubic, PI), funded!
2006	Oct	RAND project starts on interdisciplinary research center (Rantz, PI)
2007	Jan	Annual meeting for NSF ITR project with UVa. Problem solving and planning.
2007	Feb	NIH proposal submitted with GE subcontract (Rantz, PI), scored but rejected
2007	March	Ninth sensor network installed in TigerPlace
2007	May	NSF ITR Co-PI from UVa leaves academia
2007	June	Alzheimer's Association proposal submitted (Tyrer, PI), funded!
2007	July	NSF R21 project starts on video network for eldercare (He, PI)
2007	**Aug**	**First aging-related interdisciplinary course is offered for Fall, 2007**
2007	Sept	AHRQ K-Award (Alexander, PI), funded!
2007	Sept	NSF HCC project starts on vision-based sensing (Skubic, PI)
2007	Dec	Alzheimer's Association project starts on smart carpet (Tyrer, PI)
2008	Feb	UK collaborator comes for a 3-month visit
2008	June	NIH RO1 proposal with GE subcontract (Rantz, PI), scored, but rejected

TABLE 12.1 (continued)

Eldertech Timeline: Anatomy of an Interdisciplinary Research Team

2008	June	NIH R21 proposal early illness recognition (Rantz, PI), scored, but rejected
2009	**Jan**	**New 23 apartment addition opens at TigerPlace**
2009	**Feb**	**Twentieth sensor network installed in TigerPlace**
2009	Feb	National media blitz
2009	Feb	NIH R21 submitted adverse health events (Alexander, PI), rejected
2009	March	NIH R21 submitted on early illness (Rantz, PI), funded!
2009	March	AHRQ RO1 submitted with GE subcontract (Rantz, PI), funded!
2009	March	NSF submitted fall sensing and fall risk (Skubic, PI), funded!
2009	March	NIH R21 submitted acoustic fall sensor (Popescu, PI), rejected
2009	Aug	NIH R21 project starts on early illness detection with sensors (Rantz, PI)
2009	Sept	AHRQ project starts on fall detection and fall risk with rader (Rantz, PI)
2009	Sept	NSF CPS project starts on fall detection & fall risk (Skubic, PI)
2011	Sept	NSF SHB project starts (Popescu, PI)
2011	**Nov**	**Fortieth sensor network installed in TigerPlace**

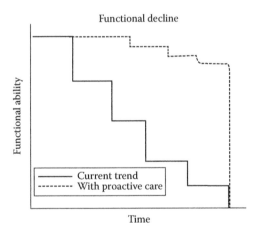

FIGURE 12.2
Squaring the life curve with detection of early illness and functional decline.

they become big health crises—and offer timely interventions designed to change the trajectory in functional decline. The result is continued high functional ability and better health outcomes. Identifying and assessing problems while they are still small can provide a window of opportunity for interventions that will alleviate the problem areas before they become catastrophic. This has become the interdisciplinary group's vision for proactive health management where the focus is on keeping people healthy instead of just intervening after they are sick.

Throughout the process, the emphasis has been on first understanding the needs and preferences of the target group and then developing solutions to address those needs and preferences. In focus groups and interviews, older adults have repeatedly shown a dislike for wearable sensing [Demiris et al., 2008a,b]. As a result, our sensing solution makes use of environmentally mounted sensors that do not require wearing anything.

12.3 In-Home Monitoring for Early Detection of Illness and Functional Decline

12.3.1 Integrated Sensor Network

Based on the shared vision described earlier, an integrated sensor network was developed to support the early detection of health changes (see Figure 12.3) [Skubic et al., 2009]. Data from sensors installed in TigerPlace apartments are logged and stored on a secure server in a mySQL database. A typical installation for a one-bedroom apartment at TigerPlace is shown in Figure 12.4. Passive infrared (PIR) motion sensors are used to capture motion in a room area and also for localized activity. For example, motion sensors are installed in the refrigerator and in kitchen cabinets to detect kitchen activity and on the ceiling over the shower to detect shower use. For convenience, a motion sensor is installed on the ceiling over the front door to detect apartment exits. Residents sometimes leave their front doors open so magnetic door sensors are not practical here. The PIR motion sensors, which use the wireless X-10 protocol for data transmission, generate an event every 7s if there is continuous motion in the sensor detection cone. This is used as an artifact to capture activity level in the home by computing a motion density as motion events per unit time [Wang and Skubic, 2008]. For example, a resident with a sedentary lifestyle may generate only 50 motion events per hour, whereas a resident with a very active puttering lifestyle may generate 400 or more motion events per hour. Changes in the motion density patterns can be analyzed and used for early detection of health changes [Wang, 2011; Wang et al., 2009, 2011, 2012].

A pneumatic bed sensor [Mack et al., 2009] is installed on the bed mattress, underneath the linens, and is used to capture sleep patterns. The bed sensor generates events

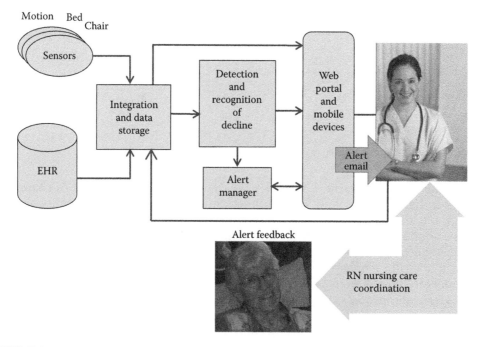

FIGURE 12.3

(See color insert.) Integrated sensor network used for early illness alerts sent via email. Nurses provide feedback on each alert as a rating on the clinical relevance.

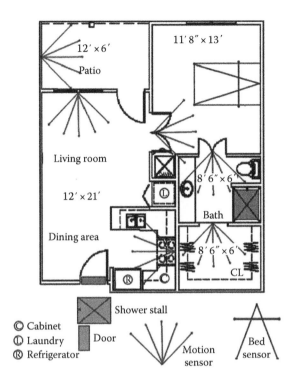

FIGURE 12.4
A typical sensor network for a one bedroom TigerPlace apartment with 10 PIR motion sensors and 1 bed sensor. The bed sensor is also used on recliner chairs for those residents that often sleep in a chair.

for restlessness in bed (four levels based on the amount of movement time) as well as qualitative events for pulse and respiration rates (low, normal, and high). Changes in these patterns can also be used for early detection of health changes. For those residents who often sleep in a recliner chair, the bed sensor is installed in the chair. An effort has been made to make the sensor installations as discrete and invisible as possible.

The sensor installations at TigerPlace also include a temperature sensor to capture use of the stove and oven. In general, there is limited use of the stove and oven by TigerPlace residents due to the excellent common dining room, so these sensor events have not been critical for early illness detection. However, in the private home setting, the use of such kitchen appliances will no doubt provide helpful insights into health changes.

12.3.2 Interactive Sensor Data Displays

A web interface has been developed for displaying the sensor data using an interactive design process that involved clinicians as target users [Alexander et al., 2008, 2011a]. Figures 12.5 through 12.7 show examples of some of the sensor data displays used in the interactive web interface. Figure 12.5 shows the basic day-to-day histogram view of restlessness events for a bed sensor installed on a recliner chair. Users are offered different views of motion and bed sensor data and have the option of displaying 24 h, daytime only, or nighttime only data, and zooming out to see more days or drilling down to see an hour-to-hour view of 1 day. Hovering over the histograms will generate a display of the number of events in the stacked histograms. The number of alerts generated per day is also shown; users can hover over the alert bar to see more detail, as shown in Figure 12.5.

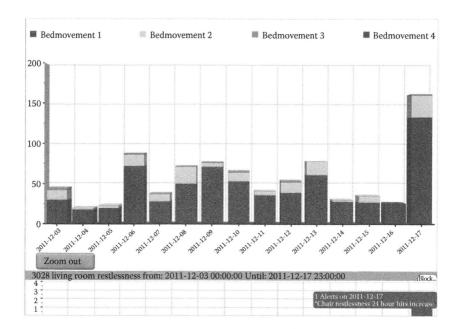

FIGURE 12.5
Sensor data displayed as histograms, in this case, restlessness events from a bed sensor installed on a recliner chair. Each histogram represents one day. An alert was generated on December 17 for increased restlessness.

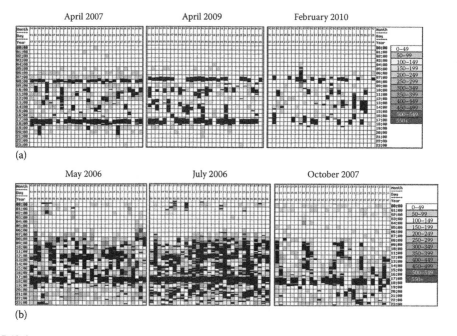

FIGURE 12.6
(See color insert.) Motion density maps from two TigerPlace residents. Each column represents one day. The vertical axis ranges from midnight at the top to 11 pm at the bottom. Black indicates out of the apartment. The color scale shows the motion density from low density (white, gray) to high density (blue). (a) A resident who was diagnosed with depression. The density maps show decreasing activity as the resident's depression increased. (b) A resident with an irregular activity pattern indicating possible cognitive problems also shows a changing pattern in the density map.

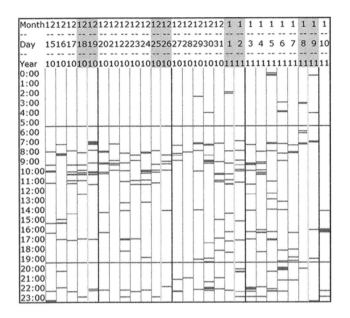

FIGURE 12.7
The bathroom activity map uses a similar format to the motion density map. Each column represents 1 day. The vertical axis ranges from midnight at the top to 11 pm at the bottom. In this example, a TigerPlace resident had increased bathroom activity at night. An alert was generated on January 1. The resident was assessed by the nurse coordinator, tested and diagnosed with a urinary tract infection, treated, and made a successful recovery.

Figure 12.6 shows examples of motion density maps generated from PIR motion sensor data. The data are first processed to determine out of the apartment time [Wang and Skubic, 2008]; these times are shown in black. Then, for the remaining time, the motion density is computed as the number of PIR events per time spent in the apartment for each 1 h block [Wang and Skubic, 2008]. The density levels are shown in color as designated in the color scale. The motion density map is organized into columns (one per day) where the top of the column corresponds to midnight and the bottom of the column corresponds to 11 p.m. Figure 12.6a shows the motion density tracked over time for a resident with increasing depression. Figure 12.6b shows the changing motion density for a resident with an irregular lifestyle pattern, indicating possible cognitive problems. A dissimilarity measure has been developed to compute the distance between one motion density pattern and another, by extracting texture features from the motion density data, much like processing of images [Wang et al., 2009, 2012]. Figure 12.7 uses a display format similar to the motion density map, but shows bathroom activity as sensed from PIR sensors. A similar format is used to display time in bed as sensed from the bed sensor. These activity maps are displayed with a default period of 6 months; the user can zoom out or select other dates to see additional time periods and track pattern changes over time.

12.3.3 Electronic Health Record

The EHR component grew out of the need to unify the residents' health data and to investigate the connection between the sensor data patterns and the residents' health conditions. Sinclair Home Care had adopted a commercially available home health EHR; however, not all of the assessments collected for the AIP project were supported. For example, the MDS (which was not supported) was needed so the clinical outcomes could be compared with nursing homes as well as home care. Supplementary databases were developed and maintained to store additional assessment information. It was necessary to develop a new EHR that could contain all of the standardized health assessments from a variety of fields and provide a link to the sensor data and medical records. No commercially available system met all of the needs of the interdisciplinary research team and health-care providers.

Clinicians typically want as much assessment data as possible to inform their medical decisions, but with technology the amount of data available can rapidly become overwhelming [Alexander and Staggers, 2009]. The vision for the new EHR was to allow the data from all of the various sources (standardized assessments, medical records, and sensors) to be synthesized and displayed in meaningful ways, making it possible to quickly and efficiently utilize the pertinent information [Rantz et al., 2010a].

A software firm was hired to develop this new integrated EHR. The interdisciplinary research team was involved from the beginning to guarantee that the system would be easy to use and the data would be displayed in a clinically meaningful way that is easy to interpret. [Alexander et al., 2008]. The resulting EHR has a web-based interface and contains all of the standardized assessments used in the AIP project as well as visit notes, orders, and other forms needed to operate a home-care agency [Rantz et al., 2010a]. Sinclair Home Care has been using the EHR as the medical record at TigerPlace since January 2011. Work is progressing on integrating the sensor data component so that it informs the medical record and is clinically relevant and easily interpreted. This integration will also facilitate automated data mining to further investigate patterns relating the sensor data to changing health conditions.

12.3.4 Early Illness Alerts

For sensor data to be clinically useful, automated processing must be included so that clinicians can be notified of potential changes in health conditions. Once notified, they also need an easy, time-efficient way to view data displays to determine clinical relevance. Clinicians caring for the elder adult with a sensor network need alerts and sensor displays that easily fold into their workflow and their busy day. With the clinician user's context in mind, we iteratively tailored the alerts and displays to maximize usability [Alexander et al., 2011b]. In the TigerPlace sensor network, the logged sensor data are automatically analyzed, looking for changes in an individual's data patterns. If a change is detected, an alert is generated in the form of an email and sent to the TigerPlace clinical staff. The alert email includes two web links. One is a link into the web portal, which facilitates fast access to the sensor data for the resident, showing a 2 week window of data before the alert. This provides context to the nurse, which helps her determine whether the alert is relevant for this resident from a clinical perspective. The second link provides access to a feedback web page that allows the clinician to rate the clinical relevance of the alert. This feedback is currently being used as ground truth to aid in the further development of the alert algorithms. The vision is to ultimately use this information for online learning and customization of alerts to the individual resident. On average, the clinician takes about 2 min to display the sensor data, analyze the alert, determine whether action is warranted, and provide feedback [Rantz et al., 2012].

The development of the alert algorithms was accomplished through an interdisciplinary collaboration funded by the NIH [Alexander et al., 2011b]. Initially, a retrospective analysis was completed around known health events such as emergency room (ER) visits, hospitalizations, and falls. A research associate examined sensor data around 74 health events from 16 participants. In 42% of the cases ($N = 31$), sensor data patterns were identified, which could serve as a basis for initial alert algorithm development [Rantz et al., 2010b]. The PI and the clinical research team (four doctorally prepared nurses and a family practice physician, all with extensive experience with older adults) confirmed the analysis, and the engineering team members

TABLE 12.2

Behaviors and Sensor Data Monitored for Early Illness Alerts

Behavior	Model
Bathroom Activity	Sum of motion sensor hits in the bathroom (bathroom, shower, laundry)
Bed Restlessness	$x_{bedrest} = \sum_{i=1}^{4} i * x_i$, where x_i is the no. of bed restlessness level i hits
Bed Breathing Low	No. of bed breathing 1 hits
Bed Breathing Normal	No. of bed breathing 2 hits
Bed Breathing High	No. of bed breathing 3 hits
Bed Pulse Low	No. of bed pulse 1 hits
Bed Pulse Normal	No. of bed pulse 2 hits
Bed Pulse High	No. of bed pulse 3 hits
Kitchen Activity	Sum of kitchen motion sensor (kitchen, fridge, etc.) hits and stove/oven temperature high
Living Room Activity	No. of living room motion sensor hits
Chair Sensor Activity	Equivalent to bed sensor behaviors above

developed the initial alert algorithms to use in the pilot study. As the study progressed, some refinements were made on the alert algorithms. The goal was to cast a wide net to ensure that critical health changes were captured even if it resulted in a high percentage of false alarms.

The team ultimately settled on an approach that looks at the sensor values per day, compared to a moving baseline of 2 weeks immediately before the day examined. That is, relative sensor values are used rather than absolute numbers. Each resident has a personalized "normal" that is reflected uniquely in the sensor data patterns, depending on the chronic health condition(s) and his or her usual lifestyle pattern as well as the size of the apartment and the number of sensors. This strategy of change detection has facilitated the testing of early illness alerts even in a diverse group of seniors with varying levels of health and chronic ailments. Table 12.2 shows the behaviors and corresponding sensor data monitored for early illness alerts. For each behavior, the system computes a mean and standard deviation for the 2 week baseline window. If the current day's values vary from the mean beyond a predetermined number of standard deviations, an alert is generated. The standard deviation multiplier was tweaked during the study and varies somewhat for different behaviors, according to the research team's view of the relative importance of the behaviors monitored. Relative changes are computed for three time periods: (1) a 24 h day, midnight to midnight, (2) daytime, 8 a.m. to 8 p.m., and (3) nighttime, midnight to 6 a.m. The alerts generated include the parameter that caused the alert, the time period of the change, the direction of change (increase or decrease), and the number of standard deviations from mean (how big is the change).

A 1 year pilot study using the alerts prospectively to detect early signs of illness was conducted from June 2010 to June 2011 [Rantz et al., 2012]. A convenience sample of 42 TigerPlace residents was recruited: 20 people living with the sensor network (intervention group) and 22 without sensors (control group). The average age of the subjects was 84.6 (range 64–96). The sample contained one Asian (control group); the remaining participants were Caucasian. Medical diagnoses including diabetes, hypertension, congestive heart failure, osteoporosis, and osteoarthritis were present in both groups. During the course of the study, three people moved to other independent housing and one control participant died shortly after baseline, so data were collected on a total of 18 intervention and 20 controls participants at the end of the study.

The intervention alerts based on the sensor data were sent to the registered nurse (RN) care coordinator at TigerPlace as well as the clinical research team. The alerts indicated potential decline in physical function, onset of acute illness, and/or exacerbation of chronic illness, allowing for further evaluation and treatment earlier than traditional health-care assessment. After receiving an alert, the RN care coordinator would access the web-based interface to determine if additional assessment was needed. The nurse would then take the appropriate actions to assess the resident, involve other health-care providers such as the participant's physician as needed, and document the assessment and interventions taken in the resident's EHR noting when the alert was received. One example of an alert that detected an impending illness is illustrated in Figure 12.7. An alert was generated on January 1 for increased nighttime bathroom activity. The resident was assessed, diagnosed with a urinary tract infection, treated, and made a successful recovery [Rantz et al., 2011]. See also Figure 12.8, which shows an example taken from the initial retrospective analysis. If the alerts had been in place for this resident, an early illness alert would have been generated 40 days before the ER visit and ultimate hospitalization.

The control participants received the normal care provided at TigerPlace. As potential problems were detected through routine assessment or participant report, the RN care coordinator assessed the resident, involved other health-care providers as needed, and documented the assessment and interventions taken in the resident's EHR.

As the clinician research team including the RN care coordinator used the web-based sensor data interface to evaluate residents after receiving alerts, they provided feedback on the clinical relevance of each alert and offered suggestions for improving the interface. The engineering team members refined the interface based on the clinician feedback. This process continued iteratively throughout the study. The clinicians also maintained logs of the time spent reviewing each alert. In addition, each month the clinicians rated the interface using seven Likert-scaled questions about the early illness sensor system.

Functional performance measures including the short physical performance battery (SPPB), the GAITRite gait analysis system, and grip strength for both hands were captured for all participants. The SPPB assesses lower extremity function using tests of standing balance, gait speed, and repeated chair stands [Guralnik et al., 1994]. The GAITRite walkway systems is a 12-ft mat that measures gait parameters such as cadence, step length, and velocity as the participant walks across it (www.gaitrite.com). Each participant walked on the GAITRite walkway once per quarter guarded by a research assistant as a safety precaution. A hand dynamometer was used to collect grip strength of both the right and left hands of each participant. Hand grip strength predicts frailty, disability, and mortality [Ali et al., 2008; Giampaou et al., 1999].

All measures were collected at baseline, before the pilot study began, and at the end of each quarter for 1 year. The Wilcoxon rank-sum was used to compare the differences in quarterly change scores for each continuous variable. Logistic regression was used to compare the differences in dichotomous SPPB component scores. The Cochran–Mantel–Haenszel test was used to compare annual differences in ER visits, hospitalizations, or falls. Adjustments were made for multiple testing.

Statistically significant results were detected in the SPPB gait speed score at quarter 3 (p = 0.030 sensor got better and control got worse), left-hand grip at quarter 2 (p = 0.024 control significantly declined while intervention remained stable), and the functional ambulation profile of the GAITRite at quarter 2 (p = 0.045, intervention improved more than control). Additional health events and routine assessments were also captured as part of the normal care at TigerPlace. ER visit, hospitalizations, and falls were totaled

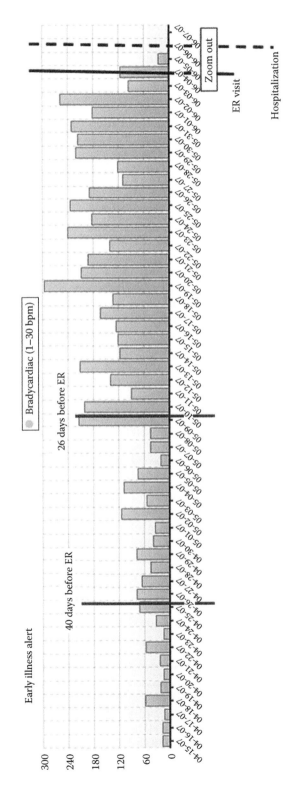

FIGURE 12.8
A retrospective example of an early illness alert that would have been generated 40 days before an emergency room visit, due to the bed sensor low pulse events.

and the GDS, MMSE, fall risk assessment, and SF-12 Health Survey were all analyzed. None of these additional measures yielded significant results.

All of the Likert-scaled questions completed each month by the clinicians improved during the study. Confidence to use the system shifted from 61% to 86%; clinical relevance of the sensor data from 52% to 83%; ease of interpretation from 43% to 70%; and confidence that the system would alert them to signs of potential decline in physical function, indicators of acute illness onset, or exacerbation of chronic illness improved from 26% to 71%. While the system was improving, the interpretation time decreased from an average of 4.3 min per alert at the beginning of the study to 2.0 min per alert at the end. The clinicians at TigerPlace seem convinced that the sensor-based alerts are providing clinically relevant information and have asked that the alerts be used for all residents who have sensor networks installed. The alerts have now been incorporated into standard care at TigerPlace.

12.5 What Do the Residents Think?

From the beginning of the sensor network studies at TigerPlace, the opinions of the residents have been gathered through focus groups and interviews [Demiris et al., 2008a,b]. An early theme that emerged was the concern about the appearance of the sensing devices. We have continued to observe anecdotally that residents can be particular about the appearance of their homes. Thus, it is important that the embedded sensors be small and blend seamlessly into the home environment. In general, we prefer that residents not consciously think about the sensors being there so that their natural behaviors are captured. Interviews with the residents have shown that indeed they do forget about the sensors after an initial period. The TigerPlace residents with in-home sensors tend to go through three stages: (1) familiarization, (2) adjustment and curiosity, and (3) full integration [Demiris et al., 2008b]. At the third stage, which typically happens within 1 month, the resident mostly ignores the sensors and follows his or her normal routine.

Acceptance of the sensing technology is related to the perceived need and perceived benefits, and privacy can be sacrificed for need and benefits if necessary. However, the interviews and focus groups have shown that seniors tend to underestimate their own needs. Residents who have lived with the motion, bed, and stove sensors described here do not report privacy concerns. However, they would like control over who has access to their data, including family members. In some cases, residents reported wanting to look at the data first before allowing access to a son or daughter. It is encouraging that seniors take ownership of their sensor data. This may be the first step toward empowering monitored residents to use the data to proactively manage their own health.

12.6 Limitations, Challenges, and Opportunities

While the early illness alerts have proven useful, there is potential for improvement in the algorithms. The simplistic alert algorithm was successful in capturing all of the critical health change events (this was verified manually); however, about half of the generated alerts were false alarms. Work is in progress to investigate additional algorithms and predictive models for refining the alerts using the collected feedback on the clinical relevance as ground truth [Guevara, 2012]. Our view is that the sensor data form a cluster for normal days with outliers representing abnormal days, for example, see Figure 12.9 [Wang, 2011]. Determining the real health outliers, however, can be complicated by added noise in the sensor data. Is the outlier

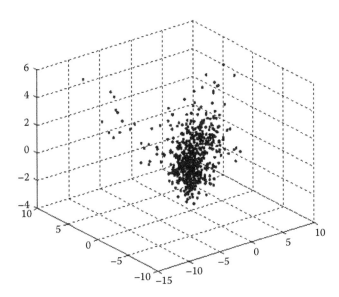

FIGURE 12.9
Sensor data collected on a TigerPlace resident with 21 features extracted from the motion and bed sensor data (projected into 3D space using principal components analysis). Each data point represents 1 day. The normal days tend to cluster; abnormal days are outliers.

due to noise, for example, visitor activity, or due to a real change in the health condition? In addition, we have seen cases in which a new cluster forms due to a change in the resident's baseline condition [Sledge and Keller, 2008]. These situations offer more challenges for early detection of health changes using sensor data.

There are also limitations in the simple sensors described here. The PIR motion sensor cannot recognize the resident, explicitly tell if visitors are present, or distinguish between two residents. Although it is possible to filter out some visitor activity, for example, using motion density and looking for sensor events in multiple locations [Wang, 2011], the approach still suffers from the limitations of the sensor. Clinicians have asked for gait information; changes in gait can be an indication of physical or cognitive problems or even mortality and provide signs of fall risk that may require early interventions to avoid falls [Buracchio et al., 2010; Studenski et al., 2011; Viccaro et al., 2011; Wennie Huang et al., 2010]. Walking speed can be acquired with an array of PIR sensors [Hagler et al., 2010]; however, other important gait parameters are still missing, such as step time, step length, stride-to-stride variability, body sway, walking paths, and posture. For these parameters, vision [Stone et al., 2010; Wang et al., 2009, 2010], depth images [Stone and Skubic 2011], and Doppler radar [Yardibi et al., 2011] offer promise as nonwearable sensing solutions.

The clinicians have also requested more resolution in bed sensing to capture quantitative pulse and respiration rates, shallow breathing episodes, as well as restlessness in bed. There are a variety of bed-sensing modalities being explored to measure respiration and the balisto-cardiogram signal [Starr et al., 1939] that yields the heart rate. Examples include piezo electric [Wang et al., 2003], radar [Droitcour, 2006], load cells [Beattie et al., 2009], pneumatic [Watanabe et al., 2005], and hydraulic [Heise et al., 2011]. The example data shown earlier in this chapter illustrate the potential impact of including bed sensing in the early detection of health changes.

Finally, there is also the challenge of clinical interpretation for all of these data, which presents important questions to be addressed. What sensor data are most pertinent to store and what is the best way to present the data trends? Some possibilities include visualizations

[Hayes et al., 2008; Wang and Skubic, 2008] and linguistic summarizations [Wilbik et al., 2011]. How should the in-home sensor data be merged with clinical data in an EHR [Grecco, 2010]? The work thus far has only begun to address these challenges. Here, we discuss monitoring activity patterns in the home, but we are not capturing activity outside the home. Intriguing opportunities exist to extend this proactive health-care approach to other, younger target populations that may benefit from both in-home and out-of-the-home approaches.

References

Ali, N.A., O'Brien, J.M., Hoffman, S.P., Phillips, G., Garland, A., Findley, J.C.W., Almoosa, K. et al. 2008. Acquired weakness, handgrip strength, and mortality in critically ill patients. *American Journal of Critical Care Medicine* 178: 261–268.

Alexander, G.L., Rantz, M., Skubic, M., Aud, M.A., Wakefield, B., Florea, E., and Paul, A. 2008. Sensor systems for monitoring functional status in assisted living facility residents. *Research in Gerontological Nursing* 1(4): 238–244.

Alexander, G.L. and Staggers, N. 2009. A systematic review of the designs of clinical technology: Findings and recommendations for future research. *Advances in Nursing Science* 32(3): 252–279.

Alexander, G.L., Wakefield, B.J., Rantz, M., Skubic, M., Aud, M., Erdelez, S., and Ghenaimi S.A. 2011a. Passive sensor technology interface to assess elder activity in independent living. *Journal of Nursing Research* 60(5): 318–325.

Alexander, G.L., Rantz, M., Skubic, M., Koopman, R.J., Phillips, L.J., Guevara R.D., and Miller S.J. 2011b. Evolution of an early illness warning system to monitor frail elders in independent living. *Journal of Healthcare Engineering* 2(2): 259–286.

Beattie, Z.T., Hagen, C.C., Pavel, M., and Hayes, T.L. 2009. Classification of breathing events using load cells under the bed. In *Proceeding Conference of the IEEE Engineering in Medicine and Biology Society*, Minneapolis, MN, September, 2009, pp. 3921–3924.

Buracchio, T., Dodge, H. H., Howieson, D., Wasserman, D., and Kaye, J. 2010. The trajectory of gait speed preceding mild cognitive impairment. *Archives of Neurology* 67(8): 980–986.

Demiris, G., Rantz, M.J., Aud, M.A., Marek, K.D., Tyrer, H.W., Skubic, M., and Hussam, A.A. 2004. Older adults' attitudes towards and perceptions of smarthome technologies: A pilot study. *Medical Informatics and the Internet in Medicine* 29(2): 87–94.

Demiris, G., Hensel, B.K., Skubic, M., and Rantz, M.J. 2008a. Senior residents' perceived need of and preferences for smart home sensor technologies. *International Journal of Technology Assessment in Health Care* 24(1): 102–124.

Demiris, G., Parker Oliver, D., Dickey, G., Skubic, M., and Rantz, M. 2008b. Findings from a participatory evaluation of a smart home application for older adults. *Technology and Health Care* 16: 111–118.

Droitcour, A.D. 2006. Non-contact measurement of heart and respiration rates with a single-chip microwave Doppler radar. PhD dissertation, Electrical Engineering Department, Stanford University, Stanford, CA.

Giampaou, S., Farrucci, L., Cecchi, F., LoNoce, C., Poce, A., Dima, F., Santaquilani, A., Vescio, M.F., and Menotti, A. 1999. Hand-grip strength predicts incident disability in non-disabled older men. *Age and Aging* 28: 283–288.

Grecco, A. 2010. Integrating new monitoring and behavioral summary metrics into standard personal health record and electronic health record systems. Oregon Health & Science University Technical Report. http://catalogs.ohsu.edu/record=b1225627

Guevara, R.D. 2012. Sensor network for early illness detection in the elderly. MS thesis, Electrical and Computer Engineering Department, University of Missouri, Columbia, MO.

Guralnik, J.M., Simonsick, E.M., Ferrucci, L., Glynn, R.J., Berkman, L.F., Blazer, D.G. et al. 1994. A short physical performance battery assessing lower extremity function: Association with self-reported disability and prediction of mortality and nursing home admission. *Journal of Gerontology* 49(2): M85–M94.

Hagler, S., Austin, D., Hayes, T.L., Kaye, J., and Pavel, M. 2010. Unobstrusive and ubiquitous in-home monitoring: A methodology for continuous assessment of gait velocity in elders. *IEEE Transactions on Biomedical Engineering* 57(4): 813–820.

Hayes, T.L., Abendroth, F., Adami, A., Pavel, M., Zitzelberger, T.A., and Kaye, J.A. 2008. Unobtrusive assessment of activity patterns associated with mild cognitive impairment. *Alzheimer's and Dementia* 4(6): 395–405.

Heise, D., Rosales, L., Skubic, M., and Devaney, M.J. 2011. Refinement and evaluation of a hydraulic bed sensor. In *Proceeding of the Conference of IEEE Engineering in Medicine and Biology Society*, Boston, MA, August, 2011, pp. 4356–4360.

Mack, D.C., Patrie, J.T., Suratt, P.M., Felder, R.A., and Alwan, M. 2009. Development and preliminary validation of heart rate and breathing rate detection using a passive, ballistocardiography-based sleep monitoring system. *IEEE Transactions on Information Technology in Biomedicine* 13: 111–120.

Rantz, M.J., Marek, K.D., Aud, M.A., Tyrer, H.W., Skubic, M., Demiris, G. et al. 2005a. A technology and nursing collaboration to help older adults age in place. *Nursing Outlook* 53(1): 40–45.

Rantz, M.J., Marek, K.D., Aud, M.A., Johnson, R.A., Otto, D., and Porter, R. 2005b. TigerPlace: A new future for older adults. *Journal of Nursing Care Quality* 20(1): 1–4.

Rantz, M.J., Porter, R., Cheshier, D., Otto, D., Servey, C.H., Johnson, R.A. et al. 2008. TigerPlace, a state-academic-private project to revolutionize traditional long term care. *Journal of Housing for the Elderly* 22(1/2): 66–85.

Rantz, M.J., Skubic, M., Alexander, G., Popescu, M., Aud, M., Koopman, R., and Miller, S. 2010a. Developing a comprehensive electronic health record to enhance nursing care coordination, Use of technology, and research. *Journal of Gerontological Nursing* 36(1): 13–17.

Rantz, M.J., Skubic, M., Alexander, G., Aud, M., Wakefield, B., Koopman, R., and Miller, S. 2010b. Improving nurse care coordination with technology. *Computers, Informatics, Nursing* 28(6): 325–332.

Rantz, M.J., Skubic, M., Koopman, R., Phillips, L., Alexander, G.L., Miller, S.J., and Guevara, R.D. 2011. Using sensor networks to detect urinary tract infections in older adults. In *Proceeding of the IEEE International Conference on e-Health Networking, Application, and Services*, Columbia, MO, June, 2011, pp. 142–149.

Rantz, M.J., Skubic, M., Alexander, G., Phillips, L., Aud, M., Wakefield, B., Koopman, R., and Miller, S. 2012. Automated technology to speed recognition of signs of illness in older adults. *Journal of Gerontological Nursing* 38(4): 18–23.

Skubic, M., Alexander, G., Popescu, M., Rantz, M., and Keller, J. 2009. A smart home application to eldercare: Current status and lessons learned. *Technology and Health Care* 17(3): 183–201.

Sledge, I.J. and Keller, J.M. 2008. Growing neural gas for temporal clustering. In *Proceeding of the International Conference on Pattern Recognition*, Tampa, FL, December, 2008, pp. 1–4.

Starr, I., Rawson, A.J., Schroeder, H.A., and Joseph, N.R. 1939. Studies on the estimation of cardiac output in man, and of abnormalities in cardiac function, from the heart's recoil and the blood's impacts; the ballistocardiogram. *The American Journal of Physiology* 127(1): 1–28.

Stone, E., Anderson, D., Skubic, M., and Keller, J. 2010. Extracting footfalls from voxel data. In *Proceeding Conference. of IEEE Engineering in Medicine and Biology Society*, Buenos Aires, Argentina, August, 2010, pp. 1119–1122.

Stone, E. and Skubic, M. 2011. Evaluation of an inexpensive depth camera for in-home gait assessment. *Journal of Ambient Intelligence and Smart Environments* 3(4): 349–361.

Studenski, S., Perera, S., Patel, K., Rosano, C., Faulkner, K., Inzitari, M., Brach, J. et al. 2011. Gait speed and survival in older adults. *Journal of the American Medical Association* 305(1): 50–58.

Viccaro, L.J., Perera, S., and Studenski, S.A. 2011. Is timed up and go better than gait speed in predicting health, function, and falls in older adults? *Journal of the American Geriatrics Society* 59(5): 887–892.

Wang, F., Tanaka, M., and Chonan, S. 2003. Development of a PVDF piezopolymer sensor for unconstrained in-sleep cardiorespiratory monitoring. *Journal of Intelligent Material Systems and Structures* 14: 185–190.

Wang, F., Stone, E., Dai, W., Banerjee, T., Giger, J., Krampe, J., Rantz, M., and Skubic, M. 2009. Testing an in-home gait assessment tool for older adults. In *Proceeding of the Conference of IEEE Engineering in Medicine and Biology Society*, Minneapolis, MN, September, 2009, pp. 6147–6150.

Wang, F., Skubic, M., Abbott, C., and Keller, J. 2010. Body sway measurement for fall risk assessment using inexpensive webcams. In *Proceeding of the Conference of IEEE Engineering in Medicine and Biology Society*, Buenos Aires, Argentina, August, 2010, pp. 2225–2229.

Wang, S. and Skubic, M. 2008. Density map visualization from motion sensors for monitoring activity level. In *Proceeding of the IET International Conference on Intelligent Environments*, Seattle, Washington, July, 2008, pp. 64–71.

Wang, S., Skubic, M., and Zhu, Y. 2009. Activity density map dissimilarity comparison for eldercare monitoring. In *Proceeding of the Conference of IEEE Engineering in Medicine and Biology Society*, Minneapolis, MN, September, 2009, pp. 7232–7235.

Wang, S., Skubic, M., Zhu, Y., and Galambos, C. 2011. Using passive sensing to estimate relative energy expenditure for eldercare monitoring. In *Proceeding of the IEEE International Conference on Pervasive Computing and Communications, Workshop on Smart Environments to Enhance Health Care*, Toronto, Ontario, Canada, March, 2011, pp. 642–648.

Wang, S. 2011. Change detection for eldercare using passive sensing. PhD dissertation, Electrical and Computer Engineering Department, University of Missouri, Columbia, MO.

Wang, S., Skubic, M., and Zhu, Y. 2012. Activity density map visualization and dissimilarity comparison for eldercare monitoring. *IEEE Transactions on IT in Biomedicine* (99): 1–8.

Watanabe, K., Watanabe, T., Watanabe, H., Ando, H., Ishikawa, T., and Kobayashi, K. 2005. Noninvasive measurement of heartbeat, respiration, snoring and body movements of a subject in bed via a pneumatic method. *IEEE Transactions on Biomedical Engineering* 52(12): 2100–2107.

Wennie Huang, W.-N., Perera, S., Van Swearingen, J., and Studenski, S. 2010. Performance measures predict onset of activity of daily living difficulty in community-dwelling older adults. *Journal of the American Geriatrics Society*, 58(5): 844–852.

Wilbik, A., Keller, J., and Alexander, G. 2011. Linguistic summarization of sensor data for eldercare. In *Proceeding of the IEEE International Conference on Systems, Man, and Cybernetics*, Anchorage, AK, October, 2011, pp. 2595–2599.

Yardibi, T., Cuddihy, P., Genc, S., Bufi, C., Skubic, M., Rantz, M., Liu, L., and Phillips, C. 2011. Gait characterization via pulse-Doppler radar. In *Proceeding of the IEEE International Conference on Pervasive Computing and Communications: Workshop on Smart Environments to Enhance Health Care*, Seattle, WA, March, 2011, pp. 662–667.

13

Quality of Life Technologies in Supporting Family Caregivers

Sara J. Czaja, Chin Chin Lee, and Richard Schulz

CONTENTS

13.1 Introduction

The population is aging at an unprecedented rate in both developed and developing countries. By 2030 there will be about 72 million people over the age of 65 in the United States who will represent about 20% of the population. Also, the older population itself is aging; in the coming decades there will be a large number of people aged 85 and older who represent the oldest old (Figure 13.1). According to U.S. projections, the number of people in this age group could increase to 19 million by 2050 and will represent 35% of the older population by 2040 (Federal Agency Forum on Aging Related Statistics, 2010). The number of centenarians is also growing.

The growth in the number of older people, especially the old–old, has important implications for society and the health-care system. The likelihood of developing a chronic disease or disability and the need for support and health-care services generally increases with age. For example, within the United States, about 80% of older adults have a chronic condition such as heart disease, diabetes, or arthritis, and about 50% have at least two conditions (Center for Disease Control and Prevention, 2010) and large numbers of older people have functional limitations that interfere with the performance of daily living tasks. Further, about 5 million Americans aged 65 and older have Alzheimer's disease (AD) and this number will increase in the coming years especially with the growth in the "oldest old" (Alzheimer's Association, 2010). The majority of older adults (~96%) live in community settings with a spouse, alone, or with other family members (Administration

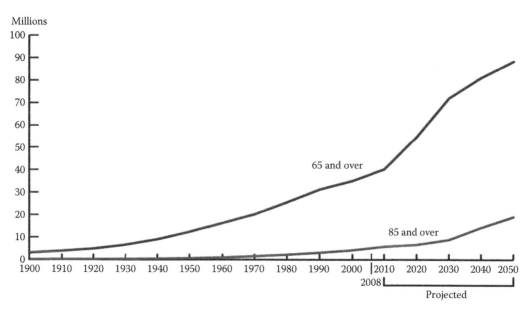

FIGURE 13.1
Population age 65 and over and age 85 and over; selected years 1900–2008 and projected 2010–2050. (From Federal Interagency Forumon Aging-Related Statistics, 2010.)

on Aging, 2011). A great number of these older people rely on family members or friends to provide needed care or some type of support to maintain their ability to live in the community. Although the estimates vary regarding the prevalence of caregiving, currently about 29% of the U.S. adult population is providing care to someone who is ill or disabled and most of these caregivers are providing care to someone over the age of 50 (Family Caregiver Alliance, 2011). Today with increased trends toward the delivery of health care in the home, outside of traditional clinical settings, patients and caregivers are being expected to assume an increasing role in the management of their own health and perform a range of health-care tasks (Figure 13.2).

As discussed in the Preface, there are a myriad of existing and emerging quality-of-life technologies (QoLT) that are designed to maintain or enhance the physical, social, cognitive, and emotional functioning of populations such as older adults or those with disabilities or chronic conditions. Examples of these technologies include monitoring devices to help with the management of chronic illness; assistive technologies that compensate for sensory, physical, and cognitive impairments; rehabilitation technologies for physical and cognitive functioning; and technologies that support resource sharing, knowledge/ learning, and social connectivity. Generally, these technologies offer great potential in terms of enhancing of the ability of older adults and those with disabilities to live in the community and receive the health care and support they need. These technologies may also be of great benefit to family caregivers. For example, computer and communication technologies may help caregivers overcome logistic barriers and have access to needed programs and services. Internet technologies can also be used to facilitate communication with family and other caregivers and health-care providers. Technology can also be used to enhance access to health-related information or information about available community resources. Monitoring technologies may also allow caregivers to maintain a check on the status or activities of their loved one while they are at work or at a distant location. In this chapter, we discuss the potential role of QoLT in providing support for caregivers and

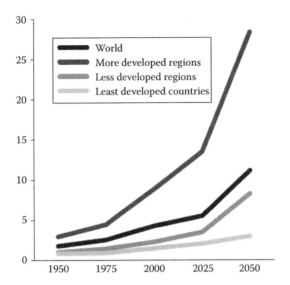

FIGURE 13.2
Parent support ratio: world and development regions, 1950–2050. (From United Nations, World population aging 1950–2050, available online http://www.un.org/esa/population/publications/worldageing19502050/, 2001. With permission.)

care recipients. We also discuss factors that affect the adoption and successful use of these technologies. Finally, we provide some suggestions for needed research in this area.

To provide a context for this discussion we begin by presenting some basic information on family caregivers. We are adopting the definition of caregiving provided by Schulz and Martire (2004, p. 240), that caregiving involves "the provision of extraordinary care, exceeding the bounds of what is normative or usual in family relationships. Caregiving typically involves a significant expenditure of time, energy, and money over potentially long periods of time; it involves tasks that may be unpleasant and uncomfortable and are psychologically stressful and physically exhausting." We recognize that there are distinct groups of caregivers such as children with chronic illness and disability who are typically cared for by young adult parents; adult children suffering from conditions such as mental illness, intellectual or physical challenges who are cared for by middle-aged parents; and older individuals who are cared for by their spouses or their middle-aged children or some other relative or friend. Because the nature of caregiving differs substantially for children versus adults, the focus of our discussion will largely be on caregivers of older adults (Schulz and Tompkins, 2010). However, much of the discussion can generalize to other caregiver populations.

13.2 Overview of Family Caregiving

13.2.1 Basic Demographics

Family caregivers have become an important extension of the health-care system and, in fact, are the largest source of long-term care in the United States. In 2011, the value of family caregiver services was $450 billion per year (Family Caregiver Alliance, 2011).

The prevalence of family members serving in a caregiving role is high and projected to increase in the future with the aging of the population, the projected shortage in geriatric health-care workers, and increased cost of formal long-term care. Veterans returning from wars such as Iraq and Afghanistan who have multiple injuries such as traumatic brain injuries and limb amputations or posttraumatic stress disorder (PTSD) will also require care and support from family members for extended periods of time.

In terms of demographics, the majority of caregivers (~66%) are females who are caring for a spouse, parent, or some other relative, and many are providing care for more than one person such as a parent and a child or two parents simultaneously. While people across the life span serve as caregivers, the current average age of caregivers is about 50 years. Most caregivers who are middle-aged are caring for parents while caregivers who are older are more likely to be caring for a spouse. Importantly many caregivers who are caring for someone aged 65+ are likely to be older themselves and many of these caregivers have health problems. For example, a typical scenario might be an older woman who had arthritis and mobility and some visual problems caring for her husband who has dementia. It has also been recognized that some informal caregivers are children. A recent survey estimated that as many as 1.4 million children in the United States between the ages of 8 and 18 provide care for an older adult (Levine et al., 2005).

Caregivers are also ethnically diverse, and although in the United States the majority of caregivers are White (~72%), the number of minority caregivers is increasing rapidly (National Alliance for Caregiving/AARP, 2009). Understanding the ethnic/culture background of caregivers is important because the expectations, roles, and impact of caregiving vary as a function of caregivers' ethnic/culture background (e.g., Belle et al., 2006; Lee et al., 2010). Finally, with respect to employment, a large number of caregivers are currently working or have worked while serving as caregivers. Simultaneously working and being a caregiver results in added stress for caregivers and also has an impact on their job performance and is costly to business/industry. Many working caregivers report that they make workplace accommodations such as absenteeism, missed opportunities for promotion, and early retirement due to caregiving. Employed caregivers have higher rates of absenteeism than other workers and most report that caregiving responsibilities interfere with their work. These types of job accommodation are more likely for female caregivers. It is estimated that these accommodations cost U.S. employers between $17 and $33 billion per year in lost productivity. For the individual, caregiving costs include losses in wages, pensions, and social security and other benefits. QoLT may be especially beneficial for caregivers who must juggle work and caregiving responsibilities (Family Caregiver Alliance, 2011). In this regard, we are currently evaluating the benefits of a multicomponent psychosocial intervention for working caregivers. The intervention is modeled after the REACH II program (Belle et al., 2006) and is delivered via a website to facilitate the ability of caregivers to access the program. The website contains videos on caregiving skills, videos from "experts" on various topics relevant to caregivers, a resource guide, information and tips, and a recommended reading list (Figure 13.3).

Demographic characteristics of care recipients are also diverse. The average age of care recipients varies across the life span and includes children as well as adults; however, in terms of adults receiving care, it is about 77 years of age. Interestingly, the average age of care recipients has increased in the last few years because of an increase in the number of people in the older cohorts. A majority of care recipients are female, and about 50% of those needing care are widowed. About 60% of care recipients live in their home and about 24% live in their caregiver's household. Caregivers who are older are more likely to report living with their care recipient. In terms of geographic proximity, according to a recent

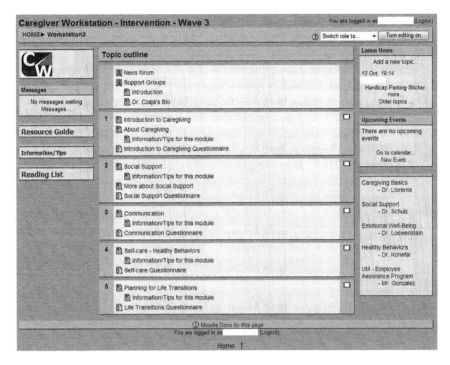

FIGURE 13.3
Working caregivers home page.

survey of those care recipients who live independent from their caregiver, 51% live less than 20 min away, 14% live 20 min to 1 h, 5% live 1–2 h, and 11% live more than 2 h away. Clearly, caregiver distance from the care recipient influences the demands and stress of caregiving. QoLT may be especially beneficial for caregivers who live far distances from their loved ones. The most common reasons for care recipient's need for care include aging, long-term physical conditions or chronic illnesses (e.g., Alzheimer's disease), and emotional or mental health problems (National Alliance for Caregiving and AAPR, 2009).

In summary, it is quite clear that people who receive and those who provide care are very diverse and possess variable skills, resources, knowledge, and experience. They also differ on a number of other characteristics such as age, cultural and ethnic backgrounds, education, health status, and living arrangements. Thus, when considering the design and implementation of QoLT for these user groups it is important to remember that, "one size does not necessarily fit all."

13.2.2 Caregiving Activities

The amount of time caregivers spend on caregiver activities varies with the age of the caregiver and the needs of the care recipient. On average, caregivers spend about 20 h per week providing care, whereas older caregivers provide about 31 h of care per week and those who live with their care recipient about 40 h of care per week. Caregivers of people with AD or another type of dementia provide more hours of care, on average, than other types of caregivers. As expected, the number of hours of care increases as the progression of the disease worsens or if the care recipient has comorbidities (Alzheimer's Association, 2009). The duration of caregiving also varies but is about 5 years. Caregivers of AD patients tend to spend longer in the caregiving role, on average 1–4 years. Also, as noted, caregivers of newly returning veterans will also likely be needed to provide care and support for extended periods of time.

Caregiving typically involves a significant expenditure of physical and emotional and economic resources and can involve unpleasant and uncomfortable tasks and interactions. Caregivers engage in a wide range of tasks and support a wide range of activities including monitoring the health and safety of the patient; assisting with complex medical tasks and treatments and medication adherence; management of physical and behavioral symptoms; assistance with bathing, dressing, and toileting, meal preparation, and eating; transfers; shopping, other errands, and transportation; and legal and financial issues. Caregivers frequently need to interact with complex medical technologies such as infusion pumps or feeding tubes when performing these tasks. Many caregivers also provide emotional and social support. They must also interact with health-care providers and other personnel from service agencies. In addition, they are often faced with complex care coordination activities and decisions about treatment and medical insurance options. Generally, caregivers of people with AD or dementia are more likely to provide assistance with basic ADLs and personal care tasks.

It is important to note that caregiving is not static and that the demands of caregiving may change over the course of a caregiver's career. For example, in the early stage of a patient's illness, a caregiver may need information about the disease and available resources, whereas in the later stages they may need assistance with the treatment of behavioral or emotional problems. Thus, designers of QoLT need to be aware of the trajectories and changing needs of caregiving when designing caregiver support systems.

13.2.3 Consequences of Caregiving

Although caregiving can be rewarding and many caregivers are proud of their role and glean positive benefits, caregiving clearly creates challenges. Many caregivers experience stress and burden, which affects their physical and mental health and ultimately their ability to provide care. The negative consequences of caregiving are well documented in the literature. Overall, caregiving has been shown to result in psychological distress, the adoption of poor health habits, and increased use of psychotropic medications; sleep disruption, psychiatric and physical illnesses, and mortality. Caregiving also often disrupts social and family relationships and employment activities (Pinquart and Sörensen, 2003a,b, 2007; Schulz et al., 1995; Vitaliano et al., 2003). Furthermore, many caregivers must adapt to a new familial role and in some cases are continually confronted with the loss of a loved one.

The extent to which a caregiver experiences negative outcomes is influenced by caregiver characteristics (e.g., gender, age), care recipient attributes (e.g., type and severity of illness), and social (e.g., available support) and environmental factors (e.g., neighborhood, housing type). For example, individuals with low socioeconomic status (SES) and with small support networks report lower levels of health than caregivers who are younger and have more economic and interpersonal resources. Family caregivers of people with AD and other dementias are more likely than other caregivers to report that their health is fair or poor (Schulz et al., 1995; Vitaliano et al., 2003) and that caregiving made their health worse (Alzheimer's Association and National Alliance for Caregiving, 2004; Bynum et al., 2004). They are also more likely to have high levels of stress hormones (Lutgendorf et al., 1999), reduced immune function (Kiecolt-Glaser et al., 1991, 1996; Lutgendorf et al., 1999), and cardiovascular disease (e.g., Vitaliano et al., 2002).

13.3 QoLT to Support Family Caregiving

13.3.1 Examples of Technology Support

The accumulating evidence on the personal, social, and health impacts of dementia caregiving has generated a broad range of intervention studies, including randomized trials aimed at decreasing the burden and stress of caregiving. Several studies have demonstrated small to moderate statistically significant effects in reducing caregiver burden, lowering depression, and delaying institutionalization (Brodaty et al., 2003; Schulz and Martire, 2004; Schulz et al., 2005) through either targeted interventions that treat a specific caregiver problem, such as depression, or broad-based multicomponent interventions that include counseling, case management, skills training, and social support. One potential reason for the limited success of these interventions is that many caregivers face difficulties in accessing available services. Barriers such as transportation problems, insufficient support from others, lack of knowledge about available services, and cultural beliefs often limit caregivers from participating in intervention programs. This is especially true for lower SES, minority caregivers. Given that the majority of caregivers provide care in the patient's home and the increased cost of care in clinical settings, there is a need for innovative strategies to provide needed support to both caregivers and care recipients. The need to develop innovative interventions for caregivers is also underscored by current demographic trends such as the increased number of women in the labor force and fewer children available to provide care.

As introduced earlier in this chapter, there are a variety of QoLT that offer this potential. Clearly, technology offers several advantages over more traditional intervention approaches such as increased ability to deliver and access information on demand, asynchronously, and over long distances; increased access to health professionals and social support; and enhanced opportunities to monitor the status and activities of care recipients and help address environmental safety concerns. Computers or mobile devices can also be an efficient means for delivering health risk assessments and health promotion material. Technology also affords the opportunity to present information in a wide variety of formats to suit the needs of the user population. For example, multimedia offers the potential of providing information in text with narration and animation. In this section, we provide examples of how QoLT can be used to support family caregivers. This is an emerging field in the caregiver literature, driven by the expanding power of computers, mobile devices such as Smartphones, and the Internet. Many caregivers are beginning to turn to technology for support in their caregiving role. In fact, a recent survey of 1000 family caregivers (National Association of Family Caregivers and United HealthCare, 2011) queried caregivers who already used the Internet or some other form of technology to support their caregiving about how various technologies might be helpful to them in terms of providing care. The findings indicated that of the technologies evaluated, the three that offered the greatest potential were: personal health record tracking, a caregiving coordination system, and a medication support system.

One basic way that technologies such as the Internet and mobile devices can aid caregivers is through the provision of information that enhances caregiver knowledge. A critical challenge facing many caregivers and requisite to providing quality care is having the necessary knowledge about the care recipient's illness or disability, how to provide care, and how to access and utilize available services. There are a vast number of websites available that can provide caregivers with information on illnesses/diseases, medications and treatments, health-care providers, and health resources. These applications can also enhance direct access to experts and professional organizations, which can also facilitate decision making by the caregiver.

Recent findings from an interview study of approximately 1500 caregivers indicated that 53% use the Internet as a source of information about caregiving (National Alliance for Caregiving and AARP, 2009). Findings from the Pew Internet and American Life Study (Fox, 2011a) indicate that 26% of Internet users caring for a loved one have looked online for someone with similar health concerns. Another recent Pew study (Fox, 2011b) queried caregivers, who said they had found the Internet to be crucial or important during a loved one's recent health crisis, about the Internet's specific role during that crisis. The findings showed that the Internet helped the caregivers find advice or support from other people (36%), helped them find professional or expert services (34%), and helped them find information or compare options (26%). Many of these websites also offer caregivers an opportunity to join support groups (Figure 13.4). There are concerns of course about the quantity and quality of health information that is available on the Internet. Caregivers and patients are able to access information from credible sources (e.g., Family Caregiver Alliance, Medline Plus) and unreviewed sources of unknown quality. Inaccurate health information could result in inappropriate treatment or delays in seeking needed support from health-care professionals.

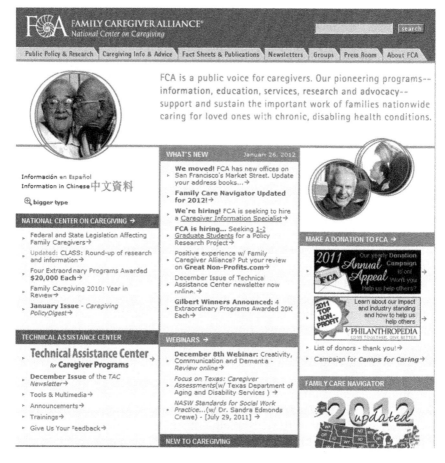

FIGURE 13.4
Family Caregiver Alliance home page.

The amount of information available can also be daunting for caregivers, especially those who have limited Internet experience, limited knowledge of credible sources of information, and low health literacy. Data from our group indicate (Czaja et al., 2008, 2010) that both caregivers and older adults trust health information on the Internet and, generally, find the Internet to be a valuable source of health information. However, data also indicated that health websites can be challenging to use (Czaja et al., 2008; Taha et al., 2009).

Networks can also link caregivers to other family members or long-distant caregivers to the person for whom they are providing care. The Internet is increasingly being used as a forum for individuals to exchange information about health difficulties, needs, and strategies for managing health challenges. Several studies have also shown that the computer networks (e.g., Bank et al., 2006; Czaja and Rubert, 2002; Gallienne et al., 1993) can increase social support for caregivers. Demiris et al. (2008) recently completed a small pilot study that evaluated the benefits and challenges of a videophone system designed to facilitate communication between long-distance family members and loved ones in long-term care facilities. Overall, the findings were promising and showed that although there were some technical challenges, the participants were enthusiastic about their ability to use the videophones and engage in videocalls and indicated that it enhanced their sense of closeness. These types of systems can also be used to connect family members with facility staff and the entire health-care team. Marziali and Donahue (2006) evaluated an Internet-based psychosocial intervention for family caregivers of older adults with neurodegenerative disease. The website included links to information, e-mail, and a video-conferencing link that enabled caregivers to participate in guided support groups. Although the sample size was small and there was a relatively high dropout rate among the participants in the control group, the results provided support for the efficacy of the technology-based intervention. Caregivers who received the intervention experienced a decline in stress and they also reported that their experience with online support groups paralleled experiences with face-to-face support group programs. Lewis et al. (2010) conducted a pilot evaluation of an Internet-based psycho-educational program designed to provide knowledge and support to caregivers of dementia patients. Caregivers in their study reported that the program was educational, convenient, and useful. They also reported feeling more confident in their caregiving skills and in their communication with other family members. However, the sample size was small (N = 47) and the participants had prior computer and Internet skills. Similarly Gallagher-Thompson et al. (2010) evaluated a cognitive behavior therapy (CBT) skill training program delivered on a DVD for Chinese American dementia caregivers. The CBT training was compared to a general educational DVD program on dementia. The results showed that it was feasible to use a DVD format to deliver the intervention and that the caregivers who received the CBT intervention reported higher positive affect and less stress in dealing with the patient's behavioral problems.

In an early study (Eisdorfer et al., 2003) we found that a computer-telephone information system (CTIS) designed for family caregivers of patients with AD was effective in reducing depression among a sample of White and Cuban American caregivers. The system was designed to enhance a family therapy intervention and facilitate the caregivers' access to formal and informal support services and information databases such as the Alzheimer's Association Resource Guide. In a follow-up study with a community agency (Finkel et al., 2007), where we used the CTIS system almost exclusively to deliver the intervention, we found that caregivers who used the system with high levels of depressive symptoms at baseline exhibited statistically significant decreases in depression at follow-up and those with high levels of support showed relatively greater capacity to maintain that support. Caregivers also reported increased confidence in their skills as caregivers and their ability to deal with difficult caregiving challenges.

More recently, we completed a study (Czaja et al., 2011) that evaluated the efficacy and feasibility of a videophone-based psychosocial intervention aimed at reducing stress and burden and enhancing the quality of life of minority family caregivers of patients with dementia. The intervention was modeled after the REACH II caregiver intervention (Belle et al., 2006) and compared to an information-only control and wellness contact control conditions. The videophone was installed in the homes of minority caregivers (Haitian, Hispanic, African, American) of dementia patients and included text and voice information features (e.g., a resource guide and information/tips) and allowed for face-to face communication between the caregivers and their interventionist and facilitated support groups (Figure 13.5). The videophone was preprogrammed so that the information was available in the preferred language of the caregivers—Creole, Spanish, and English (Figure 13.6). Preliminary data from the study are encouraging and suggest that the intervention was helpful in terms of alleviating caregiver distress. The majority of caregivers indicated that the videophone was understandable and easy to use. The caregivers in our sample were generally of lower SES and had limited experience with technology prior to this study. We also learned some valuable lessons about technology implementation. For example, none of our caregivers had Internet connections prior to the study (a requirement for the technology), and the interactions between the clinical and the technical team were sometimes challenging.

Technologies that monitor behavior and communicate with professionals and family members offer great promise for enabling older adults to age in place, and provide support for family caregivers especially those who are working or long distance. Such systems could, for example, know how well a person slept the previous night, identify potential health problems before they become serious or catastrophic, know whether they are able to carry out daily routines, and assure a daughter who lives in a distant city that they are doing well today. Various monitoring systems for older adults and their caregivers are

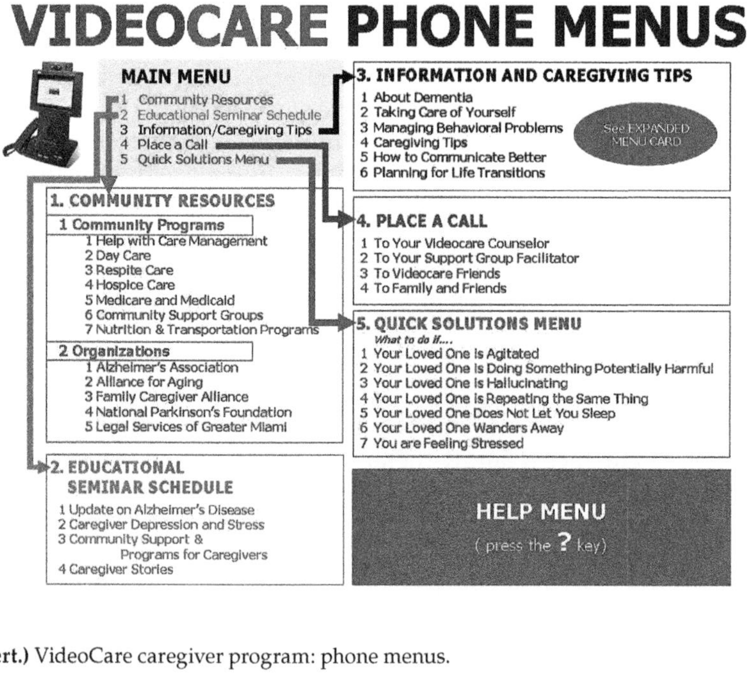

FIGURE 13.5
(See color insert.) VideoCare caregiver program: phone menus.

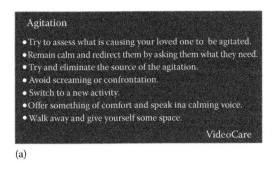

(a)

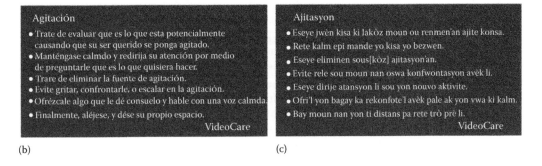

(b)   (c)

FIGURE 13.6
Selected information from VideoCare caregiver program in (a) English, (b) Spanish, and (c) Creole.

already on the market, and many more are being developed. These include systems such as fall detection and prevention systems, wearable activity monitors, non-wearable embedded sensor activity monitors, medication compliance systems, and safety monitors such as smoke and temperature monitors. A more recent development is the design and implementation of smart home applications. These involve integrated networks of sensors—which may include a combination of safety, health and wellness, and social connectedness technologies—installed into homes or apartments to simultaneously and continuously monitor environmental conditions, daily activity patterns, vital signs, sleep patterns, etc. over the long-term. The goal is to capture physical and cognitive behavioral patterns and develop algorithms to detect deviations from normal patterns in the hopes of early detection of health problems and prevention of health declines (see Chapter 12 and Czaja, Beach, Charness, and Schulz [in press] for a more complete discussion of monitoring technologies). Health and wellness monitoring may benefit family caregivers by enabling them to be more informed about their loved one's health, improved health-related communication, opportunities for prevention and early detection and intervention, and reduced burdens and strains of care. However, issues related to data integration, privacy, and user interface design may outweigh some of the potential benefits of these technologies.

Overall, the findings from our research and that of other investigators indicate that it is feasible to use technology to deliver intervention programs and support to family caregivers. However, as discussed in the next section, there are a number of factors that influence the success of these applications. These factors include issues pertaining to training needs and technical support, reliability, access to technology, the adaptability of technology to individual needs, the extent to which a technology undermines individual autonomy, control, and dignity, and privacy issues as well as possible legal or liability issues raised by some technological applications.

13.4 Factors Influencing Technology Adoption

The previous section provided examples of various technologies and their potential benefits for family caregivers and care recipients. In order for the benefits of these technologies to be realized by caregivers, patients, and health-care providers, it is important that the technology is useful and useable by these populations and that systems are reliable and responsive. If a system is unavailable, it cannot be used, and if it is unreliable, users will become frustrated and avoid using the technology regardless of potential benefits. All technology involves potential barriers to acceptance that must be overcome to facilitate widespread acceptance, adoption, and continued use. These include a broad range of user characteristics (socio-demographics, health status, social support, experience with and attitudes toward technology) and resources (sensory, cognitive, psychomotor); system characteristics (user interface, instructional support, aesthetics, engagement, functionality); and the fit between the user and the system (see Chapters 2 and 11). An issue particularly important for caregivers and older care recipients is access to technology. Although the rate of technology adoption is increasing across age groups, existing data indicate that there are still age-related gaps in usage. For example, in the United States in 2010, about 42% of people age 65+ were Internet users as compared to 78% of people age 50–64 and 87% of those 30–49 years old (U.S. Census Bureau, 2011). Older adults using computers and the Internet tend to be better educated and White, and have greater social resources and fewer functional impairments than non-adopters. Home broadband adoption is also lower among older people. In 2010, only 31% of people aged 65+ had broadband access at home, which limits the scope and potential of the online experience and the ability to use many health applications (Smith, 2010). Also, although caregivers use technology such as the Internet to support caregiving activities, the rate of using this technology among caregivers is still relatively low (Czaja et al., 2010; National Alliance for Caregiving and AARP, 2009).

A number of studies have examined factors influencing technology adoption among older adults and caregiver populations. For example, Mahoney (2010) recently completed a meta-synthesis of adoption of four technology systems that provided support to family caregivers. The results indicated that factors critical to technology adoption included the targeted end users' perceived value of usage, training sufficiency, reliability and stability of the systems, and concerns about having too many technologies. We (Czaja et al., 2006) have shown that technology self-efficacy and anxiety about use are also important predictors of technology adoption. Chiu and Eysenbach (2011) examined factors influencing caregiver's use of a Web-based intervention. The intervention was designed for caregivers of dementia patients and included information on the disease and caregiving strategies, community resources, and a personalized e-mail support system. They found that the three main factors that influenced use of the intervention were as follows: (1) caregiver needs that are influenced by personal capacity, social support available, and caregiving beliefs; (2) technology factors such as accessibility barriers and perceived effort in using the technology; and (3) style of the technology such as degree of interactivity. Importantly, they found that the new caregivers needed a different type of support than experienced caregivers.

With respect to monitoring technologies, concerns about uptake were related type of information being recorded, how it is recorded, and with whom it is shared. A recent national web-based survey of 1518 disabled and nondisabled baby boomers (age 45–64) and older adults (65+) found significant variations in attitudes toward adoption (Beach et al., 2009, 2010) as a function of the type of information being recorded (e.g., vital signs, moving about the home, driving behavior, taking medications, toileting), methods of recording (video with sound, video without sound, sensors only), and the target recipient of the information (self, family, doctor, researchers, insurance companies, government). The results showed that potential users were less accepting of the use of video cameras, either with or without sound, than of sensors; less accepting of sharing information about driving or toileting behavior when compared to other types of behavior; and less willing to share information with insurance companies and the government when compared to other groups such as family members or physicians. The other major finding of the study was that both baby boomers and older adults reporting higher levels of disability were more accepting of having information recorded and shared than those with lower levels of disability or no disability.

Other important issues related to the acceptance and use of technology are perceived need and perceived usefulness of the technology. Caregivers and older adults are much more willing to be monitored if they perceive it as providing clear benefits. System design features such as the complexity of the technology and difficulty in learning how to use it and remembering how to use it and maintain it are also critical factors with respect to adoption. Generally, adoption is enhanced if the system is relatively easy to use, has an intuitive interface, and requires minimal training of end users and other stakeholders. The issue of interoperability is also becoming increasingly important with the expanding power of networks and smart applications. Of course, another crucial system "demand" is the cost of the system. The results from the survey conducted by the National Association of Family Caregivers and United Healthcare (2011) indicated that the most prevalent potential barriers to use of technology among caregivers included perceived expense, the belief that technologies do not address caregiver needs, and fears that the care recipient would resist acceptance of new technologies.

13.5 Conclusions

While information technologies hold the promise of improving the quality of life for caregivers and care recipients, there are a number of issues that must be addressed before the full benefits of these technologies can be realized for these populations. Existing barriers to widespread adoption for current cohorts of caregivers and care recipients include large and diverse user groups with varying needs and abilities; caregivers' lack of knowledge about the potential benefits of technology; low technology self-efficacy and anxiety about using technology among caregivers and care recipients; cost and accessibility; training opportunities; and system design characteristics. For example, much more research is needed regarding the relative advantages of more advanced technologies such as multimedia and smart mobile devices when compared to simpler technologies. What is the optimal combination of low- and high-tech strategies that best serve a particular caregiver group?

Monitoring devices are likely to play a central role in caregiver technology applications, and we are beginning to learn about end-user preferences with respect to people's willingness to be monitored, but we know relatively little about caregivers' preferences for how data should be presented to them and how they should be designed to promote effective caregiving. Inherent in this question are many others concerning effective interface designs for both caregivers and care recipients as well as questions about access and training requirements. Developing systems that integrate caregivers with patients and their health-care providers into an effective communication network should be given high priority. Ideally, such a system would enable the exchange of all types of information, including monitoring of vital signs, behavior, and functioning of the patient, along with verbal and visual communication. It is also essential to investigate sources of potential harm inherent in some technologies such as privacy intrusions, false perceptions about the capabilities and safety of technology systems, the proliferation of too much and inappropriate information and miscommunication among caregivers, patients, and health-care providers.

Finally, the widespread adoption of technologies to support caregiving will depend on powerful demonstrations that these technologies are not only effective but are cost-effective; that is, they improve the quality of life of caregivers and their care recipients at a lower cost when compared to alternative strategies.

Acknowledgments

Langeloth Foundation, AT&T, Cisco, NIH/NINR.

References

Administration on Aging 2011. A profile of older Americans. Available online http://www.aoa.gov/aoaroot/aging-statistics/Profile/2011/docs/2011profile.pdf

Alzheimer's Association and National Alliance for Caregiving. 2004. Families care: Alzheimer's disease caregiving in the United States. Accessible at: www.alz.org

Alzheimer's Association. 2009. Alzheimer's disease facts and figures. *Alzheimer's Dementia* 5: 234–270.

Alzheimer's Association. 2010. Azheimer's disease facts and figures. Available online http://www.alz.org/documents_custom/report_alzfactsfigures2010.pdf

Bank, A. L., Arguelles, S., Rubert, M., Eisdorfer, C., and Czaja, S. J. 2006. The value of telephone support groups among ethnically diverse caregivers of persons with dementia. *Gerontologist* 46: 134–138.

Beach, S. R., Schulz, R., Downs, J., Matthews, J., Barron, B., and Seelman, K. 2009. Disability, age, and informational privacy attitudes in quality of life technology applications: Results from a national web survey. *Trans Access Comput (TACCESS)*, Special issue on Aging and Information Technologies, 2(1), Article 5: 1–21.

Beach, S., Schulz, R., Downs, J. et al. 2010. Monitoring and privacy issues in quality of life technology applications. *Gerontechnology* 9: 78–79.

Belle, S. H., Burgio, L., Burns, R. et al., 2006. Enhancing the quality of life of dementia caregivers from different ethnic or racial groups: A randomized, controlled trial. *Ann Intern Med* 145: 727–738.

Brodaty, H., Green, A., and Koschera, A. 2003. Meta-analysis of psychosocial interventions for caregivers of people with dementia. *J Am Geriatr Soc* 51: 657–664.

Bynum, J. P. W., Rabins, P. V., Weller, W., Niefeld, M., Anderson, G. F., and Wu, A. W. 2004. The relationship between a dementia diagnosis, chronic illness, Medicare expenditures and hospital use. *J Am Geriatr Society* 52:187–194.

Center for Disease Control and Prevention. 2010. Improving and extending quality of life among older Americans: At a glance 2010. Available online http://www.cdc.gov/chronicdisease/resources/publications/AAG/aging.htm

Chiu, T. M. L. and Eysenback, G. 2011. Theorizing the health service usage behavior of family caregivers: A qualitative study of an internet-based intervention. *Int J Med Inform* 80: 754–764.

Czaja, S. J., Beach, S., Charness, N., and Schulz R. (in press). Older adults and adoption of healthcare technology: Opportunities and challenges. In A. Sixsmith and G. Gutman (Eds.), *Technology for Active Aging*, New York: Springer Press.

Czaja, S. J., Charness, N., Fisk, A. D. et al., 2006. Factors predicting the use of technology: Findings from the center for research and education on aging and technology enhancement (CREATE). *Psychol Aging* 21: 333–352.

Czaja, S. J., Lee, C. C., and Schulz, R. 2010. The use of the Internet to support family caregivers of older adults. Presented at the *International Society of Gerontechnology* 7th *World Conference*, Vancouver, British Columbia, Canada.

Czaja, S. J., Perdomo, D., Nair, S. N., and Schulz, R. 2011. A technology-based psycho-educational intervention for minority AD caregivers. Poster presentation at the *International Conference on Alzheimer's Disease*, Paris, France.

Czaja, S. J. and Rubert, M. P. 2002. Telecommunications technology as an aid to family caregivers of persons with dementia. *Psychosom Med* 64: 469–476.

Czaja, S. J., Sharit, J., and Nair, S. N. 2008. Usability of the Medicare Health Web Site. *JAMA* 300: 790–792.

Demiris, G., Parker Oliver, D. R., Hensel, B., Dickey, G., Rantz, M., and Skubic M. 2008. Use of videophone for distant caregiving: An enriching experience for families and residents in long-term care. *J Gerontol Nurs* 34: 50–55.

Eisdorfer, C., Czaja, S. J., Loewesnstein, D. A. et al. 2003. The effect of a family therapy and technology-based intervention on caregiver depression. *Gerontologist* 43: 521–531.

National Alliance for Caregiving and AARP. 2009. Caregiving in the US: A focused look at those caring for someone age 50 or older. Available online http://www.caregiving.org/data/FINALRegularExSum50plus.pdf

Family Caregiver Alliance. 2011. Selected caregiver statistics. Available online http://www.caregiver.org/caregiver/jsp/content_node.jsp?nodeid=439

Federal Agency Forum on Aging Related Statistics. 2010. Older Americans 2010: Key indicators of well-being. Available online http://www.agingstats.gov/agingstatsdotnet/Main_Site/Data/2010_Documents/Docs/OA_2010.pdf

Finkel, S. I., Czaja, S. J., Schulz, R., Martinovich, Z., Harris, C., and Pezzuto, D. 2007. E-Care: A telecommunications technology intervention for family caregivers of dementia patients. *Am J Geriatr Psychiatry* 15: 443–448.

Fox, S. 2011a. Peer-to-peer healthcare. Pew Internet and American Life Project. Available online http://pewinternet.org/Reprots/2011/P2PHealthcare.aspx

Fox, S. 2011b. Health topics. Pew Internet and American Life Project. Available online http://pewinternet.org/Reports/2011/HealthTopics.aspx

Gallagher-Thompson, D., Wang, P-C., Liu, W. et al. 2010. Effectiveness of a psychoeducational skill training DVD program to reduce stress in Chinese American dementia caregivers: Results of a preliminary study. *Aging Mental Health* 14: 263–273.

Gallienne, R. K., Moore, S. M., and Brennan, P. F. 1993. Alzheimer's caregivers. Psychosocial support via computer networks. *J Gerontol Nurs* 19: 15–22.

Kiecolt-Glaser, J. K., Dura, J. R., Speicher, C. E., Trask, O. J., and Galser, R. 1991. Spousal caregivers of dementia victims: Longitudinal changes in immunity and health. *Psychosom Med* 53: 345–362.

Kiecolt-Glaser, J. K., Glaser, R., Gravenstein, S., Malarkey, W. B., and Sheridan, J. 1996. Chronic stress alters the immune response to influenza virus vaccine in older adults. *Proceedings of the National Academy of Science*, National Academy of Science, Washington, DC, Vol. 93, pp. 3043–3047.

Lee, C., Czaja, S. J., and Schulz, R. 2010. The moderating influence of demographic characteristics, social support, and religious coping on the effectiveness of a multicomponent psychological caregiver intervention in three racial ethnic groups. *J Gerontol B Psychol Sci Soc Sci* 62B: 185–194.

Levine, C., Gibson Hunt, G., Halper, D., Hart, A. Y., Lautz, J., and Gould, D. A. 2005. Young adult caregivers: A first look at an unstudied population. *Am J Public Health* 95: 2071–2075.

Lewis, M. L., Hobday, J. V., and Hopburn, K. W. 2010. Internet-based program for dementia caregivers. *Am J Alzheimers Dis Other Dem* 25: 674–679.

Lutgendorf, S. K., Garand, L., Buckwalter, K. C., Reimer, T. T., Hong S.-Y., and Lubaroff, D. M. 1999. Life stress, mood disturbance, and elevated interleukin-6 in healthy older women. *J Gerontol A Biol Sci Med Sci* 54A: M434–M439.

Mahoney, D. F. 2010. An evidence-based adoption of technology model for remote monitoring of elders daily activities. *Ageing Int* 36: 66–81.

Marziali, E. and Donahue, P. 2006. Caring for others: Internet video-conferencing group interventions for family caregivers of older adults with neurodegenerative disease. *Gerontologist* 46: 398–403.

National Association of Family Caregivers and UnitedHealthcare. 2011. E-Connected family caregiver: Bringing caregiving into the 21st Century. Available online http://www.caregiving.org/data/FINAL_eConnected_Family_Caregiver_Study_Jan%202011.pdf

Pinquart, M. and Sörensen, S. 2003a. Differences between caregivers and noncaregivers in psychological health and physical health: A meta-analysis. *Psychol Aging* 18: 250–267.

Pinquart, M. and Sörensen, S. 2003b. Associations of stressors and uplifts of caregiving with caregiver burden and depressive mood: A meta-analysis. *J Gerontol B Psychol Sci Soc Sci* 58: 112–128.

Pinquart, M. and Sörensen, S. 2007. Correlates of physical health of informal caregivers: A meta-analysis. *J Gerontol B Psychol Sci Soc Sci* 62: P126–P137.

Schulz, R. and Martire, L. M. 2004. Family caregiving in persons with dementia: Prevalence, health effects, and support strategies. *Am J Geriatr Psychiatry* 12: 240–249.

Schulz, R., Martire, L., and Klinger, J. 2005. Evidence-based caregiver interventions in geriatric psychiatry. *Psychiatr Clin North Am* 28: 1007–1038.

Schulz, R., O'Brien, A. T., Bookwala, J., and Fleissner, K. 1995. Psychiatric and physical morbidity effects of dementia caregiving: Prevalence, correlates, and causes. *Gerontologist* 35:771–791.

Schulz, R. and Tompkins, C. A. 2010. Informal caregivers in the United States: Prevalence, characteristics, and ability to provide care. *The Role of Human Factors in Home Health Care: Workshop Summary*, Steven Olson, (Ed.) Washington, DC: National Academies Press, pp. 117–143.

Smith, A. 2010. Home broadband 2010. Pew Internet & American Life Project. Available online http://pewinternet.org/Reports/2010/Home-Broadband-2010.aspx

Taha, J., Czaja, S. J., and Sharit, J. 2009. Use of and satisfaction with sources of health information among older internet users and non-users. *Gerontologist* 46: 82–88.

Vitaliano, P. P., Scanlan, J. M., Zhang, J., Savage, M. V., Hirsch, I. B., and Siegler, I. 2002. A path model of chronic stress, the metabolic syndrome, and coronary heart disease. *Psychosom Med* 64: 418–435.

Vitaliano, P. P., Zhang, J., and Scanlan, J. M. 2003. Is caregiving hazardous to one's physical health? A meta-analysis. *Psychol Bull* 29: 946–947.

United Nations. 2001. World population aging 1950–2050. Available online http://www.un.org/esa/population/publications/worldageing19502050/

U.S. Census Bureau. 2011. Information and Communications. Statistical Abstract of the United States: 2011. Available online at http://www.census.gov/prod/2011pubs/11statab/infocomm.pdf

Part IV

Transforming Education and the Market Place

14

Developing Future Generations of QoLT Researchers through Education, Outreach, and Diversity Initiatives

Mary Goldberg, Maria Milleville, Dan Ding, Reid Simmons, Shelly Brown, and Diane Collins

CONTENTS

14.1 Introduction

QoLT is an emerging field that focuses on the use of intelligent technology to support those in need by enabling them to more independently perform activities of daily living and giving them opportunities to participate in society longer and more fully. QoLT is not just a set of new technologies. It promises a fundamental shift from traditionally more intelligent and more autonomous systems to person–system symbiosis in which people and engineered components are mutually dependent and work together. The unique focus of this emerging field demands integration across diverse disciplines including engineering, robotics, design, clinical, and social sciences, as well as a systems perspective on creating socially constructive products for human communities. Existing training programs fail at providing this interdisciplinary integration of fields by isolating the engineering and technical domains from the medical and rehabilitation sciences. In contrast to traditional training programs, because integration across several disciplines is inherent in QoLT research, the QoLT Center Education, Outreach, and Diversity (EOD) team has created an environment where faculty, students, practitioners, and consumers from multiple disciplines collaborate on hands-on projects that address real-world problems.

The QoLT EOD mission is aligned with the QoLT Center's agenda of creating and supporting a community of intellectually prepared and motivated engineers, scientists, practitioners, and consumers. This is accomplished through a comprehensive education overhaul that starts early with K-12 outreach, and continued through undergraduate and graduate education, with a focus on increasing the enrollment and retention of students with disabilities, and consumer and continuing education (CE) initiatives. Though we have distinct strategies for recruitment, facilitation, and evaluation at each level, the core goal of engaging people in QoLT, especially those from underrepresented groups, is constant. Exciting a young student about a career in STEM, assisting a disabled veteran in his/her transition to college, or inspiring a consumer to use emerging technologies to be able to live independently for a longer period of time are direct outcomes of the QoLT EOD team's efforts.

The sections that follow detail methodologies and example programs at each level of the academic pipeline: K-12, undergraduate (including veterans' reentry), graduate, continuing, and community education. Lastly, an evaluation section details our strategies for monitoring the effectiveness of our initiatives.

14.2 K-12 Education

Many students are not aware that academic decisions they make during their K-12 years have long-term impact on their future career. For example, the traditional perception of scientists and engineers does not include women, so it is not surprising that middle school girls tend to eschew the science and math path, even though their academic skills are at the same level as boys' (Weinburgh 1995). Role models from the world of science do not include many women, ethnic minorities, and people with disabilities (Fancsali, Froschl, 2006). The QoLT Center's EOD team is determined to counteract that trend in its K-12 activities. In our educational efforts at the K-12 level we ensure that we achieve the following goals: participants of our K-12 programs view other people and themselves through the prism of their abilities, rather than their disability, gender, or race; expose K-12 students to academic research and to encourage them to explore academic and industry career paths by pursuing internship opportunities in STEM; and prepare K-12 students for careers in STEM, specifically, in QoLT-related disciplines. The QoLT Center's EOD team has been especially successful in reaching those goals at the middle-school and high-school level.

Taking advantage of available resources and developing new tools have allowed us to become successful in reaching our goals. QoLT's strong ties to the medical and scientific communities in Pittsburgh and state-of-the art facilities at the affiliated institutions enable K-12 students to participate in research alongside "real" scientists, as well as graduate and undergraduate students.

The QoLT Center's EOD team chose not to reinvent the wheel and instead infuses existing programs with QoLT elements. We have established partnerships with youth-serving agencies whose mission is to increase the STEM pipeline. Our partners include universities, non-profits, and corporations in Western Pennsylvania and beyond. Such partnerships allow us to maximize resources by building on existing programs at different educational levels. See Table 14.1 for a listing of our partnerships.

The EOD team participates in and manages several initiatives at the middle school level. "Creative Technology Nights for Girls" at the School of Computer Science at CMU is an

TABLE 14.1

Outreach Partnerships

Partnering Organization	Population Served
Boy Scouts of America's TrailBlazer District	K-12 students with disabilities
National Society of Black Engineers Pre-college Initiative (NSBE PCI)	K-12 students from underrepresented backgrounds
Carnegie Science Center	K-12 students from local schools
NSF Disability Alliances	Students with disabilities
Abilities Expo	Adults and children with disabilities
"Entry Point" with AAAS	Undergraduate students with disabilities
American Association of Persons with Disabilities	Adults and children with disabilities
Paralyzed Veterans of America (PVA)	Veterans
United Cerebral Palsy (UCP)	Adults and children with disabilities
Easter Seals	Adults and children with disabilities
Disability Resource Centers	Adults and children with disabilities
National Collaborative on Workforce and Disabilities	Adults with disabilities
HealthSports	Adults and children with disabilities
Hiram G. Andrew Center	Adults with disabilities
Local disability support groups	Adults and children with disabilities
Three Rivers Center for Independent Living	Adults and children with disabilities
Office of Vocational Rehabilitation Counselors	Adults and children with disabilities
Woodlands Foundations	Children with disabilities
The Children's Institute	Children with disabilities
Learning Research and Development Center, Pittsburgh	Teachers in Pittsburgh public schools

established weekly program that introduces middle school girls to STEM. The QoLT Center contributes to the program by hosting special sessions in which women engineers and students from the Center share their experiences with program participants. Another example of a partnership that benefits middle school students is our partnership with the Boy Scouts of America's TrailBlazer District. The TrailBlazer District targets scouts with disabilities and provides adapted options for earning merit badges. The QoLT Center's EOD team designed a curriculum that outlines the requirements for merit badges in engineering and disability awareness, which would be earned through participation in a series of workshops. Currently, we are developing a QoLT merit badge that encompasses disability awareness and understanding of QoLT for various merit badge-earning entities (Boy Scouts, Girl Scouts, 4H).

Unlike the aforementioned initiatives, Tech-Link is a truly unique robotics program coordinated entirely by the QoLT Center's EOD team. The program celebrates the strengths of every student by creating an environment of mutual collaboration. Yet, it educates students about benefits of healthy competition as they prepare to participate in the FIRST Lego League tournament at the end of the program. Over the past 10 years, Tech-Link has attracted a diverse group of middle schoolers, including girls, students with disabilities, and underrepresented ethnic minorities.

The QoLT Center's educational programs at the high-school level stem from partnerships with organizations committed to diversity in STEM. Our partnership with the Junior Achievement Program led to the establishment of the Job Shadow Day Program, which provides 9th and 10th grade students with an opportunity to learn about career opportunities in assistive technologies and QoLT by touring the QoLT Center's research laboratories and shadowing QoLT faculty, staff, and graduate students. The program's focus on

9th and 10th graders ensures that students interested in STEM have enough time to make academic choices that support their career goals.

The QoLT Center is also the site for School2Career, a local agency, affiliated with Pittsburgh Public Schools that exposes high school students to a variety of career experiences through hands-on research projects. Students from private, suburban, and charter schools work with QoLT research scientists on projects that range from developing sensitive cloth covering for a robotic arm to building custom hardware. For example, an all-girls private school has added QoLT to their science curriculum: their mini-course in QoLT includes a tour of our laboratories and students' participation in a current research project.

14.3 Undergraduate Education

The QoLT Center's educational efforts at the undergraduate level focus on developing an undergraduate curriculum in QoLT, providing research opportunities in QoLT to undergraduate students in STEM disciplines, and designing a reentry program for veterans.

14.3.1 Curriculum

At the undergraduate level, opportunities to learn about QoLT come in many forms including formal coursework, project-based classes, research experiences, as well as activities facilitated by campus services and local, regional, and national organizations serving students with disabilities and veterans. The QoLT curriculum should be built across multiple disciplines such as robotics, human–computer interaction, rehabilitation science and technology, and engineering.

An "Introduction to Quality of Life Technology" course serves as an introduction to QoLT principles. Such a course should include students' visiting a client's home to perform an environmental assessment that generates ideas for products that can help the user. In addition to QoLT problems, students should be educated on underlying QoLT research principles. Participatory Action Design (PAD) is one such principle. It is essential to the QoLT research. PAD involves QoLT stakeholders's participation in the entire product development process, including the complete feedback cycle of ideation, interaction design and ethical consideration, technology development and integration, prototype deployment and evaluation and, finally, design refinement and iteration. The "Introduction to Quality of Life Technology" course has received positive feedback in the QoLT center and improved student participation in other QoLT Center's educational and research activities.

Project-based courses included in the QoLT undergraduate curriculum include service learning and capstone classes. Such classes allow us to link community partners (e.g., long-term care and other clinical partners) with faculty and students from multiple disciplines. For example, undergraduate students at the QoLT Center have worked on a variety of projects, including a tracking system for assistive technologies equipment at the Western Pennsylvania School for Blind Children and a "no-mess hair apparatus" to make beauty salon stations more accessible. To introduce more undergraduate students from traditional engineering disciplines to the PAD process, we recommend partnering with Rapid Prototyping courses that teach students to realize the design, including the iterative process of prototyping and evaluation. For example, by partnering with a Rapid Prototyping course at CMU, students have worked on the QoLT Center's health kiosk and self-tuning environment projects for persons with traumatic brain injuries and other disabilities. For both projects, the students worked with QoLT faculty to develop a system consisting of a computer interface, hardware, and physiological sensors. Similar opportunities may exist within senior capstone courses that extend to two semesters allowing students to experience the entire design life cycle to deliver useful, usable, and desirable products to their clients. In the first semester of the capstone course, student teams should be matched with clients (individuals with disabilities or older adults) and assigned a technical and clinical faculty mentor.

A Quality of Life Technology Certificate (16–18 credits) program can be designed to help undergraduate students from multiple disciplines to become better versed in QoLT. A similar certificate program has been developed by a QoLT partner at Penn State University Greater Allegheny (PSUGA; McKeesport, PA). This program focuses on information space, or ways in which the information needs of people with disabilities and the elderly can be satisfied. PSUGA works with its industry partner Blueroof Technologies to enhance the educational process with real-world experiences. The curriculum of this certificate program focuses on residential information technology systems and involves designing smart homes; designing and integrating innovative technologies; developing user-friendly interfaces for older adults and their caregivers; creating entertainment technology that promotes play, physical movement, and mental stimulation; understanding of telemedicine systems and decision-making support for financial and personal needs, networking, network security, and telecommunications; and creating databases to store and analyze large amounts of data.

A minor in QoLT at the undergraduate level can be designed to provide an even greater insight into QoLT discipline. Curriculum for the minor should include the core Introduction to Quality of Life Technology course, along with classes related to research methodologies, medical aspects of disability, the social experience of disability, funding and policy, and design. The minor can fit well in the computer and rehabilitation science domains and can also be marketed to students in the engineering departments.

14.3.2 Research Opportunities

The QoLT Research Experience for Undergraduates (REU) program, sponsored by the NSF, aims to excite undergraduate students about QoLT; engage them in cross-disciplinary research; expand their knowledge of emerging technologies; and prepare them for graduate studies or professional careers in QoLT. In addition, the REU program can serve as an excellent mechanism to enhance diversity. Because the focus of the QoLT REU program is on serving underrepresented populations (specifically, people with disabilities), the program attracts a high number of students from underrepresented populations. The ratio of underrepresented students (students with disabilities, females, African American, and Hispanic students) participating in the QoLT REU program is significantly higher compared to other engineering programs and reflects the overall U.S. population. This in itself constitutes an excellent outcome.

All QoLT REU students should participate in workshop series that covers areas such as fabrication, electronics, design practices, research methods, and statistics. Seminars on scientific writing and oral presentation skills should supplement research activities. In addition, throughout the REU program, students should have ample opportunities to learn about clinical and social aspects of aging and disability. A research symposium should be held at the end of the internship where students present their research findings to faculty, peers, and industry representatives. Faculty and mentors from students' home institutions should be invited to attend the symposium, which strengthens research collaborations and helps with intern recruitment. Students who exhibit a strong interest in pursuing advanced education in QoLT should be encouraged to work further with their mentors after the internship to submit research papers to related professional conferences.

The QoLT REU program has had a very positive impact on its participants. 87% of the students stated that this internship increased their knowledge of both the field and the research process; 57% of former QoLT REU students are currently pursuing graduate degrees. We hope that by replicating the format of the QoLT REU program, other academic institutions with a focus on QoLT achieve similar results.

Because the QoLT undergraduate curriculum is still in development and a limited number of students can participate in the QoLT REU program, an additional program was created to promote undergraduates' involvement in QoLT. Coordinated by the Student Leadership Council (SLC) and the QoLT Center's EOD team, the semester-long QoLiTy program allows undergraduates at Pitt and CMU to gain research experience by participating in a QoLT project. The program is open to sophomores and juniors, as well as freshmen who already have some research experience. Similar to the REU program, QoLiTy program matches undergraduates with mentors from Pitt and CMU faculty, graduate students, industry partners, and practitioners. At the end of the semester, QoLiTy students present their work at a poster session and submit a summary of their work to program organizers. Participants of the program are encouraged to apply to graduate programs affiliated with the QoLT Center.

14.3.3 Funding Educational Programs at the Undergraduate Level

Opportunities to fund educational initiatives with a focus on QoLT lie in three different areas: program development, research related to educational outcomes, and scholarships and fellowships for students. The NSF REU program and National Institute of Health (NIH) research training programs provide funding to programs that engage students in interdisciplinary research outside of their home institutions. The NSF Research to Aid Persons with Disabilities solicitation provides funding to support courses that involve students in the assistive technologies design process. NSF Research in Engineering Education grants support design, development, and evaluation of innovative interventions that make engineering education more accessible to underrepresented groups, including students with disabilities.

14.3.4 Special Initiative in Undergraduate Education: Veterans

Students with disabilities, especially veterans with disabilities, encounter significant obstacles in completing a university STEM education. A recent study conducted at the University of Minnesota's Institute of Technology with 65 students with disabilities identified three major barriers common to STEM undergraduate and graduate students with disabilities: (1) faculty attitudes regarding certain accommodations, (2) financial aid, and (3) the disability itself and its limitations (Seymour and Hunter 1998). In designing a successful veterans' college reentry program, affiliated faculty should be trained in disability and veterans' issues; students should be provided with information about accommodations and other helpful campus services; networking opportunities should be utilized to facilitate interaction between veteran students from different disciplines and to connect them to those veterans in the community who have already completed similar academic programs.

While undergraduate engineering education in the United States is reaching a critical shortage, only 6% of high school SAT takers are expressing an interested in engineering, down from 9% in 1998 (Cook 2009), statistical data demonstrate that active duty service members and veterans returning to school may not follow the same trend.

Education transition programs like Experiential Learning for Veterans in Assistive Technology and Engineering (ELeVATE), facilitated by the QoLT center, provide veterans with year-long program support, internship experiences, innovative networking, and opportunities for building lasting relationships with professionals in the community.

University bureaucracies, the uncertainty of transfer of credits, and the complicated GI Bill present barriers for veterans in higher education. Educators can use many support systems to ensure the success of wounded, injured, and ill (WII) veterans in academic programs (NSF 2009). Such support systems include mentors, veteran student cohorts, and rehabilitation support. A formal needs assessment conducted by the QoLT Center concluded that a support structure that includes undergraduate students (e.g., peers in engineering and technology), graduate students, faculty (e.g., research faculty and academic mentors), and veterans in the community matched to the participants' interests can improve the retention of veteran students. Transition programs should provide housing and hourly stipends, in addition to existing educational benefits. To assist veterans with the application process and financial aid paperwork, reentry programs are encouraged to collaborate with the campus veterans' office. It is also important to establish partnerships with veterans' services organizations to create a support system that extends beyond the university into the community. Many veterans may relocate to attend college. Therefore, it is important to connect them to the network of veteran community members, mentors, etc., with whom they can consult regarding benefits, family issues, and employment.

When the support structure is in place, the appropriate personnel must be identified to assist with the program. It is important to include other veterans as role models, mentors, or program directors. Beyond the focus of the program, additional opportunities for vocational counseling, goal setting, and career exposure should be provided.

Recruitment for veterans' reentry programs does not pose a challenge. Though military medical transition programs like Warrior Transition Units (Army) and Wounded Warrior Brigades (Marines) cannot officially endorse nonmilitary programs, establishing relationships with coordinators of such programs ensures access to a pool of prospective participants who are preparing for transition. By demonstrating that the relevant support activities and networks are in place, nonmilitary veterans' reentry programs can gain an unofficial stamp of approval from the military personnel, which translates into assistance with recruitment. It is also beneficial to reach out to several national veteran organizations that have local chapters such as Paralyzed Veterans of America (PVA) and Disabled American Veterans (DAV). Local support services such as Offices of Vocational Rehabilitation at the state level are also good sources for recruitment. Social networking platforms such as Facebook and Twitter should be used to connect with individual veterans and veteran organizations. A workshop series co-facilitated by campus veterans' services offices can also be used to inform veterans about educational options in addition to serving as a recruitment mechanism for specific programs.

Based on results from the first cohort of our ELeVATE program, participants should be instructed on the academic and research culture, yet engaged in some of the military-like procedures such as reporting to a chain of command to provide a sense of familiarity and avoid confusion. Providing rehabilitation and counseling support is essential to success of reentry programs. While participants are improving their self-efficacy through experiential learning, a comprehensive rehabilitation plan should be implemented for each participant to coach him/her on how to manage the stress of academic life. A rehabilitation plan should be based on functional, neuropsychological, interest, and aptitude and assistive technology assessments designed to identify an academic goal as well as the service, support, and accommodation needs of the participant. Career counseling should also be incorporated into the planning process. A rehabilitation support team should establish and implement a monitoring strategy to guarantee that should the participant encounter difficulties, they will be addressed through modifications to their rehabilitation plan.

Supplemental training activities are what make programs like ELeVATE a unique educational opportunity rather than just a one-time research experience. ELeVATE participants fine-tune general writing, math, and statistics skills and become accustomed to an academic setting. They are tasked with concrete and achievable assignments that correspond with a concrete timeline and goals, all related to the research project they have been assigned.

There are three main areas related to funding in veterans' education: (1) program development, (2) research related to educational outcomes, and (3) additional funding for students in the form of scholarships and fellowships. NSF Research in Engineering Education has solicitations for the first two areas. Nonprofit organizations such as DAV and PVA also have funding opportunities related to veterans' education and training for employment.

14.3.5 Special Initiative in Undergraduate Education: Research Partnerships

EOD has developed successful partnerships with institutions that have evolved into concentric circles of collaboration to introduce students to QoLT systems and connect graduate students with research and doctoral studies opportunities, including underrepresented minority students. One such partnership is with PROMISE: Maryland's Alliance for Graduate Education and the Professoriate (AGEP). The PROMISE AGEP is part of an alliance between the historically diverse University of Maryland, Baltimore County (UMBC: The Honors University in Maryland); the University of Maryland, College Park; and the University of Maryland, Baltimore, with UMBC being the lead institution. Our partnership with the PROMISE AGEP has lead to students from UMBC participating in QoLT REU cohorts and QoLT hosting Dissertation House, a dissertation preparation workshop for doctoral students facilitated by Dr. Renetta Garrison Tull and Dr. Wendy Carter, leadership faculty from the PROMISE AGEP program. Continued efforts are being developed to increase joint university opportunities for collaboration in areas of QoLT focused recruitment, curricula development, and research.

14.4 Graduate Education

The goal of the QoLT graduate education program is to produce a new generation of researchers and industry practitioners who are prepared to work at the interface of multiple seemingly disparate disciplines, thereby being able to integrate basic understanding of human functions (psychological, physiological, physical, and cognitive) and behaviors in everyday living and socioeconomics in the design of intelligent devices and systems that aid, interact, and work in symbiosis with people with disabilities and older adults.

The process of creating such an interdisciplinary graduate program has been challenging due to the organizational and cultural differences between disciplines and little flexibility in existing graduate programs. For example, practitioners of these disciplines have stereotypical differences over many areas, for example, expectations for graduate students, curriculum design, lecturing style, and also social beliefs. We have designed our educational program with these challenges in mind.

It is important to first define the educational qualities that differentiate QoLT from other engineering disciplines. We consider those to be the centrality of (1) person–system symbiosis, (2) the societal aspects of technology, (3) multidisciplinary approaches to technology development, and (4) the complete life cycle, systems approach to technology development. Based on these qualities, we then derive the core competencies that we expect a QoLT student to acquire during the course of graduate studies. The QoLT Center has used the following competencies to guide the development and evaluation of its graduate curriculum and other educational activities:

Understanding the Problem

Understanding of medical, social, legislative aspects of disability and aging

Understanding and assessment of personal/clinical needs for technology

Understanding and assessment of the promises and limitations of technology to solve clinical problems

Developing the Solution

Understanding of the complete design life cycle of QoLT systems

Understanding of funding and policy impact on QoLT systems

Understanding of the process of developing new QoLT systems and incorporating it into new products, processes, and services

Evaluating the Technology

Ability to prepare and conduct human subject testing of QoLT systems

Understanding of qualitative and quantitative research methods

Appreciation of ethical principles to guide the design, development, and implementation of new intelligent systems

Promulgating the Approach

Communication skills for cross-disciplinary collaboration

Leadership skills

Prior to designing a formal curriculum, we first communicated with the course instructors at CMU and Pitt to assess how the existing courses contribute to the students' competencies. We have the opportunity to infuse these courses with QoLT content (see Table 14.2). For example, Pitt's "Rehabilitation Engineering Design" course teaches students the complete design life cycle of assistive technologies, including the complete feedback cycle of ideation, interaction design and ethical consideration, technology development and integration, prototype deployment and evaluation, and design refinement and iteration. The course also introduces the commercialization process for innovative technologies. In this course, graduate students from different academic backgrounds work in teams to identify, formulate, and solve problems confronted by people with disabilities. The course

TABLE 14.2

Core Competencies Covered by a Sample of QoLT-Relevant Courses

Core Competency Course	Medical Aspects	Clinical Needs	Technology Needs	Design Life-Cycle	Funding and Policy	Development Process	Subject Testing	Research Methods	Ethical Principles	Communication Skills	Leadership Skills
Rehabilitation Engineering Design		X		X	X					X	
Ethical Issues in Healthcare	X			X	X				X		
Assistive Technology Funding and Policy				X	X	X					
Medical Aspects of Disability	X	X		X							
Individual and Social Experience of Disability	X	X		X	X						
Ethnography: How Context Affects Tech Use	X	X		X			X	X	X	X	
Robot Ethics							X		X	X	X
Adaptive Control			X	X		X		X			
Biomechanics and Motor Control			X	X		X	X	X			

provides student teams with opportunities to work with QoLT industry partners. This course addresses the core competency requirements in many ways, and is thus listed as one of the core courses recommended to QoLT students.

This assessment process not only resulted in a list of existing courses recommended to QoLT graduate students, but revealed missing elements in the existing curriculum, which has led to the development of new QoLT courses. For instance, "Ethnography: Analyzing How Context Affects Technology Use" is an immersive course, cross-listed between the partnering universities and taught by two instructors with different areas of expertise (namely, human–computer interaction and clinical/rehabilitation sciences) from CMU's Robotics Institute and Pitt's Department of Rehabilitation Science and Technology. The course teaches students how to apply qualitative ethnographic methods to understand the end user for whom new technology is intended. By covering topics such as field-work, passive and active observation, secondary analyses, and novel computer-assisted approaches, the Ethnography course helps students characterize and understand the practices, preferences, and needs of end users, the surrounding environment, and the associated societal factors that will affect technology success. A formative evaluation was conducted on the first-run course where an external evaluator interviewed the two instructors separately to determine the course goals and surveyed the students to evaluate attainment of these goals. By comparing the course goals stated by the two course instructors, and the agreement between the instructors' stated goals and student feedback on learning outcomes, the evaluator generated a detailed report, which provided a basis for course revision and future planning. A similar evaluation process is being carried out for "Robot Ethics," another QoLT course.

In addition to courses offered at CMU and Pitt, we observed uniquely designed interdisciplinary courses from other centers and institutions. One such course is "Rehabilitation

Medicine for Scientists and Engineers" at Case Western Reserve University. The course exposes scientists and engineers-in-training to the broader medical, psychological, and social issues relevant to the rehabilitation of persons with limb amputation, spinal cord injury, stroke, traumatic brain injury, and neuromuscular diseases. The course includes (1) introductory clinical didactics, (2) attendance and participation in inpatient clinical rounds and outpatient clinics, and (3) preparation and presentation of a paper identifying a clinical problem and proposing a novel technological approach to addressing the problem. Students are required to register for four consecutive semesters to complete this comprehensive course and can choose any three of the five topics for both the didactic sessions and their related clinical rotations to enhance their training in the areas that they find relevant and interesting. This comprehensive course not only provides engineering students with content, but enhances communication and problem-solving skills. The course allows patients to achieve their individual goals of becoming independent participants in our society.

Credentialing through certificates or minors helps to identify a graduate student's interdisciplinary training. This credential may also aid in communicating both disciplinary depth and interdisciplinary breadth to potential employers. Building upon existing courses and programs, we created a Gerontechnology track under the existing Graduate Certificate Program in Gerontology at Pitt, which focuses on fitting technological solutions to support changing life goals and lifestyle preferences into advanced age. The QoLT Ethnography course is one of the required courses for this track.

Given the multi-institutional nature of the QoLT Center, students in each program have to fulfill their program's requirements and thus have few opportunities to take additional courses. In addition, QoLT students come from diverse disciplines and their interests in each phase of the design life cycle of the QoLT systems may vary based upon their backgrounds. To ensure that QoLT students have the breadth and depth of knowledge essential to the QoLT field, we have designed and implemented the educational activities that provide more flexible learning options and supplement classroom learning:

1. Short Course Series
2. Practicum Series
3. Innovation and Commercialization Workshop Series

Short courses have several advantages. They can offer students the ability to obtain knowledge and skills in a chosen area that are more relevant to their research interest. Short courses are effective in facilitating cross-training where students in one field learn the essentials from other fields. For example, the QoLT Center has developed a short course series including two online modules on medical aspects of disabilities for students in engineering and computer science, and is developing another course series on machine learning for non-computer science students. We suggest that QoLT students be required to take each module, in order to provide a minimum common baseline for all QoLT students, regardless of discipline. Because the course content is available online, students can learn at their own pace and test their learning outcomes by completing the posttest at the end of each module.

Students in QoLT disciplines must have first-hand knowledge of clinical problems and social issues encountered by people with disabilities and older adults in order to learn how to develop technological solutions. Our students have an opportunity to observe patient care in outpatient and inpatient settings at our partnering clinics. For example, a QoLT student at CMU's Human Computer Interaction Institute spent 1 month at the Pitt's Center for

Assistive Technology observing the process of evaluation and prescription of wheelchair seating components before designing the virtual seating coach, a device that encourages safe and healthy use of wheelchair seating functions by detecting seating activities, analyzing user behaviors, and responding accordingly to provide suggestions or reminders. Another example was a 1 day practicum at a local nursing facility where students had a team conference with the staff members, observed different areas of care, and interviewed the residents. We suggest making such clinical observations mandatory for all QoLT graduate students.

In order for QoLT systems to have direct impact on stakeholders, it is critical to teach QoLT students entrepreneurial skills. Although our graduate students participate in the innovative process and learn innovation skills through coursework and research, their interaction with industry and exposure to real-world scenarios are limited. Through partnership with the QoLT Foundry, we have designed a workshop series covering various topics related to innovation and commercialization. The workshops have covered topics such as assessment of commercial potential of a discovery, development market analysis, intellectual property protection, regulatory and reimbursement considerations of QoLT, structuring a company, financing, and possible roles and responsibilities of founders. The annual industry practitioner panel, hosted by the QoLT SLC enhances the workshops by providing students with an opportunity to discuss careers in industry and entrepreneurship with industrial practitioners in an open forum.

14.5 Continuing Education

CE is ongoing education that promotes workplace or professional competence and is targeted at adults with a high school education or higher. CE allows professionals to remain competent by providing them with opportunities to learn about newly adopted technologies and treatment interventions in a formal setting. CE does not replace, but rather complements, fundamental knowledge.

The need for CE can result from needs assessment, changes in laws or regulations, adoption of new technologies, or requirements by credentialing organizations. A CE needs assessment can be conducted for the target population: Employees may be asked directly about which work tasks or topics for which they would request more training, or employee knowledge can be tested to determine whether they need additional information in certain areas of their jobs. Once the need for CE has been identified, the CE program should be planned and measureable learning objectives that would serve as the foundation for the CE program should be identified. Based on our needs assessment, the QoLT Center designed its CE program with two distinct purposes in mind: (1) to supply QoLT affiliates (including students, faculty, and staff) with basic knowledge on disability and disability-related issues and (2) to educate the clinical (e.g., physical and occupational therapists, physicians, nurses, and others who will implement QoLT in their professions) and scientific (e.g., researchers in QoLT-related fields) community about the QoLT Center's goals and accomplishments.

CE programs vary in format and may include in-person presentations, video of in-person presentations, and reading of relevant publications followed by posttests. The QoLT Center's CE initiatives are not limited to one format. They include online modules, including "Demystifying Disability," "Disabilities Related to Aging," "Fall Prevention Through the Use of Assistive Technology," "Progressive Neurological Conditions that Benefit from

QoLT Technology," "Non-Progressive Neurological Conditions that Benefit from QoLT" (all available on MediaSite Live); the annual QoLT Symposium, held in conjunction with the Rehabilitation Engineering Society of North America (RESNA) conference; and the State of the Science Symposium, held quarterly at Walter Reed Military Medical Center. Interested students, faculty, healthcare professionals, and physicians have opportunities to learn about latest developments in QoLT-related fields and earn Continuing Education Units (CEUs) by participating in any of these programs.

14.6 Community Outreach

The main goals of the QoLT Center's community outreach efforts are to (1) increase public awareness of the innovative research in QoLT and (2) systematically change the thinking of all individuals reached by (a) raising public awareness of the QoLT Center's mission and vision, (b) ensuring that the community is aware of the QoLT Center's educational programs and outreach events, and (c) ensuring that individuals and organizations actively seek out opportunities to participate in such programs and events.

Prior to developing outreach programs, constraints must be identified and available resources must be assessed. Typically, in-house resources are limited. To augment these resources, one can turn to external funding from grants and other sources. In addition, it is important to utilize existing resources for community outreach. The resources that have been essential to the success of the QoLT Center's outreach efforts are dedicated volunteers with experience in STEM education, multi-institutional expertise in QoLT research and services, and the QoLT Center's partnership with community organizations and centers.

Good, widespread communications is key to any successful outreach effort. It is essential to ensure sufficient web presence, including on social media sites. For instance, we have developed a QoLT Center presence on major social media platforms including YouTube, Facebook, Twitter, Flickr, Picasa, LinkedIn, and explored new opportunities as new social media outlets become available. Specifically, we have linked existing project-level social media communications to better integrate QoLT Center-wide communications and worked on leveraging the social media aspects of YouTube, Picasa, and Flickr by "favoriting" related research videos at other organizations and selecting "friends" and "subscribers" in YouTube. We have also created QoLTient, a biweekly news digest designed to share information about QoLT-related research and activities. The QoLTient is distributed to all QoLT affiliates and partners, including community organizations and individual subscribers.

The most effective way to communicate the QoLT Center's mission to the public is to reach out to the community itself. QoLT Ambassadors are the indispensable link connecting the QoLT Center and the community. QoLT Ambassadors are volunteers with experience in STEM fields and education (e.g., former teachers, engineers). They work alongside the EOD team at outreach events and assist during educational programs including the aforementioned SciTech Festival at the Carnegie Science Center and tours to groups ranging from middle school students to special interest groups across all levels. They attend EOD meetings, where they have an opportunity to contribute to the development and assessment of outreach programs. The lead Ambassador coordinates and keeps track of Ambassador involvement in outreach events and reports on Ambassador activities to the rest of the QoLT Center. The QoLT Ambassador program gives committed members of the community an opportunity to be part of the QoLT team and to spread the word about QoLT's research and mission. At the same time, it ensures that the QoLT EOD team has additional help at large outreach events.

The high level of expertise and innovation of QoLT scholars and availability of state-of-the-art research facilities at Pitt, CMU, and partnering organizations (e.g., Blueroof Technologies) has allowed us to conduct age-appropriate tours of our laboratories, where individuals have an opportunity to interact with QoLT and communicate with the scientists (faculty and graduate students) behind each project. By giving tour participants an opportunity to interact with QoLT (e.g., persons without disabilities can try on a prosthesis or they can try to navigate the lab space in different wheelchairs), the tours provide a glimpse of the challenges a person with a disability might face on a daily basis. The tours are conducted by the QoLT Ambassadors, who were trained by the project researchers themselves. The QoLT Center also participates in community events and science fairs at local and national levels, such as Carnegie Science Center's SciTech Festival, Allegheny Green + Innovation Festival, Pittsburgh Regional Science & Engineering Fair, the National Girl Scout Convention, and National Veterans Wheelchair Games and continues to explore new venues for participation.

More in-depth outreach can be accomplished through formal courses targeted to the community. For instance, "Technology for Smart Living" is a course designed specifically for the Osher Lifelong Learning Institute at CMU. In this course, researchers at CMU and Pitt work with retirees to define their needs and the possibilities of technologies to provide assistance in the home, thereby enabling elders to continue to live independently. The students learn about products on the market and in development, gain an understanding of the underlying technologies, and then conceptualize new products. This course provides QoLT researchers with invaluable information for new QoLT projects and empowers older adults by giving them information on available and future technologies that can potentially enhance their personal lives.

14.7 Evaluation

The evaluation of QoLT education programs should include both a process and an outcome evaluation with yearly (pre-/post-data collection) and longitudinal (multiple years data collection) follow-ups. A logic model, a visual representation of inputs, activities, outputs, and outcomes, should be used to define the program's proposed processes. A process evaluation helps monitor the implementation of the program as proposed, to capture any revisions that were made to address obstacles, and to determine the efficacy of services provided to the participants. Surveys completed by participants at the end of each activity and end-of-the-year surveys completed by participants (and, if applicable, their mentors) help determine which activities should be retained, revised, or discontinued. An outcomes evaluation determines the impact of the activities on participants in terms of changes in knowledge, skill, attitudes, behaviors, and status. A triangulation of methods and sources ensures that the collected data are encompassing and accurate. An evaluator should interview participants at the beginning, middle, and end of year to measure changes in awareness and other defined program outcomes. A follow-up survey should be designed to track participants' graduation and employment dates. Facebook has proven to be an effective tool for identifying former participants' academic and/or employment status. Changes in knowledge, skills, and self-efficacy toward QoLT education and careers should be measured for short-term outcomes, while change in behavior and status and condition should be measured mid- and long-term, respectively.

As QoLT graduate students are deeply entrenched in QoLT educational initiatives, we use additional methods to evaluate their learning. We assess short-term and intermediate outcomes (e.g., disability awareness, knowledge of QoLT methodologies and commercialization process, assessment skills, motivation, and attitude toward QoLT interdisciplinary education) through artifacts such as presentations, written reports, and research. We also track progress of QoLT students who attend activities outside their departments, who participate in the QoLT Foundry or other entrepreneurial activities, whose dissertation committee includes faculty from different disciplines, whose publications include authors from multiple disciplines, and citations of such publications. It is also important to track student publications in QoLT-related journals and conference proceedings as well as student job placement post-graduation. Special attention must be paid to positions that imply interdisciplinary approach to technology and/or entrepreneurship.

Specific initiatives have individual evaluation needs. For example, to evaluate the success of general outreach activities, appropriate assessment mechanisms need to be developed. Some important ways of evaluating outcomes of the QoLT Center's outreach efforts include conducting satisfaction surveys of event participants; tracking the hours spent on participation in outreach activities; tracking the number of individuals receiving the QoLT Center's promotional materials; tracking the number of individuals who follow up with the QoLT Center's staff after an outreach event; monitoring web traffic; tracking the number of references in popular media outlets; and tracking the number of individuals who contact the QoLT Center. The data collected through such assessment mechanisms allow the QoLT EOD team to assess the effectiveness of specific activities and to identify directions for future outreach efforts.

Similarly, to determine the effectiveness and timeliness of the QoLT Center's CE offerings, it is required that additional evaluation metrics be used in the form of posttests that are completed with each QoLT module. Evaluation forms are always collected for each of QoLT's CE programs. The forms are used to determine whether the speaker covered the specific learning objectives of the program, to establish the timeliness and value of the topic, as well as to solicit ideas for additional topics participants would like to see offered by the QoLT Center.

14.8 Conclusion

Our aspiration is that students, consumers, and practitioners who have participated in QoLT initiatives at any educational level will possess a higher degree of social awareness and intellectual preparedness to implement QoLT principles in creating enabling solutions for persons with disabilities and older adults. The interdisciplinary nature of QoLT will continue to inspire healthcare practitioners, social scientists, computer scientists, and engineers to work together on solutions to some of society's greatest problems, such as social isolation and loss of independence for persons with disabilities and older adults.

References

Cook, B. 2009. *From Soldier to Student: Easing the Transition of Service Members on Campus*. Y. Kim, Ed. American Council on Education: Washington, DC.

Fancsali, C. and Froschl, M. 2006. Great science for girls: Gender-equitable STEM & afterschool programs. *Science Books and Films* May/June: 99–105.

National Science Foundation. 2009. Veterans' education for engineering and science. Arlington, VA. Available at http://www.nsf.gov/eng/eec/VeteranEducation.pdf [Accessed 15 December 2011].

National Science Foundation, Division of Science Resources Statistics. 2011. Women, minorities, and persons with disabilities in science and engineering: 2011. Arlington, VA. Available at http://www.nsf.gov/statistics/wmpd/ [Accessed 15 December 2011].

Seymour, E. and Hunter, A. 1998. *Talking about Disability: The Education and Work Experience of Graduates and Undergraduates with Disabilities in Science, Mathematics and Engineering Majors* (AAAS Publication No. 98-02S). American Association for the Advancement of Science: Washington, DC.

Weinburgh, M. 1995. Gender differences in student attitudes toward science: A meta-analysis of the literature from 1970–1991. *Journal of Research in Science Teaching* 32: 387–398.

15

Innovation, Commercialization, and Start-Ups

James F. Jordan

CONTENTS

15.1 Introduction

Nine out of 10 companies fail to make it to venture capital (VC) funding sources, even after passing technical feasibility hurdles and developing working prototypes [1]. This chapter illustrates the steps and resources needed to grow a start-up company out of academic research. In it we outline general concepts of beginning and maintaining a successful start-up company, and through the use of three case studies, we will show how these guidelines directly relate to quality of life technology (QoLT).

Discussions of innovation frequently exclude commercialization. By our definition the processes of research, development, and commercialization are all part of the broader topic of innovation. Thus, innovation involves the systematic pursuit of all three steps involved in bringing a product to market:

- Research: a studious inquiry or examination. Discovery and interpretation of facts, the revision of accepted theories or laws in light of these new facts, or practical application of such new or revised theories or laws
- Development: the act of creating that which is unknown; a gradual and focused process by which anything is developed in a series of progressive steps
- Commercialize: to make something available to be exploited for profit

The end result of commercialization is the availability of the innovation to be exploited for profit, which creates both jobs and wealth. So it appears we have numerous embedded processes in innovation. The inclusion of commercialization and its required steps are a necessity in order to get an innovation to market.

These steps include having the time, money, and other resources necessary to prepare a product or service for "launch" and the activities necessary for the company to become self-sufficient. This chapter provides a systematic overview of the processes and pitfalls of launching a successful start-up.

15.2 Innovation Is a Process of Connected Steps

The process begins with *research*, the primary goal of which is the discovery and interpretation of new facts. In general, the government, academic institutions, and large industries perform the majority of the research in the United States.

Frequently, one research project does not yield one result applicable to a specific market situation. It can take many research chapters to yield a development story.

Development is the step in which the research chapters are converted into a practical, applicable idea. Development generally occurs in academic and government institutions, within an existing company, or is handled by an individual or group of individuals.

Commercialization is a process of connected steps to bring a product to market. Progressive commercialization techniques embrace integration, concurrence, and/or overlap with the development process to ensure proper downstream execution. Commercialization is executed primarily through two organizational forms: corporations and start-ups (Figure 15.1).

Corporations generally have more specialized personnel and have access to public financing. As a result, their commercialization teams have less of a focus on obtaining financing to fund the endeavor. The team's main focus is developing a quality product that meets product specifications.

Although there are numerous commercialization processes and philosophies, they all contain a common series of steps and reviews often referred to as "gates." The "gate" process typically starts with screening development ideas and scoping the objectives and deliverables of the project. A business case is documented and a prototype developed. The prototype is tested and validated at which point the product is launched. Successful conclusion of this process is generally considered to be the final phase of new product development.

Start-up companies typically do not have access to public financing. Thus, private financing is required and comes in the form of founder self-investment, organic growth

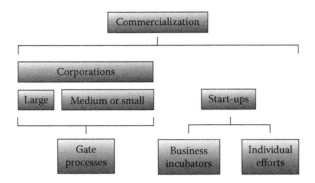

FIGURE 15.1
Commercialization executed through two organizational forms: Corporations and start-ups.

(invest more when you sell more), and angel or VC investment. As a result, raising funds frequently consumes as much, or more, management time for a start-up as commercializing the product.

An example of the process and the programs at the Pittsburgh Life Sciences Greenhouse (PLSG) is given in the following. The PLSG is a nonprofit incubator that offers programs and funding to help companies progress.

Figure 15.2 articulates, on the left, the sources of innovation. The investment continuum is highlighted at the bottom of the graphic representing the funding sources for each phase. The specific programs of the PLSG are identified in their Concept to Commercializaton™ Model (blue circles). The company's objectives are to provide capital, connectivity, people, and space to move client companies from pre-seed to early-stage funding.

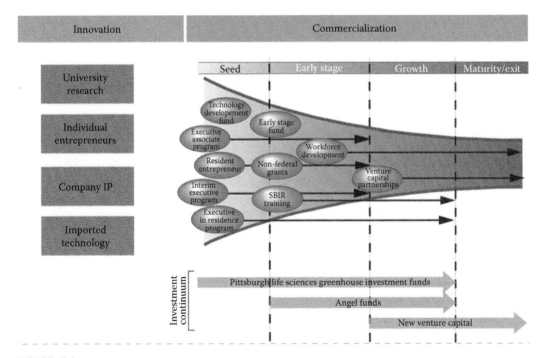

FIGURE 15.2
(See color insert.) Innovation and commercialization in start-up companies.

15.3 Domain Experience Personnel Reduce Risk

Domain experience means that the company's founders or their management have worked in the industry before and have specific knowledge of the industry and the tasks at hand. Private investors have learned that successful start-up ventures are led by those who have lived in the industry. In short, domain experience is the experience that an employee has acquired by virtue of their employment at another successful firm in a particular industry or industry segment.

This concept becomes intuitive when you consider that the first step in product development requires a thorough understanding of the "voice of the customer" and the customer problem you are solving. From that foundation, the product specifications are built: If you get it wrong, the entire business foundation is flawed.

Start-ups with limited budgets for market research must make assumptions on the "voice of the customer." Who has a higher probability of making better assumptions, someone with 20 years of domain experience or someone from a different industry?

In addition to understanding the customer's voice, domain experience brings relationships and an understanding of the connectivity within the industry.

Many products are part of a broader value chain that creates the ultimate customer solution. For example, a steering wheel for an automobile is important but without the entire car, its value is relatively trivial. Frequently the product may be part of a bigger customer system or may need to go through a particular channel partner. Those who have domain experience have relationships and knowledge about how to access these systems and channels.

The concept of domain experience is evidenced in the franchise industry. Why would one pay five or six times more to open a Dunkin Donuts than one would pay to open his own coffee shop? This is done because it is understood that much of a start-up company's initial dollars are spent (wasted) finding a profitable business model. Those who franchise recognize this and are willing to invest more money in a proven model to reduce their investments risk of failure.

Additionally, continuing our Dunkin Donuts example, the company brings its entire supplier network to the franchisee. As Dunkin Donuts has greater buying power than a local coffee shop, the franchisee has access to a broader amount of products at a better price. Dunkin Donuts analyzes best practices on what the store should look like, how the kitchen is planned, how the receipts are prepared—these are all done to ensure franchisee success. What works is known and therein lays the value.

Another example almost states the obvious; Queen Isabella funded Christopher Columbus's four voyages of exploration an attempt to colonize the "New World." Christopher Columbus had significant sailing experience. Would Queen Isabella have sent an inexperienced person into uncharted waters? You would not send someone who has just learned to navigate the local harbor to discover the "New World." These examples illustrate the feeling investors have regarding the importance of domain experienced personnel, particularly when funding a start-up company.

15.4 Match Your Strategy to the Product Life Cycle

Successful commercialization requires alignment with your target market's life cycle. Innovation is successful when matching the appropriate strategy with the appropriate product life cycle. Different tactics are deployed at each phase to affect change. The four

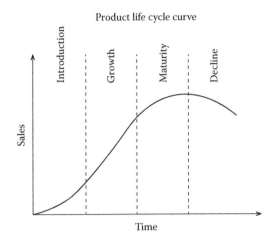

FIGURE 15.3
Revenues at different stages of a product life cycle.

stages of the product life cycle are introduction, growth, maturity, and decline. The graphic depicts the evolution of revenue with time (Figure 15.3).

Innovation is defined as introducing something new to affect change. From a business perspective, a marketing specialist would state that the desired effect of innovation is either to

- Create a new, differentiated, and protectable market category
- Collapse the value steps in an existing category, resulting in decreased cost or an increased benefit

As demand declines, industry consolidation is necessary to adjust supply with demand while maintaining declining pricing.

At the introduction stage of the product life cycle, the product is initiated into its market. The priority at this time is to create awareness of the offering through promotional efforts. It is noteworthy that frequently competitors are few or nonexistent at this point. If there are competitors, promotional efforts are oriented toward growing the category to the benefit of all versus competitive attacks.

At the *growth stage*, sales are generally escalating due to product awareness. This growth, with its corresponding cash, attracts competitors. Incumbent companies reinvest their cash windfalls to maintain position and hold off competitors. It is at this stage that promotional efforts change focus toward differentiating from the competition.

At the *maturity stage*, the market is established and sales tend to plateau: weaker competitors struggle for market share and ultimately leave the market and the remaining players intensely compete for market share. At this point, large cash profits are available for investors as product reinvestment is not as attractive based upon the market maturity.

At the *decline stage*, sales growth ceases and there are fewer players in the marketplace. As demand falls, companies either eliminate product lines or seek to extend life spans through new product line extensions or repositioning the products to new markets.

15.5 Start-Up Must Tell a Compelling Story

A start-up must be mindful of the need to pull together a compelling story that satisfies multiple constituencies. Naturally, the start-up and its product must have a story that is appealing to its customers: those who would purchase the product. However, to obtain a liquidity event (going public or a sale), a start-up must be attractive to the public markets, the private markets, and the company's potential acquirers. You could call these multiple constituencies the company's "publics."

Figure 15.4 demonstrates that the complexity of the start-up company trying to define a voice to its "publics." The company must tell a compelling story to obtain funding and advance through the investment continuum. Each subsequent round of investors (seed, early stage, growth, and later stage) is interested in different aspects of the story.

Achieving a "liquidity event" (the method by which investors get their money returned and hopefully profit) may require one story for an acquirer that may be an entirely different story needed for sustainability (public capital). Given the vast amount of "publics," the process can be difficult and complex. However, the best companies have the capability to create a simple story that is compelling for all.

15.6 Story Must Be Supported with an Evidentiary Investor Pitch

An investor pitch is a comprehensive plan that can be communicated according to the "rule of three." There are moments where you must communicate your story in less than 3 min. There are times when you have 30 min to communicate your plan and then there are occasions during final negotiations for fundraising where you may have up to 3 h to communicate your message. Creating a presentation that can be used for all three occasions (3 min, 30 min, and 3 h) requires some planning.

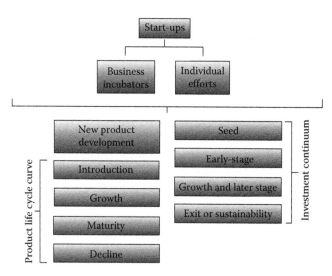

FIGURE 15.4
Product life cycle and investment continuum for start-ups.

The best pitches contain a concise preview of the company and a compelling story of success for the "publics." The market need is defined, the product offering is expressed, and the market opportunity is quantified. Competition is expressed and the business model is articulated. There is a commercialization plan with future milestones and their corresponding funding needs. The skill of the management team is communicated, and the presentation is closed with an opportunity summary.

"The Pitch" Workshop presented in the following demonstrates the type of content that should be included in your presentation.

"The Pitch" Workshop

Development Plan

Page 1 *Date: 1-10-06*

Table of Contents

- The Preview
- The Venture Concept
- The Market Need
- The Product Offering
- The Market Opportunity
- The Competition
- The Business Model

- The Commercialization Plan
- Future Milestones
- The Management Team
- Funding Needs
- Opportunity Summary

Page 2 *Date: 1-10-06*

The Preview

- A concise summary message of the opportunity
- If you have only 3 minutes, this slide & the Venture Concept slide would be your entire presentation

Page 3 *Date: 1-10-06*

The Venture Concept

- 30 second pitch
- Funding past & future
- Strength of the team

Page 4 *Date: 1-10-06*

The Market Need

- Has the company identified a clear need/ problem in the market
  - The solution & economic need (customer pain)
- How it is addressed today
- What gaps exist
- The primary & secondary customers

Page 5 *Date: 1-10-06*

The Product Offering

- Near-term product/service offering
- How it works
- How is it protected
- Current status of the technology
- Demonstrated outcomes of the concept
- The long-term opportunity

Page 6 *Date: 1-10-06*

The Market Opportunity

- Patient profile, prevalence, incidence, treatment methods
- Market size: growth rates of industry & target market
- Creation of new/untapped market demand
- Describe external factors driving growth
- Is the competitive advantage sustainable

The Competition

- Macro: what companies play in these segments
- Micro: what product lines do each company play with
- What competing technologies are under development
- Is the company positioned to compete effectively

The Commercialization Plan

- Intellectual property
- Market selection rationale
- Adoption drivers
- Performance data
- Reimbursement
- Regulatory
- Sales channel & pricing strategy

The Business Model

- Market strategy
- Mfg, market, sales, distribution strategy
- Anticipated market share
- Anticipated revenues 1yr/5yrs
- If too early provide a sense of scale
- Price of product/CAGS

Future Milestones

- Product development milestones
- Regulatory milestones
- Product launch dates
- New hire schedule
- Other significant milestones

The Management Team

- Management team
- Scientific advisory board
- Board of Directors
- Express the domain experience
- Identify special skills that will help you win
- Communicate special relationships

Funding Needs

- Money raised to date
- Money currently being sought/use of funds
- Anticipated future funding needs
- How will investor realize profit/exit strategy

Page 13   Date: 1-10-08

Opportunity Summary

- How fundable is the company in the venture capital community
- What are the likely sources of follow-up funding
- Does the company have a clear understanding for finding f/u funding
- What are the companies "fundable milestones" are how are you tracking to them.

Page 14   Date: 1-10-08

15.7 Great Pitches Constantly Undergo the Plan–Do–Check–Act Cycle

Plan–Do–Check–Act (PDCA) was made popular by Dr. W. Edward Deming, who is considered by many to be the father of quality control.

The "Plan" cycle is the establishment of objectives and the processes necessary to deliver the results are specified. In the "Do" cycle, the process is implemented, preferably in a small scale. In the "Check" cycle, the process is reviewed to determine if it met its expected output. The "Act" process determines if there was a difference between the desired output and the actual output. If there is a difference, the steps to apply changes are designed to meet the "plan." The process is then repeated.

15.8 Revisit Your Value Drivers after Each PDCA Cycle

15.8.1 Create an Unfair Advantage

Great start-ups are constantly attending to their "unfair market advantage," which is composed of characteristics the company possesses that favors its success.

This unfair advantage can be had by creating new categories or markets, collapsing the value steps of an existing market, seeking team members with proprietary customer relationships or know-how, or seeking first-mover advantage.

Venture capitalists particularly enjoy the creation of new categories or markets that are protected by intellectual property. Start-up companies that seek to create new, differentiated, and protectable areas frequently cause displacement of an existing market player and are acquired early. Venture capitalists find that these investments have shorter life cycles from creation and to acquisition. This process is something they can continually deploy with great success.

Start-ups that seek to collapse the value steps in the market offer a decreased cost as one aspect of new customer benefit. Destruction of the existing market results in the start-up firm connecting new components of the value chain or completely removing components of the value chain. Private investors also prosper from this particular tactic: However, collapsing value chains is not a continuously repeatable tactic as it takes time for the industry to standardize on your chains.

Private investors also seek teams with proprietary customer relationships or know-how. This tactic is particularly attractive when large players decide to outsource whole categories of businesses previously performed internally. Management teams departing from these large businesses generally enjoy intimate relationships with the outsourcing company and can quickly grab revenue contracts. The start-up businesses either eventually are acquired as the industry consolidates or becomes self-sustaining. Sustaining models generally are not attractive to venture capitalists; however, they are attractive to angel investors.

Frequently, seeking first-mover advantage can suffice. Sometimes an industry-incremental improvement, not capable of enjoying intellectual property protection, can still be significant. Even though a major player could eventually copy the idea, they may find it more cost-effective to acquire it. Why? Because acquiring new customers is expensive and it may be cheaper to just buy the ones you already have. These models may not be as attractive to venture capitalists; however, they are attractive to angel investors.

15.8.2 Differentiate Yourself Early and Plan to Evolve for Distance

Many companies fail to be planful when it comes to positioning. Positioning is an investment to influence the perception of a branded product. The objective of a brand is to occupy a unique space in the consumer's mind. The intention of this investment is that the product enjoys a higher sales volume and/or price than the product would have if it stood without a particular brand attribute. Careful consideration to positioning is frequently overlooked by start-up companies. If a start-up company is the first into the market category, they may not see the importance of this as their initial positioning speaks not to their product but to the category in general. (See the product life cycle management discussion.) When this occurs, followers enter the market and either copy the incumbent's positioning and/or create a differentiated positioning to steal market share. It is therefore advisable to "stake a position that is impervious to competitive advancement™." This can be done through alignment with the company's intellectual property or by capturing some other meaningful category symbol/message that others cannot replicate.

Lastly, it is important to recognize in the innovation cycle that the market will evolve through growth and maturity and will eventually decline. Therefore, positioning must evolve over time to continue to distance you from the competition. Considering each phase of the future market and setting your initial positioning for that evolution is prudent and cost-effective.

15.8.3 Domain Experienced Management Is the Key to a Successful Enterprise

We have spoken of the importance of domain-specific management upon the formation of a start-up company. The company must remember that each new hire is an opportunity to gain additional domain experience and specific know-how.

Start-up companies also require different management skills at different sizes of revenue and in different product life cycles phases. It is, therefore, critical that the start-up companies not only look at each new hire as an opportunity to gain domain experience and specific know-how but an opportunity to bring in personnel who match the particular product life cycle that the company is either in, or intends to be in, in the foreseeable future. A caution: it is also common for companies to make mistakes at this phase by hiring personnel too early. For example, the CEO or marketing executive skilled at the maturity or decline phase is not likely to be as effective in the introduction or growth phase.

15.8.4 Follow the Norms of the Start-Up Capital Market

Start-up companies begin without revenue and thus traditional discounted cash-flow valuation methods do not apply for valuations. Start-up companies must be aware of the norms associated with those private investors who frequent their particular market. Each specific market has certain steps that are associated with an increase in the value of the company. These steps and their associated value points must be known and are frequently called "fundable milestones." Figure 15.5 provides examples of milestones and investment at different stages of development.

Private investors generally equate a funding series with a particular stage in the investment continuum. Pre-money refers to the value given to the company before it raises a round of capital. Once the capital is raised, it is added to the pre-money valuation to obtain post-money valuation. You will notice that the post-money for Series A is not the pre-money of Series B. This is due to the premium awarded to the previous investors in Series A for success. It is noteworthy to comment that there can also be a "down round" which means that the Series B pre-money could be less than the Series A post-money. This happens when the previous "fundable milestones" were not met efficiently and the new investors are not going to pay for that inefficiency.

15.8.5 Plot Your Funding Syndicate

Start-up companies generally receive their initial funding from "Family and friends," followed by angels and then perhaps venture capitalists. "Family and friend" investors are exactly that—people the founders know personally who are willing to invest in their venture. Angel investors are high net-worth individuals. Frequently, they are accomplished business leaders. Other times, they are individuals whose wealth is gained through a

Series A—in millions		
Pre-money	Capital raise	Post-money
0.5	1.5	2

Fundable milestones:
+ Create proof of concept
+ Hire technical team
+ Demonstrate the viability
  of the commercialization plan

Series B—in millions		
Pre-money	Capital raise	Post-money
2.4	4	6.4

Fundable milestones:
+ Create prototype
+ Hire domain CEO
+ Attain regulatory approvals

Series C—in millions		
Pre-money	Capital raise	Post-money
7.68	10	17.68

Fundable milestones:
+ Launch product
+ Scale sales team
+ Initiate brand
+ Complete Mgmt team build-out

Exit in millions		
Minimum	Average	High
20	45	70

Fundable milestones:
+ Demonstrate brand value
+ Growth Mgmt talent in place
+ Demonstrate sustainable
  high growth revenue
+ Attain cash-flow positive

FIGURE 15.5
Fundable milestones and investment at different stages of development.

nonbusiness means (like a sports figure) or their wealth is inherited. More recently, angel investors have joined together and formed angel groups.

A venture firm is simply an investment firm that gives money to growing companies for a return. The VC firm generally receives their money from institutional investors and high net-worth individuals. These funds are pooled together to create a dedicated firm whose core skill is to identify start-up companies with the potential to generate high returns. VC firms generally focus in a specialty area such as healthcare or information technology. Many are even more focused such as those who invest only in the medical device or the pharmaceutical segments of healthcare. Those who place their money in a venture firm are counting on the expertise and specialized knowledge of the firm's investment partners to gain a high return.

A syndicate is a group of investors who come together to fund a particular company. Funding syndicates are not formal or permanent entities; however you will frequently notice groups of individuals, angels, or VC Funds that collaborate on financing.

Most likely each round of funding in a start-up will not be from one individual but from a group. This can be considered a syndicate. However, consider broadening that concept. If you combined all the people involved in financing the company from inception to cash flow positive, is that also not a syndicate? We will discuss this more later.

Angel investors can be the most important role in your start-up company as they are generally the first non-founder Board of Director members and nonfamily and friend stockholders. Experienced angels can offer advice based upon their experience and can be invaluable to helping you obtain future financing rounds.

Recall our discussion regarding where angel investors obtain their money. Would not you expect to receive better advice from an Angel Board of Directors member with significant business results in your specific industry than from someone who inherited his or her wealth? As money is power and influence, an inexperienced angel could unintentionally and adversely impact the company.

Frequently, the term "smart money" is used to refer to investors with industry experience. "Smart money" investors not only offer domain experience, they also offer other industry connectivity to suppliers, as well as relationships with potential management candidates and potential acquirers. Some offer VC connectivity as they may have had successful VC endeavors themselves. All of this domain experience is needed as the company progresses.

Depending on how much money the start-up company may require, they may need to involve VC. The VC industry has several different types of firms that are distinguished by the timing and the purpose of an investment. VC firms are generally broken into seed, early-stage, growth, and later-stage firms. There are further distinctions but they are beyond the scope of this discussion.

Each type of VC firm is skilled at their particular phase of development (i.e., seed) and they frequently offer domain experience and industry connectivity. By design and necessity, they also have relationships with the next level of VC firm. For example, early-stage venture firms have relationships with growth venture firms. One can appreciate that the VC is by design built on syndicates.

One will also hear the term "smart money" used in VC. An investment partner who has had several successful start-up ventures offers more operational experience than someone with an investment banking background at the seed stage. Yet the opposite would be true at the later stage venture firm. As later-stage firms are focused on providing funding toward a liquidity event, an investment banking background would be more cherished at this phase.

Figure 15.6 to the right depicts the path a start-up company needs to navigate.

As those involved in your company have downstream relationships (i.e., seed to early-stage), it is important to understand how the next potential investors can improve

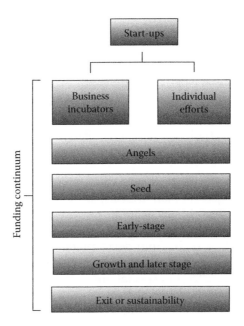

FIGURE 15.6
Funding continum for start-ups.

your connectivity and reduce your firm's risk. It therefore is critical to plot, to the best of your ability, a syndicate of relationships from business incubators right through to your final exit.

15.8.6 Consider Your "Exit Candidates" When Plotting Your Business Model

Often, start-up companies will excitedly communicate that a large number of potential companies could acquire them. This is frequently as much a burden as it is an opportunity.

The reason for the burden is that acquiring companies are interested in products that deliver their value in a manner that is consistent with the acquiring company. By its nature, the acquiring company has scaled its business model and become efficient by following specific steps to satisfy their customers.

Start-up companies can make an egregious error when their process of satisfying the customer's need is significantly different from that of the potential acquirer. Acquirers are looking to put new products through their existing customer value pipeline. This is how they gain leverage over their existing cost infrastructure. If the start-up company's new product also requires an investment in infrastructure, the acquirer must decide if the incremental investment is worthwhile. The necessity of new infrastructure can add an unnecessary level of risk to your company: a risk that may not have been necessary to add. Therefore, start-up companies who may have more than one acquirer may develop a business model that tends to satisfy no one.

15.8.7 Every Dollar Invested Should Focus on the Removal of Risk

Your *business plan* expresses your vision, defines the opportunity, articulates necessary funding, and delineates the major steps associated with achievement. Your *commercialization plan* is a further refinement and contains all the tactics associated in achieving your business plan. To simplify our discussion, the word product will be used to describe either a manufactured product, software, or a service.

The International Organization for Standardization (ISO) defines risk as the effect of uncertainty on objectives. Risk management is asking what could fail during the planning cycle and creating defensive processes to inhibit risk. Contingency plans define what you will do if the risk does occur: a "Plan B." Risk management and contingency planning are designed to address areas of predictable failure.

Your business plan is essentially the expression of customer expectations with an understanding of the product specifications and process investment necessary to achieve the projected results.

Your commercialization plan, being a more comprehensive document, should contain a risk and contingency management plan to anticipate how bad benchmarks or poor conformance could enter your system. Let us detail this a little further.

Benchmarks are the external customer specifications that you are targeting. For example, the product must do "A" and "B." Your development team must translate those benchmarks into something that can be measured so that design personnel can numerically define when they have met customer expectations.

When the design team is satisfied that they have a system configuration that meets R&D benchmarks, they have developed their product specifications. Next you need to communicate to the organization all the activities that need to be followed to deliver the product. These are called the process specifications. In attempting to deliver that plan, two things can go wrong: bad benchmarks (targets) or bad conformance (adherence to processes).

There are numerous types of risk items and their specific discussion is beyond the scope of this chapter. However, for start-ups to obtain funding, they must articulate their understanding of risk areas and express their plans to manage or remove the risk. By identifying these areas and demonstrating that the risk has been removed from the system, the company is advancing and thus its valuation should increase.

15.8.8 Build Creditability and Knowledge through Third Parties

As every industry contains standards in one form or another, planful utilization of these standards can communicate the removal of risk, which increases investor and customer confidence.

Before a company is formed, value points can occur. For example, if the technology started in a university and the university professor received a research grant—that has value. The grant award states that the granting organization (which has an independent assessment committee) saw the project as differentiated and viable. In early company formation, Small Business Innovation Research (SBIR) and Small Business Technology Transfer (STTR) grants are highly valuable. These programs provide qualified small business concerns with money to develop and commercialize an innovative idea. The details of these programs can be found at http://www.sbir.gov.

The value of an SBIR/STTR to the start-up company is that scientific experts have vetted the technology and the approving panel sees the commercial potential in the project. The funding for this program goes toward the development of the product and because it is a grant it is basically free money in the eyes of the investor. Investors recognize that the dollars invested by the grant reduces the need for the company to raise additional equity. As grants are not paid back they reduce the need to raise additional equity. This is referred to as "non-dilutive funding."

Patents communicate value. For example, submitting a patent application and having a "patent pending" designation expresses that the technology is at a specific phase. An issued patent is the government issuing the right for the company to be the only one to perform that patent—this is very valuable.

Before a product is launched many companies must adhere to some form of industry regulatory process. In regulated industries, ISO certification is valuable. It communicates that your product specifications meet industry standards and that your internal processes are designed to a certain standard of excellence. In healthcare, FDA approval is required before a company can commercialize its product and is therefore very valuable. Audited financial systems provide investor confidence that the financial systems adhere to certain standards and are a fair representation of the company's status.

Having an article published in a peer-reviewed journal can also provide the investor with confidence that the technology is unique. That same article can also communicate confidence that your customer (being the peer) has also vetted the technology and finds it valuable.

15.8.9 Consistently Deliver to Your Documented Plan

Developing a comprehensive plan from the beginning is difficult. This difficulty is natural, as it is nearly impossible to conceive of every aspect of a commercialization plan from the start-up phase to cash flow positive to exit. Understating or overstating the cost of your plan is a major risk. Benchmarking is a valuable mechanism to guard against this frequent error and a tool to assist you in managing risk.

Benchmarking against large companies and other start-ups in your industry helps you gain insight into the total cost of other such endeavors. When you match your particular business plan to certain benchmarks and find variance, this leads the writer of the business plan to either investigate for what is missing or make a dollar assumption on the effort.

Misaligned investor expectations are one of the biggest challenges for a start-up CEO. Benchmarking is a great tool to defend your plan against investors who are always looking to drive down the pre-money value of a deal in the motivation to own more of the company with their investment.

Once invested, that same investor is motivated to have the company spend as little as possible to minimize future funding needs so they can maximize their ownership and return.

For example, if every other company in the category took $25–$35 million to build, how is it reasonable that your start-up can do it with $5 million. Databases such as Venture Source™ (www.venturesource.com) and Hoovers (www.hoovers.com) are great tools.

15.8.10 Exit Wisely

There is a saying that goes, "pigs get fed and hogs get slaughtered." The intention of this idiom, as it relates to our subject, is that one should exit at a reasonable price given the company's progress and funding environment.

Frequently start-ups get overexuberant once they start having success and overstate the value of their company. Previously, we discussed the value of benchmarks and here again valuation and exit comparatives keep one realistic. Understanding historical benchmarks is valuable. Awareness of the immediate environment is also critical. Four to 6 months into our last recession, Venture Source data suggested that medical device company valuations decreased by 25% due to the lack of availability of money. Those investors who did have money to invest saw this as a great opportunity to invest in companies at low valuations. So at that moment, if your start-up needed more capital and you were offered an exit at the 25% discount, would you wait or would you exit? This question needs to be answered within the context of a particular company. If the company was cash flow positive and not in need of further cash, perhaps waiting for a change in economic cycle with the chance of regaining the lost 25% makes perfect sense. However, if your company had an exit opportunity and also was in need of more capital, then an analysis would need to be completed.

If the current stockholders could not continue to invest in the company, then new investment money would dilute the current stockholders (to dilute means that the current stockholders would own less of the company). As a result, it is conceivable that the cost of dilution would offset the 25% valuation increase at a future date. Under this scenario, considering risk, the company should sell now.

These are complex analytical considerations and require analysis beyond the mathematical. Understanding the voice of the exit company is as important as understanding the voice of your customer. The details of a target exit company should be well understood. What are their strategies, business tactics, and cycles of their exit targets? Start-up CEOs should know as much as possible about their target companies. The following examples, with details changed and embellished to protect the companies, make this point.

This start-up company had a technology that addressed a specific industry problem. As the start-up company's product did not touch the customer, it was part of a bigger company system. (Think of a steering wheel vendor selling to an automotive company). As a result, the bigger companies controlled access to the market.

The industry with access to the company saw this problem as minor and therefore did not want to address it. The start-up company faltered because it could not obtain an industry relationship for distribution. Just before faltering, the industry regulatory body determined that this problem was a major issue and asked the industry what it was going to do about the problem. All of a sudden, the company was bought. This was pure luck and had nothing to do with the actions of a thoughtful CEO.

Another example is a company that was negotiating with the industry market share leader (>55% market share) to buy their start-up company. The industry leader used their size to intimidate the start-up in an attempt to drive the acquisition price down. This intimidation was not without evidence as the industry leader had done this before.

However, the start-up CEO knew the industry well. He knew the industry leader was concerned over the announcement that its largest competitor in Europe intended to launch into the United States the following year. The industry leader knew that if the competitor had access to this technology it would provide them with a significant cost advantage. This was of great concern to the industry leader. The result—the start-up company was acquired at a premium.

15.9 Applications to Quality of Life Technologies

Throughout this book we have described technologies that have the potential of improving the quality of life of older individuals and persons with disability. These technologies are in various stages of development, but the long-term goals for each technology are to develop helpful products that are commercially viable. With this goal in mind, it is useful to view the status of some of the key technologies of the center through the lens of innovation and commercialization.

In Tables 15.1 through 15.3 we identify three such technologies—a personal mobility and manipulation appliance (PerMMA), first-person vision system, and the community-based health kiosk—and for each system we address key questions relevant to the

TABLE 15.1

Case Study: Personal Mobility and Manipulation Appliance (QoLT Specific)

Problem being solved:	Many people with disabilities depend on a human attendant who assists them with ADLs (activities of daily living, i.e., eating, hygiene, transfers between seating surfaces, etc.) and IADLs (instrumental activities of daily living, i.e., meal preparation, household chores, shopping, etc.)
Technology solution:	A robotic power wheelchair with appended manipulators and multiple control modes (automatic, local user, remote controlled from a distance) can perform many of the functions of a human attendant

Market applications:	• People who rely on attendants
	• Subdivide along dimensions of
	  • Diagnosis (e.g., spinal cord injury, ALS, MS, etc.)
	  • Employed/unemployed

Commercialization priorities:	• Detailed understanding of
	  • Target population ADL and IADL priorities (to define functional requirements of the robotics)
	• Residual capabilities of users
	• Developed business models of
	  • Constituent parts: power wheelchairs, robotic manipulators for wheelchair users
	  • Human attendant service providers
	  • Remote delivery of services, e.g., computer troubleshooting
	• Regulatory barriers
	• Applicable reimbursement codes

Market selection rationale:	• Veterans market • Non-dilutive grants available from federal and philanthropic sources
Management team selection:	• Entrepreneurs in assistive technology industry • Hire management with regulatory and reimbursement experience and proprietary business relationships, especially as a supplier to the Department of Veterans' Affairs • Have world-recognized scientist
Initial fund raise	$25 million
Compelling story	• Wounded warriors (Iraq and Afghanistan conflicts) are in the news regularly and high priorities for both DOD and VA; appeal to "grateful nation" sentiment • Cost of providing a PerMMA veterans and other people with disabilities into the workforce can be offset by reduction in human attendant costs • General humanitarianism
PDCA cycle	• Unfair advantage—current devices on the market are not integrated; management team connections • Following the norms of start-ups in medical device markets • Invested dollars should focus on removing risk to users • Build creditability and knowledge through third parties. Exploit CMU's reputation in robotics and Pitt's reputation in rehabilitation, specifically world-leading reputation in wheelchair technology

TABLE 15.2

Case Study: First-Person Vision (Adjacent Market)

Problem being solved	Facial recognition systems have already demonstrated their benefit in military and security operations. The challenge with today's systems is that they are based on cameras at fixed locations, hence recognition performance is limited by distance and viewing angle
Technology solution	Image registration of faces is achieved via a wearable system removing impediments to field situations
Market applications	• What is the fastest path to commercial success with the least amount of risk • Military and Security • Media fields • Customer relations management • Sports and entertainment
Commercialization priorities	• The first priority market would ideally posses: 　• A developed business model 　• An existing infrastructure 　• Minimum regulatory barriers 　• Opportunities for non-dilutive funding 　• An existing digitized facial database
Market selection rationale	• Military and border security markets • Non-dilutive funding grants available • Numerous exit candidates
Management team selection	• Utilize QoLT incubator to increase the probability of success • Hire personnel with previous software entrepreneurship experience • Hire management with proprietary customer relationships • Have world-recognized scientist
Initial fund raise	• $10 million
Compelling story	• Terrorism and border security are issues in the news daily and the subject on numerous grants • Sports broadcasters are constantly seeking to implement novel approaches to deliver content
PDCA cycle	• Create an unfair advantage and differentiate—current devices are not mobile • Following the norms of start-up capital market • Funding syndicate interested in military and security • Build creditability and knowledge through third parties. Exploit CMU's general reputation as major player in computer vision and specifically world-leading reputation in face recognition technology

commercialization process: (a) What is the problem being solved? (b) what is the technology solution? (c) what are the market applications? (d) what are the commercialization priorities? (e) what is the rationale for market selection? (f) how should the management team be selected? and (g) what are the initial funds needed to launch this enterprise?

As noted in Table 15.1 and described in Chapter 10, PerMMA is a robotic power wheelchair with appended manipulators and is designed to perform many of the functions of a human attendant assisting a person with spinal cord injury with limited upper body mobility. It is designed to provide assistance with basic activities of daily living such as eating as well as other daily activities such as meal preparation, household chores, and shopping. The target market for this appliance is relatively

TABLE 15.3

Case Study: Community-Based Health Kiosk (QoLT Specific and Adjacent)

Problem being solved:	Many people with chronic diseases need frequent, often daily measurement of vital signs. Many do not have access to devices to make those measurements and many, particularly older adults, lack the technical skills to properly use them. As a consequence, neither of those groups is able to provide their clinicians with such data
Technology solution:	An integrated suite of vital sign sensors with a fool-proof user interface that guides people through the steps of proper use. A clinician/caregiver interface provides on-demand access to patient data in user-specified formats on a number of computer and smartphone platforms
Market applications:	• Which chronic disease presents the fastest path to commercial success with the least amount of risk? • Diabetes • Heart disease • Hypertension • Obesity

Commercialization priorities:	• The first priority market would ideally possess:
	  • A developed business model, e.g., disease management organizations (DMO), or an emerging business model, e.g., accountable care organization
	  • An existing infrastructure
	  • An "open" (or easy to connect to) electronic medical record (EMR) system
	  • Minimum regulatory barriers
	  • Opportunities for non-dilutive funding

Market selection rationale:	• Disease management organizations (a developed business model) • Accountable care organization (an emerging business model) • Numerous exit candidates • Non-dilutive funding grants available (e.g., NCHIT, AHRQ)
Management team selection:	• Utilize QoLT incubator to increase the probability of success • Hire management with (1) proprietary customer relationships, (2) prior DMO or EMR company experience • Hire personnel with previous software entrepreneurship experience
Initial fund raise	$10 million
Compelling story	The rising cost of healthcare is unsustainable. The coming wave of retirees brings with it a dramatic increase in chronic disease prevalence
PDCA cycle	• Unfair advantage—current devices are not usable • Following the norms of start-up capital market • A funding syndicate interested in disease management • Exit candidates, DMO and EMR companies, considered when plotting the business model • Invested dollars should focus on data security and integrity • Build creditability and knowledge through third parties. Exploit CMU's general reputation as major player in computer science and human–computer interaction and Pitt's reputation in nursing. Secure a major player as a reference customer

small—persons with severe mobility limitations—when compared to the population at large; however, the costs of supporting this population with human assistance are extremely high both in terms monetary costs and in the autonomy and self-determination afforded to the person with mobility limitations.

Developing a successful product in this domain requires a detailed understanding of the target population and its needs, preferences, and abilities, and since this device will likely be classified as a medical device, the business plan needs to address regulatory barriers as well as reimbursement scenarios as the cost of such a system will be too high for most individuals to afford through private pay. As a result, having a management team with experience with regulatory agencies and private and federal reimbursement systems would be highly desirable. The costs of launching a start-up in this domain would be considerable, given the relatively high costs of the constituent technologies required.

Additional examples are provided in Tables 15.2 and 15.3. Although none of these technologies have come to fruition in terms of launching successful start-ups, they are all on paths aimed at achieving this goal. A key feature of all three examples is that they are based on core technologies that potentially have many other applications. For example, PerMMa could be developed into a kitchen robot for normal functioning individuals, and the health kiosk technology could be exported to computers in the home for self-monitoring of individual health and functioning. The ultimate value of these technologies will likely come in the form of spin-off products that take advantage of the core capabilities being developed by the QoLt ERC.

15.10 Conclusion

Innovation is a process of connected steps. Measuring and incorporating best practices would ultimately perfect the system. One of the most documented and measured steps today is in the area of incubation. Incubation improves company survival and those companies that have succeeded have impacted the economy. There are numerous forms of incubators but they all share a common goal—find viable companies and progress them to early-stage capital or sustainment.

Finding capital consumes the total start-up management team far more than the management teams of larger companies. Having domain-experienced personnel reduces start-up risk as these CEOs have "navigated these waters before." Domain-experienced start-up CEOs should match the product life cycle and the start-up company must tell a compelling story, which must include the start-up company's exit candidates.

Every time the story is told, there is an opportunity for improvement. Using Dr. Deming's PDCA cycle is one method and we offered 10 checkpoints to consider during every improvement cycle.

Successful start-up personnel do not necessarily know it all; however, they benchmark to ensure that they are reasonable in their planning and they frequently adjust their plans through a type of PDCA Cycle upon every new gain in knowledge.

"Be smart, move fast, and correct often" is the motto of the successful start-up.

References

1. Mid-session review budget of the US government, fiscal year 2009, http://www.gpoaccess.gov/USbudget/fy09/pdf/09msr.pdf
2. Wikipedia, PDCA, http://en.wikipedia.org/wiki/PDCA
3. International Organization for Standardization, ISO 31000:2009, http://www.iso.org/iso/catalogue_detail.htm?csnumber=43170
4. Internal analysis, Pittsburgh Life Sciences Greenhouse, Pittsburgh, PA.

Index

Printed and bound by CPI Group (UK) Ltd, Croydon, CR0 4YY

18/10/2024

01776253-0008